An Atlas on the Comparative Anatomy of the Retinae of Vertebrates

By

David T. Yew

Maria S. M. Wai

Winnie W. Y. Li

CONTENTS

CHAPTERS

FOREWORD

The retina is a light sensitive portion of the eye. It contains the rods and cone. The rods are responsible for white and black vision and vision in the dark, while the cones are for color vision. In this book the authors reported a comparative study on the retinae and the visual cells from the primitive fish to mammalian species (chapter 1). Some of the species featured in this chapter are rare and the comparison between species across the major groups in the animal kingdom will provide interesting insights in evolution. For example, the double cones which were originally thought to be present only in birds are demonstrated in the retinae from fish all the way to primates. Then using the chicken model as an example they describe the development and maturation of other layers (chapter 2). The third chapter is on the development of retinae in several mammalian species. The most interesting chapter is the last chapter that describes the degenerative retinae in different animal models adapting to different environments. The function and degeneration of the retinae in different environmental situation provides a better insight on the roles, functions and capabilities of the retinae. The degeneration of the retinae is also reported in a special pathological situation such as ketamine toxicity. This serves as an example on how drug abuse may affect the nervous system. This book will be useful to visual scientists, zoologists and ophthalmologists alike, and to those who are interested in eye research in general. This is one of the few atlases on the eye that includes micrographs from many different species.

I have known Prof David Yew, the senior author since 70s when we both just joined the Faculty of Medicine, The University of Hong Kong. He was trained in anatomy and is now Chair Professor of Anatomy in the Chinese University of Hong Kong. He has worked in the field of neuroscience (brain and retina) all his academic life. He has wide research interests and the visual system and effects of drug abuse on the nervous system are two of his many interests. David is a real scholar as reflected by his active scholastic activities - over 260 research papers and over 20 book chapters and /or books. In recognition of his achievement, he has been elected fellows of the Society of Biology (UK), the Zoological Society (London) and the Royal Society for the promotion of public health (UK). He is also a fellow of the American Association of Anatomists (USA). He is on the editorial boards of several textbooks and many journals.

Dr Wai and Dr Li have both worked in the field of neuroscience for many years and have published many papers on animals and humans.

TM Wong

Former Professor and Head of Department of Physiology, and
Deputy Director and Head of College of Life Sciences and Technology, The School of
Professional and Continuing Education,
The University of Hong Kong

PREFACE

In the last century, two exhaustive and interesting books have been published on the retina, Walls's (1942) *'The vertebrate eye and its adaptive radiation*' and Polyak's (1941) *'The retina'*. These two volumes of world famous literature on the eyes have stimulated the thoughts of numerous vision researchers across the globe. With the establishment of national funding agencies in eye research around the world, the 20th century has been the most productive era of eye research, with many excellent papers published in the field, including those on the comparative anatomy of the eye. In spite of these advances, comparative atlases on the vertebrate retina, a region of the eye which is mostly explored in research, remains lacking. This atlas tries to amend some of these problems. In this volume, the authors have attempted to enlist as many as 27 specimens of different animals as well as human. All figures in the book are micrographs, either light microscopic or electron microscopic figures. For the latter, both transmission and scanning electron micrographs are included. These figures can amend information illustrated in both Walls's and Polyak's books which contained mainly hand drawn figures. This book here is divided into several chapters – with a longest chapter on the comparison between the retinas of different vertebrates. It starts with the fish retina all the way to the primate. To those interested in comparing ontogeny with phylogeny, observation of, for example, the oil droplets in the eyes of different vertebrates may be intriguing, as oil droplets in the retina are seen in the oldest fish – the sturgeon.

Comparison between different mammals – cows, pigs, dogs, cats, and monkeys give a possibility of looking at these mammals of different habitat and diet. To us, the authors, we found the cat and the monkey to be most interesting. The layers of the retinas, on the other hand, display different patterns between the fish and the mammals and are worth noting. This atlas also has other chapters on the inner layers of the retina (exclusive of the visual cells or photoreceptor cells) and discusses inner retinal layers from their morphogenesis to maturation. There are further chapters to illustrate the development of the retina in general and examples of retinal degeneration. In the acquisition of all these different specimens, especially for the rarer one (crocodiles, humans etc.), the fixation may not always be optimal due to time lapse in securing the specimens. The authors of this atlas also have a special interest in the types of visual cells and, therefore these cells may receive more coverage than others.

The book aims to at least give an introduction to the ophthalmologists, zoologists, comparative anatomists, evolutionary biologists, embryologists and vision researchers, to trigger their interest in the retina in general or in specific species. The atlas, like all others, is not meant to be exhaustive. It is hoped that a basic knowledge on the comparative retinal structures presented here would lead to further scientific enquiries and discoveries by others.

The corresponding author of this atlas, David. T. Yew would like to dedicate this work to Professor David Bernard Meyer who introduced him to the beauty of the retina many decades ago, to the late Professors Roger Warwick (author of Gray's Anatomy) and late Professor Ronald Fearnhead for their help and encouragement during periods of difficulties, to Professors M.C. Yu and Amy Yu and Professor David Randall for their everlasting friendship and unfailing support for the past twenty years.

In the course of preparation of the book, Mr. Wai-Man Chan and Miss Lai-Yin Yeung had offered much assistance and comments in the draft of the manuscript. Without their help, the completion of the book would be impossible. We are also much indebted to Dr. Bushra Siddiqui and the staff in the very detail editing of the book.

David T. Yew
Maria S. M. Wai
Winnie W. Y. Li

ACKNOWLEDGEMENT

All members of the laboratory of the authors have helped in different ways to make this atlas a reality. These include particularly WP Lam, LH Lam, HC Tang, YW Wong, YM Tsui and especially to WS Cheung who helped in the technical and scientific work.

LIST OF ABBREVIATIONS

A-A	Amacrine-amacrine
A	Amacrine cell/Artery
AB	Arciform body
Ac	Accessory cone
AC	Accessory cone pedicle
AcN	Accessory cone nucleus
AcI	Accessory cone inner segment
AcO	Accessory cone outer segment
AP	Amacrine cell process
BM	Basement membrane
BP	Bipolar cell
BV	Blood vessel
C	Cone cell/Cone cell body/Central retina
Cap	Blood capillary
CB	Cone bipolar
Cc	Chief cone
CC	Chief cone pedicle
CcN	Chief cone nucleus
Ce	Centriole
Ch	Layer of Chevitz
Ci	Cilium
CcI	Chief cone inner segment
CcO	Chief cone outer segment
CI	Chief inner segment
CP	Cone pedicle
CS	Cone synaptic body
D	Distal region
DB	Dense bodies
Dc	Double cone
DCV	Dark-cored vesicle
De	Debris
DJ	Dense junctions
DP	Dense particles
E	Nucleated red blood cell
EF	End foot
ELM	External limiting membrane
GA	Golgi apparatus
GL	Ganglion cell layer
G/GP	Ganglion cell/ Ganglion cell process
Ho	Horizontal cell
HP	Horizontal projection

Hp	Horizontal process
I	Inter-receptor synapse/Inner segment of visual cell
ICR	Institute for cancer research rat
ILM	Internal limiting membrane
INL	Inner nuclear layer
IPL	Inner plexiform layer
L	Landolt's club
Mc	Multiple cone
Mi	Microvillus
M	Mitochondria
Mü	Müller cell
NDV	Non-dark-cored vesicle
NL	Nuclear layer
Nt	Neurotubule
Nu	Nucleus
O	Outer segment of visual cell
OD	Distal outer segment
ONL	Outer nuclear layer
OPL	Outer plexiform layer
OP	Proximal outer segment
Os	Ora serrata
P	Peripheral retina/Proximal region
PAS	Periodic acid-schiff staining
PE	Pigment epithelium
PEc	Pigment epithelial cell
PG	Pigment granule/Pigment cell
PPT	Postsynaptic thickenings
Pr	Projections
PS	Photoreceptor synaptic body
PTAH	Phosphotungstic acid hematoxylin
RCS	Royal college of surgeons rat
RER	Rough endoplasmic reticulum
Ri	Ribosome
R	Rod/Rod spherule
RI	Rod inner segment
RN	Rod nucleus
RS	Rod synaptic body
S	Optic stalk
S/Sc	Single cone
SC	Single cone pedicle
ScN	Single cone nucleus
SR	Synaptic ribbon
T	Tumor cell

Tc	Twin cone
Tr	Twin rod
V	Vein
VCL	Visual cell layer

CHAPTER 1

Comparative Retinae and Visual Cells

Abstract: During evolution, the eyes of vertebrates develop different adaptations in order to fit into the different habitats. In this chapter, 27 vertebrates, both rare and common, from different animal groups were selected to illustrate the histological differences in their retinae. For example, it is interesting to compare vertebrates between groups e.g. fish and amphibians. It is also interesting to compare vertebrates that are herbivores with those that are omnivores. In addition, comparing between species is also enlightening. A cat, which is an agile and fast moving animal, has a lot more types of visual cells than other slow moving species, while bottom living Chinese soft shelled turtles have visual cells that are rudimentary. In other cases, the Japanese eels, which inhabit both ocean and freshwater streams during their life-cycle, have retinae with highly packed and numerous visual cells while the goldfishes, which live in freshwater streams and ponds, have retinae with scattered visual cells. The differences in the retinae among different groups of vertebrates demonstrate a significant increase in visual cells in the mammalian retinae.

Key Words: visual cell layer, outer nuclear layer, outer plexiform layer, inner plexiform layer, inner nuclear layer, ganglion cell layer, rods, double cone, chief cone, accessory cone, single cone, twin cone, pigment epithelium, various animals

VISUAL CELLS

In almost all animals, except the primitive mammals, there is a central region of the retina - the fovea centralis - where the retina is pitted, the inner nuclear layer merges with the outer nuclear layer, and there is a marked increase in the density of visual cells with the exclusion of rods and the presence of many cones [1-3]. In the deep sea fish, the density of photoreceptor cells is about 3:1 from the central region to the periphery [4]. The optic nerve is divided into two bundles, one from the fovea and the other from the periphery [4]. The birds of prey – hawk, falcon, and peregrine - all have very deep foveae [5, 6]. They look at the prey straight for short distances but look at the prey sideways and circle the prey for long distances. They often move their heads in several directions to obtain the best view via the deep foveae. In monkeys, cones predominate in the fovea but the cell numbers drop to 1/4 of its quantity only 750 μm from the fovea [7]. Cone density is higher in the nasal and inferior retina while rod density is higher in the superior retina. This arrangement is similar to that of humans and other mammals [7, 8]. For the human retina, the cones are usually divided into 3 types: long and medium wavelengths, with blue sensitive cones at only 7% of the total [9]. There are, however, still cones near to the ora serrata (refer to this atlas). Cone cells are present even in primitive fishes [10] and there is often an asymmetry of these cells in the dorsal-ventral retina of higher vertebrates [11]. The peripheral retina, on the other hand, mainly consists of rods, reducing spatial resolution but increasing sensitivity [1]. In the archer fish, half of the eye is below water and they have differentially tuned their rods and cones across the retina [12]. Convergence in the retinae of deep sea fishes is similar to noctural mammals; in some species have tubular eyes with multiple foveae, e.g. scopelarchid retina [13]. Another peculiar point about cones is the presence of twin cones (two identical cones), as documented by Walls [14]. This is also known in a number of books as twin rods Double cones, another type of special cones, are frequently found in, amphibians, reptiles and birds [15]. These cones distinctively consist of one tall chief and one short accessory component which have been suggested to play roles in sensing movements [16] and polarization vision [17]. Cones in general are for color vision [18] and activation involves isomerization of all trans retinal to 11 cis retinal [18]. It has also been suggested that in the last ten years in some animals, including a few fishes, there are multiple cones adhering together (e.g. triple, quadruple cones) [19]. Apart from double cones and triple cones, many of these multiple cones are restricted in number and limited to the central retina [19]. In many of the lower species, notably the goldfish, the retina is under continuous renewal. Neurons die via apoptosis and are replaced by new cells at the margins [20].

In the salamander, rods outnumber cones (roughly 62% to 38%) [21]. So-called red rods are the most numerous and are sensitive to middle wavelengths while the relatively scanty green rods are sensitive to short wavelengths [21]. Salamanders also have single and double cones [21], with prominent glutaminergic transmission in the horizontal/bipolar/visual cell contacts [22]. In the reptile (e.g. snake), there were two cone opsins, the short wavelength (SWS1) and the long wavelength (LWS) for color vision, together with a Rh1 rod opsin [23]. In the fish

David T. Yew, Maria S. M. Wai and Winnie W. Y. Li

(e.g. eel), Rh2 cone opsin and SWS2 opsin are the visual pigments [24]. In the chameleons, oil droplets are frequently seen in the cones [25] and are seen as well in fish and the chicken (refer to this atlas). There are no rods [25] in the chameleon, with double cones for long wavelengths of 555 nm to 610 nm and three single cones of 480-505 nm, 440-450 nm, and 375-385 nm [25]. In the xenopus, red and green rods are observed. In this animal, there are three cones including a UV sensitive cone [26]. In the literature, the absence of rods in lizard and turtle has been documented [27].

The snake, a fast moving prey-seeking reptile, has a rod and two single cones – a large and a small cone. The visual pigment of the rod is of 495 nm, the large cone of 549 nm while the small cone is of 357 nm (at the UV range) [28, 29]. In the crocodile retina, like those of the deep-sea fish and the cat, a tapetum full of aligned pigments is located outside the pigment epithelium [30] to maximize vision particularly in dim light.

RETINAL LAYERS

There are three main elements in the outer plexiform layer of the retina, the synaptic bodies of photoreceptors and the processes of bipolar and horizontal cells. The synaptic terminals of the photoreceptors are called pedicles for cones and spherules for rods; all of them are invaginated by horizontal and bipolar cell processes that form synapses. These synapses have dense junctions with synaptic ribbons and vesicles on the presynaptic (photoreceptor) side [31]. Ladman and Soper [32] have described the cone-bipolar synapse in the pigeon and Herring gull, and Shiragami [33, 34] has further elucidated four different types of visual cell synapses in the chicken. Interreceptor synapses between synaptic terminals of photoreceptors [35] are also observed in many animals; they are characterized by dense junctions and no synaptic ribbons.

The inner nuclear layer contains four types of cell bodies: horizontal, bipolar, Müller and amacrine cells. In addition, it receives the termination of the specialized efferent system of the centrifugal fibers. The terminations of these fibers are characterized by their large size and are densely packed with synaptic vesicles [36]. They usually end on the soma of amacrine and other cells of the inner nuclear layer [37].

Horizontal cell bodies are oval in shape and occupy the most choroidal position within the inner nuclear layer. These cells have short processes which extend horizontally into the outer plexiform layer. The cytoplasmic content of these cells includes mitochrondria, nucleus, rough endoplasmic reticulum, dense bodies and neurotubules, but not Kolmer's crystalloid – an inclusion body with parallel-oriented tubular structures and ribosomes – as observed by Yamada and Ishikawa [38] in the human. With the use of the Golgi technique, Ramón y Cajal [29] differentiated two types of horizontal cells in the chicken retina: the brush-shaped horizontals with numerous short and dense protoplasmic processes, and the stellate horizontals which appear as flat stellate cells with longer but less dense processes. Unfortunately, these two cell types have not yet been distinguished on an ultrastructural basis in the chicken, nor in any other avian retina.

The bipolar cell bodies constitute the second row of cells in the inner nuclear layer. These cells possess dendrites that extend into the outer plexiform layer and axons that extend into the inner plexiform layer. Their perikarya contain mitochondria, rough endoplasmic reticulum, Golgi apparatus (only in inner bipolars, see below), neurotubules and ribosomes, all of which are essentially the same components as reported by Missotten [40] in the human. Ramón y Cajal [39] found two variations of the bipolar cells in the chicken: outer bipolars and smaller, inner bipolars. The outer bipolars had many short dendrites immediate to their cell bodies, whereas each of the inner bipolars had a single, long dendritic trunk which became heavily branched in the outer part of the outer plexiform layer. A single, long dendrite branch that is continuous through the external limiting membrane forms the so-called Landolt's club which has been verified in the pigeon retina [41]. In contrast to Ramón y Cajal's findings [39], Dowling and Boycott [42] were unable to distinguish two different types of bipolar cells in the chicken retina by electron microscopy.

Müller cells, or fibers as they are sometimes called, are the most prominent neuroglial cells found in the chicken retina [39]. Their cell bodies occupy the third stratum of the inner nuclear layer and send a perpendicular process toward the outer and inner retina. The outer process intervenes between the photoreceptor cells and forms desmosomes between them (the external limiting membrane). From their ends, microvilli are projected into the optic ventricle. The inner process projects to the vitreal surface where it participates in the formation of the internal limiting membrane.

Within the retina, lateral branches arise from each process and fan out between the cells and processes of the outer plexiform, inner plexiform, ganglion cell and nerve fiber layers. Visualized by electron microscope, these processes possess neurotubules, a few apically located mitochondria, rough endoplasmic reticulum and ribosomes, similar to those reported in higher vertebrates [43,44]. As in the pigeon [45], glycogen particles are found only sparsely in the Müller cell cytoplasm of the chicken retina.

The innermost stratum of the inner nuclear layer is occupied by the bodies of the amacrine cells which, according to Ramón y Cajal [39], are divided into two main groups (diffuse and stratified) with numerous subgroups. The diffuse amacrine cells have processes that descend into the different zones of the inner plexiform layer and break up to form clusters of delicate branches; the stratified amacrines have processes which end in a specific layer of the inner plexiform layer.

Ultrastructurally, all types of amacrine cells possess the same cytoplasmic contents, namely, mitochondria, rough endoplasmic reticulum, ribosomes, dense bodies, some Golgi bodies and centrioles. No reliable criteria have been established to identify the various amacrine cell types under the electron microscope. An indented nucleus, characteristic of amacrine cells in higher animals [35], is rarely observed in the chicken.

Ramón y Cajal [39] was the first to gain insight into the complex organization of the inner plexiform layer in the chicken retina. He described in detail the processes of bipolar cells and the branching systems of the processes of amacrine, ganglion and Müller cells in this region. Although he had also indicated a possible synaptic relationship between bipolar axons and dendritic processes of ganglion cells, accurate details of these cytological associations had to wait for more sophisticated techniques (e.g. electron microscopy) that permit better resolution. Recently, studies of a variety of vertebrates [46-48], including chickens [42], have shown that bipolar axons synapse with amacrine and ganglion cell processes to form a complex called "dyad". Bipolar axons are characterized by a densely stained cytoplasm with numerous parallel neurotubules, mitochondria, synaptic ribbons and synaptic vesicles, whereas amacrine cell processes are characterized by a moderate amount of neurotubules, some mitochondria, dense bodies and some synaptic vesicles. According to Cowan [34], the morphology of the avian amacrine cells is essentially similar to that found in amphibian and mammalian retinas [36, 42] . In addition, the ganglion cell processes are readily distinguishable by an absence of synaptic ribbons and synaptic vesicles. They possess a clear cytoplasm, a few neurotubules, groups of ribosomes and dense bodies.

The Golgi technique [39] reveals that the retina contains many types of ganglion cells that can be divided into two main groups: single layered and multilayered. Single layered ganglion cells send dendrites to only a single sublayer within the inner plexiform layer and are subdivided into further subgroups. The multilayered ganglion cells have processes that terminate in more than one sublayer of the inner plexiform layer. Ramón y Cajal [39] described three subtypes in the latter group.

The cytoplasmic fine structure of ganglion cells in the chicken, a typical model, resembles that of higher species [35, 49]. Nissl bodies, ribosome groups, mitochondria, a few neurotubules and some dense bodies are present. Unfortunately, different subtypes do not show morphological differences in cellular content under the electron microscope.

The nerve fiber layer contains the axons of ganglion cells, Müller fiber components and centrifugal fibers [39]. Electron microscopy shows the ganglion cell axons with numerous neurotubules and mitochondria. Some nerve fibers are myelinated, as reported by Villegas [50] in the chicken and by Cowan and Powell [51] in the pigeon, and apparently represent the centrifugal (efferent) fibers. The majority are non-myelinated centripetal (afferent) fibers. Astrocytes are observed in this layer in some mammalian species (e.g. rodents).

The internal limiting membrane consists of the end feet of Müller cells and a basement membrane [52, 53] with a structureless space between. Salzmann [54] and Polyak [55] were the first to investigate this region extensively, followed much later by Wolff [56].

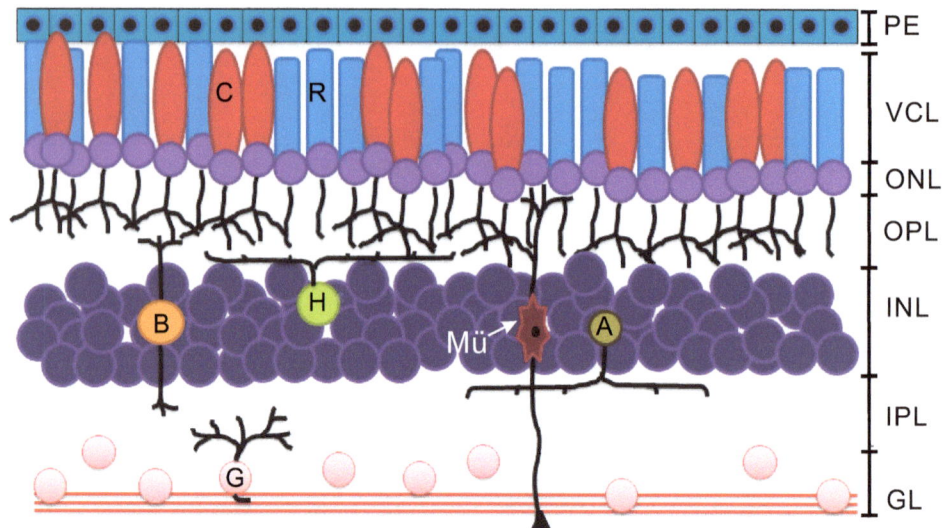

Figure 1.0.

A simplified diagram showing a retina composed of several layers including visual cell layer (VCL), outer nuclear layer (ONL), outer plexiform layer (OPL), inner nuclear layer (INL), inner plexiform layer (IPL) and ganglion cell layer (GL). In general, there are two major types of visual cells, rods (R) and cones (C) in the visual cell layer. The nuclei of the visual cells form the outer nuclear layer. Composing the inner nuclear layers are amacrine (A), bipolar (BP), horizontal (Ho) and Müller cell (Mü) bodies. Nerve processes of the retinal cells make up the two plexiform layers (i.e. OPL, IPL). The innermost layer consists chiefly of ganglion cell bodies and fibers which ultimately become the optic nerve.

1. STURGEON

The oldest fish, the sturgeon, is the only fish with oil droplets in their visual cells in the retina. The outer nuclear layer of the sturgeon's retina is quite thin and usually composed of two cell layers, implying that there is only small number of visual cells present. The inner nuclear layer has fewer cells which are loosely packed together. The ganglion cells are also very few in number. Differentiation between the rods and cones is easy because of their distinct structures.

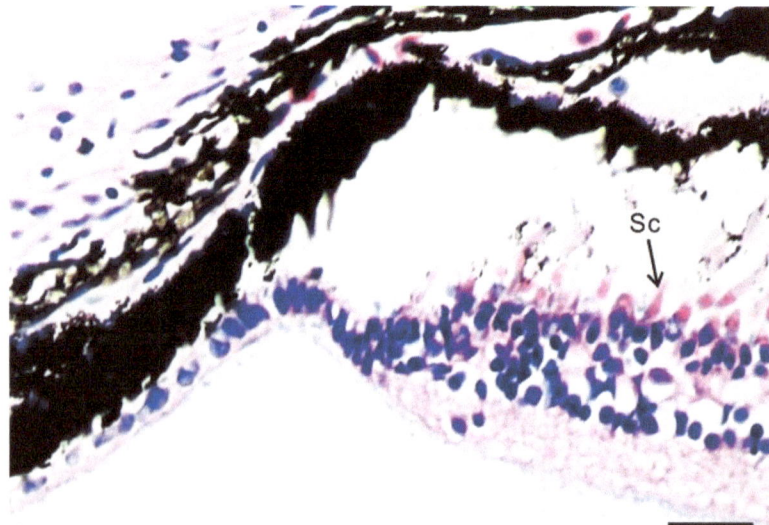

Figure 1.1a. *Ora Serrata.*

This figure shows the presence of cone cells around the ora serrata of a sturgeon. "Sc" denotes a single cone. Bar = 50 μm.

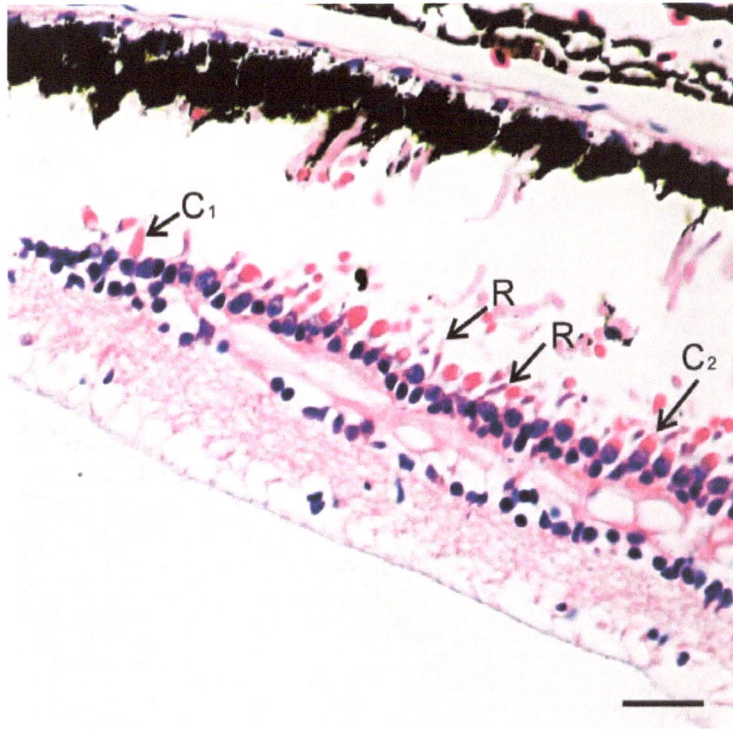

Figure 1.1b. *Anterior retina, near ora serrata.*

A gradual change of retinal thickness is seen in the anterior region. The density of visual cells in this region is low; however, rods (R) and different types of cones (C1 and C2) can be identified. Bar = 50 μm.

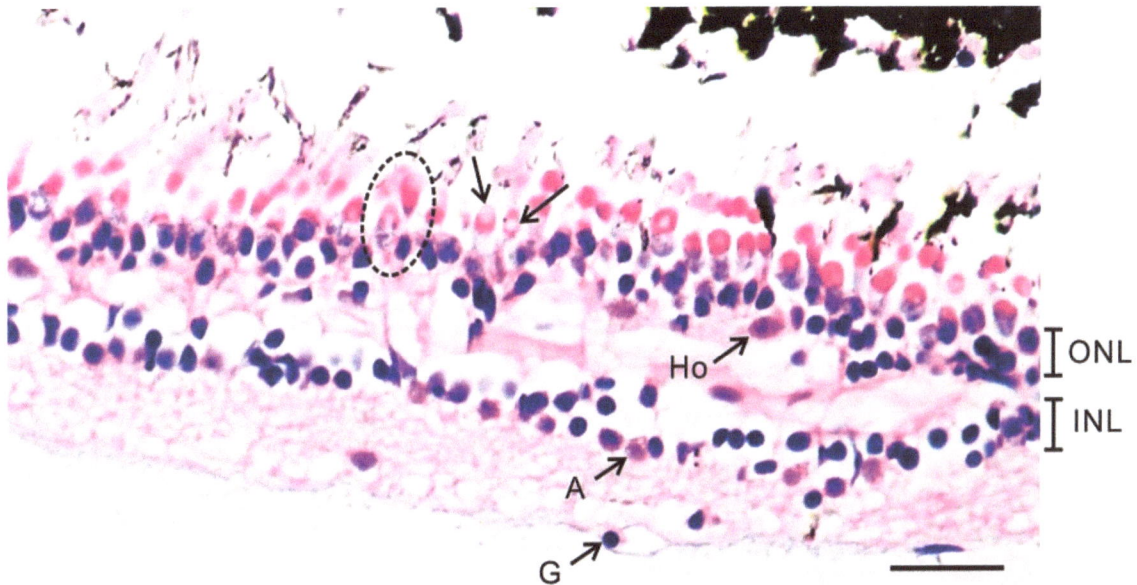

Figure 1.1c. *Anterior retina.*

Another part of the anterior retina is shown. A double cone (circle), composed by a tall chief cone and a short accessory cone is identified. The nucleus of the chief cone is located inferior to that of the accessory cone in the outer nuclear layer (ONL). Some cone cells appear to have oil droplets occupying the inner segment (arrows). In the inner nuclear layer (INL), "Ho" denotes a horizontal cell, "A" denotes an amacrine cell, and "G" denotes a ganglion cell. The ganglion cells are sparsely placed in this fish. Bar = 50 μm.

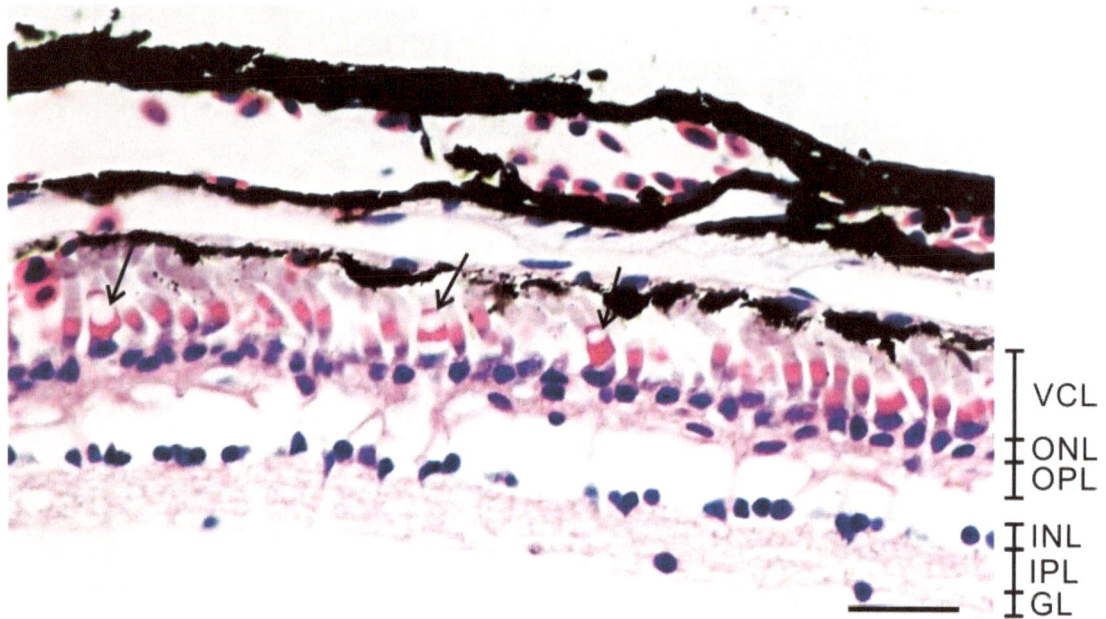

Figure 1.1d. *Peripheral retina.*

This figure indicates several layers of the retina. In the visual cell layer, oil droplets (arrows) are noted in some cone cells which have a pyramidal shaped inner segment. Bar = 50 μm.

(GL - Ganglion cell layer; INL - Inner nuclear layer; IPL - Inner plexiform layer; ONL - Outer nuclear layer; OPL - Outer plexiform layer; VCL - Visual cell layer).

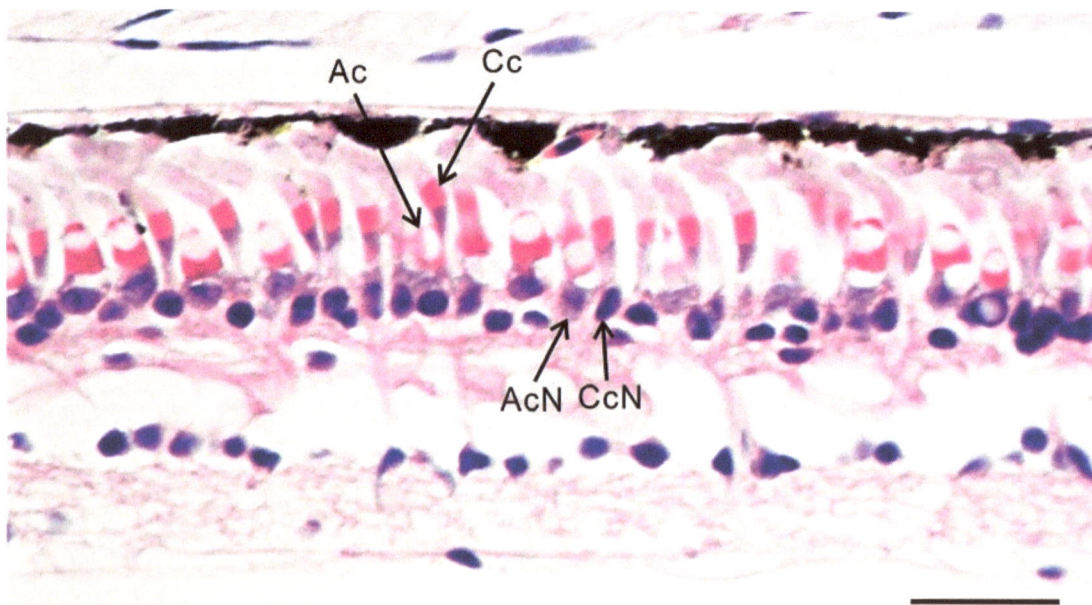

Figure 1.1e. *Peripheral retina.*

A pair of double cone comprised of a chief cone (Cc) and an accessory cone (Ac) is shown. The chief cone (Cc) usually has an inner segment with a very narrow stalk and a more rectangular distal inner segment. Bar = 50 μm.

(CcN - Chief cone nucleus; AcN - Accessory cone nucleus).

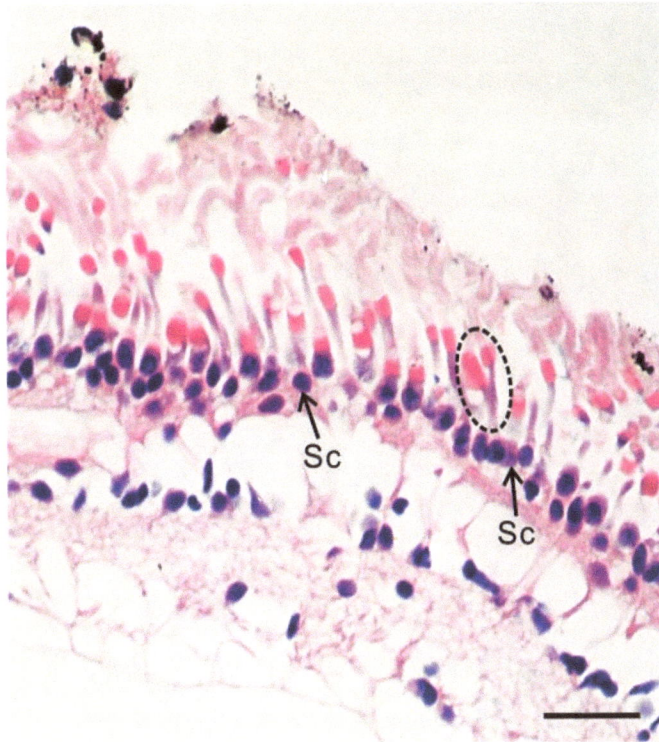

Figure 1.1f. *Peripheral retina.*

In this peripheral retina, single cones (Sc) with tapered outer segments and oil droplet- containing inner segments are noted. Moreover, a double cone pair (circle) is also identified. The inner segment of the accessory cone appears to be pear shaped whereas the inner segment of the chief cone is slender and long. Bar = 50 μm.

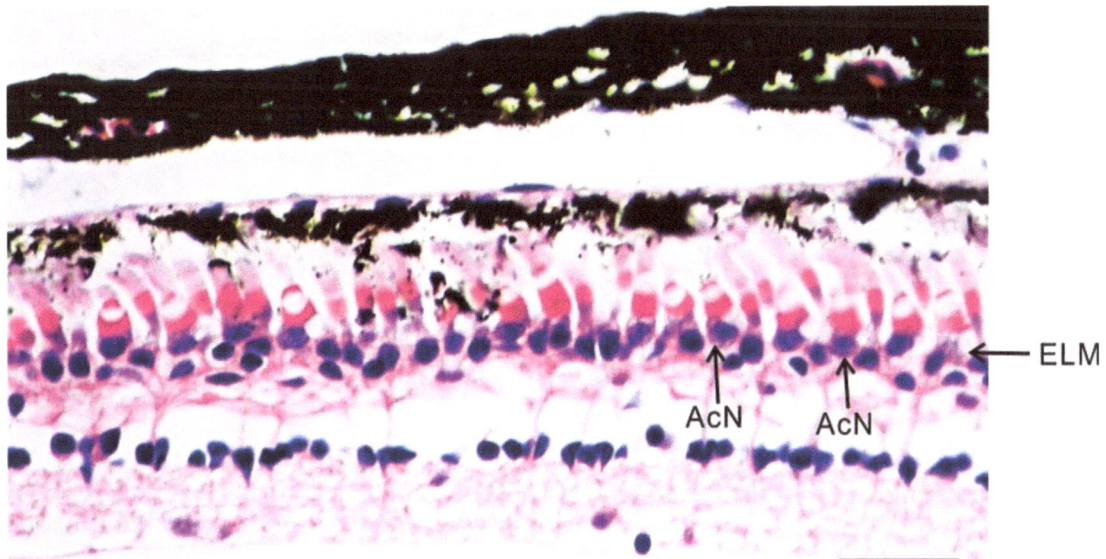

Figure 1.1g. *Mid-peripheral retina.*

A chief cone and an accessory cone with different nuclei. Note that the accessory cones have ellipse shaped nuclei (AcN) above the external limiting membrane (ELM). Bar = 50 μm.

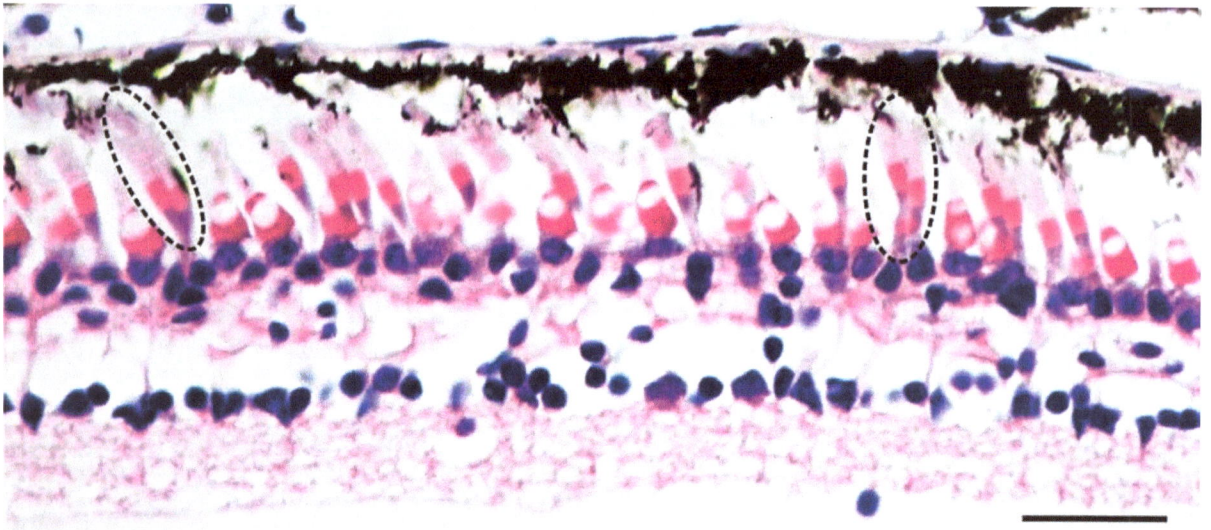

Figure 1.1h. *Mid-peripheral retina.*

In this figure, two pairs of possible twin cones (circles) are indicated. Members of the twin cones are characteristically similar in appearance and in height. Bar = 50 μm.

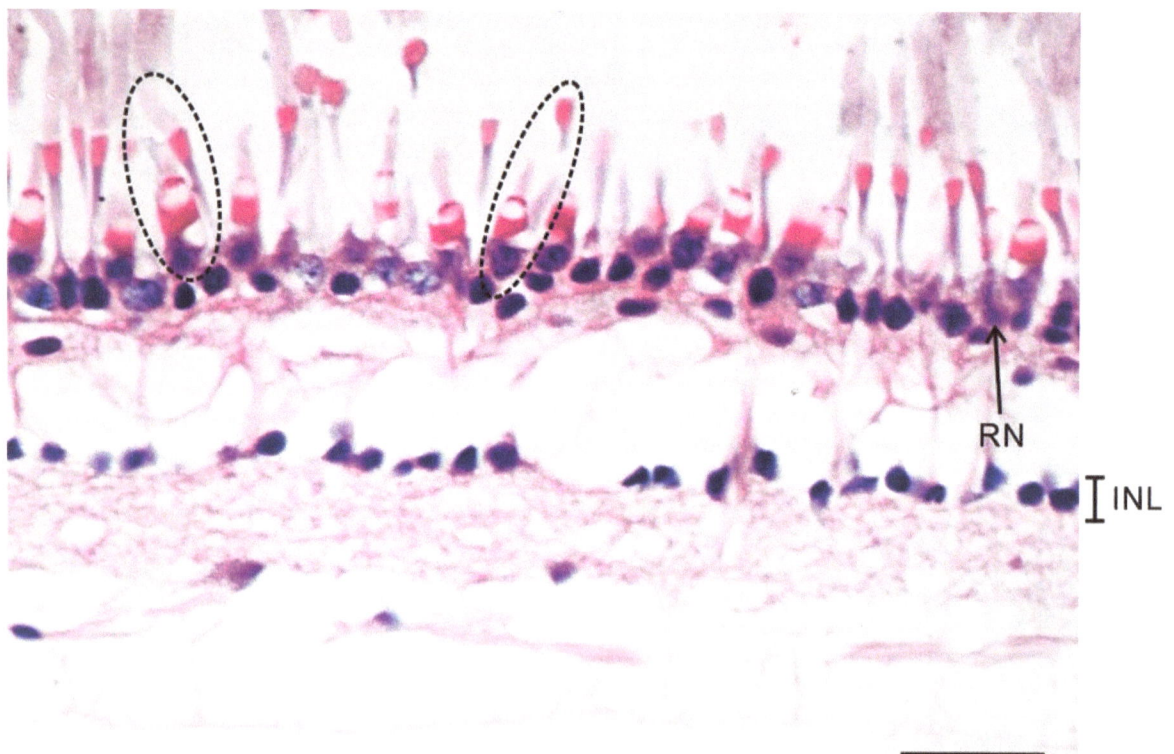

Figure 1.1i. *Central retina.*

The density of visual cells is similar in both peripheral and central regions. Visual cells are shown to be loosely packed together. Moreover, the retinal cells in the inner nuclear layers (INL) of this region are also few in number as in the peripheral. Circles indicate standard double cones with larger accessory cones and slender chief cones. A rod with an elongated nucleus (RN) is also noted in this figure. Bar = 50 μm.

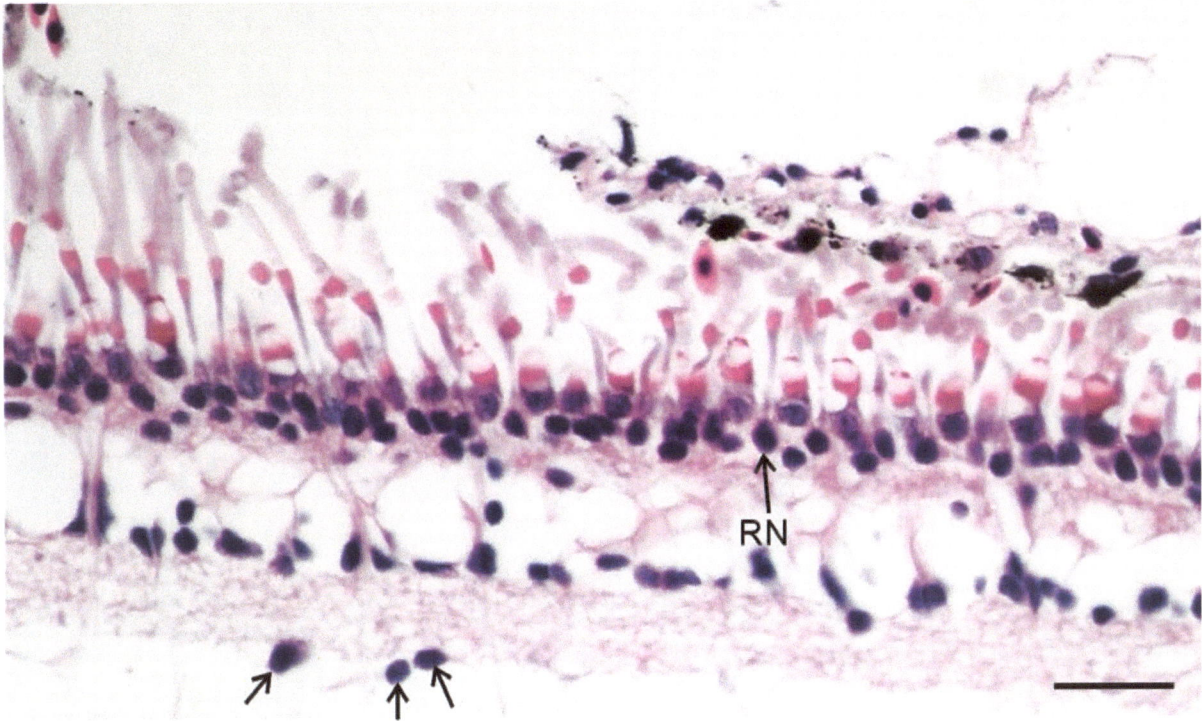

Figure 1.1j. *Central retina.*

More rods with elongated nucleus (RN) is shown. The retina of this sturgeon is noted to have very few ganglion cells (arrows) placed consistently in different regions. Bar = 50 μm.

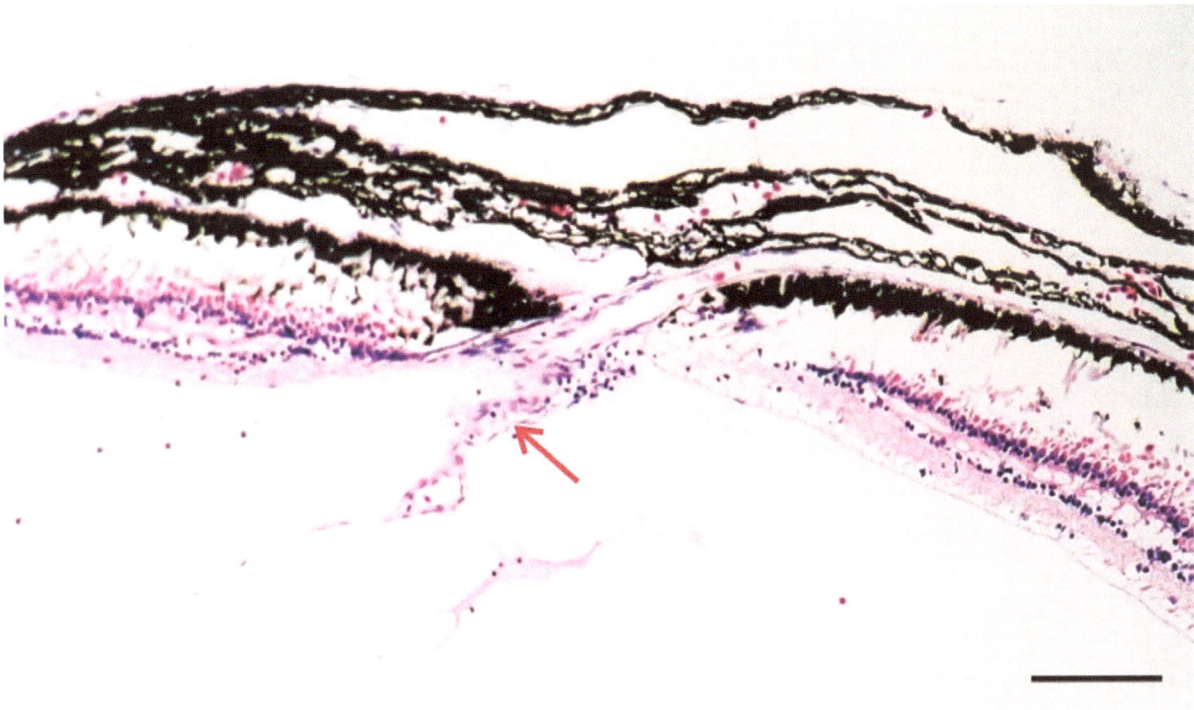

Figure 1.1k. *Fovea.*

A process with blood vessels (red arrow) sticks out from the fovea centralis of the sturgeon. Bar = 200 μm.

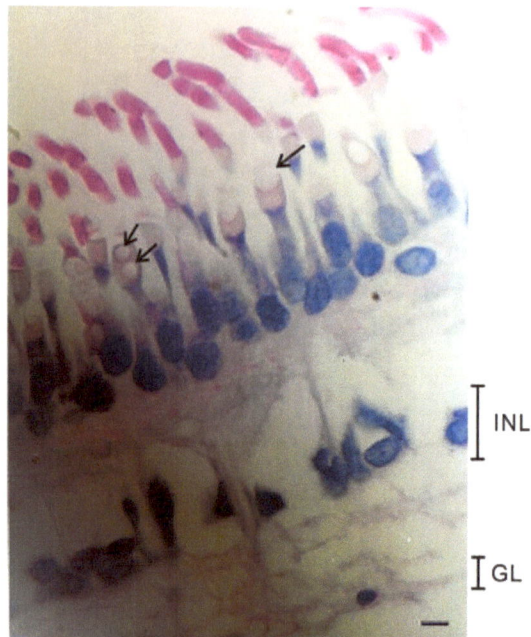

Figure 1.1l. *Periodic acid-schiff/Hematoxylin staining.*

The visual cells of the sturgeon retina show single (arrows) or double oil droplets (arrows) in the cone cells. Note the retina is not very cellular and is comprised of a simple inner nuclear layer (INL) and ganglion cell layer (GL). Bar = 50 μm.

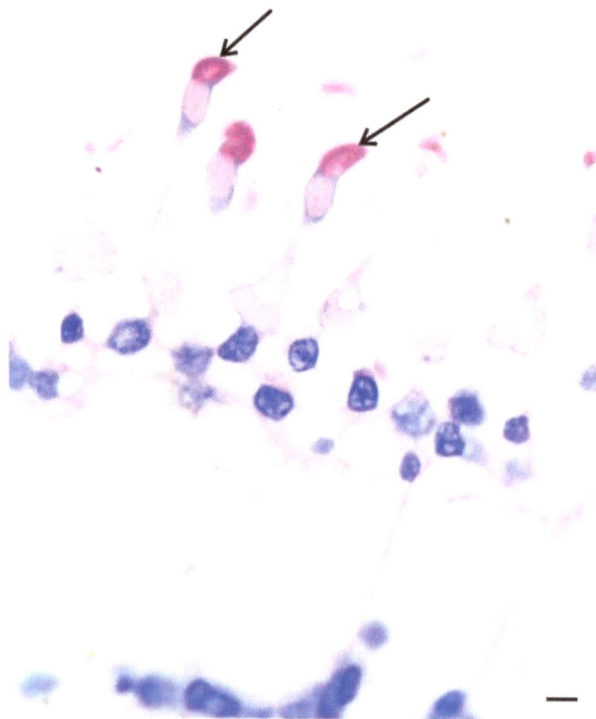

Figure 1.1m. *Periodic acid-schiff/Hematoxylin staining.*

The anterior segment of the sturgeon retina (i.e. near the ora serrata) shows mucopolysaccharide (PAS positive) surrounding the small cones (arrows). Bar = 50 μm.

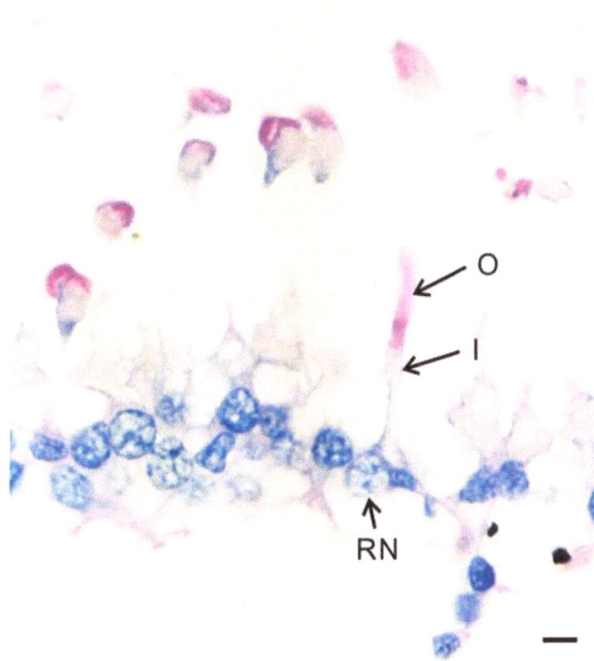

Figure 1.1n. *Periodic acid-schiff/Hematoxylin staining.*

The anterior segment of the sturgeon retina shows a rod with a vesicular nucleus (RN) and its outer (O) and inner segments (I). Bar = 50 μm.

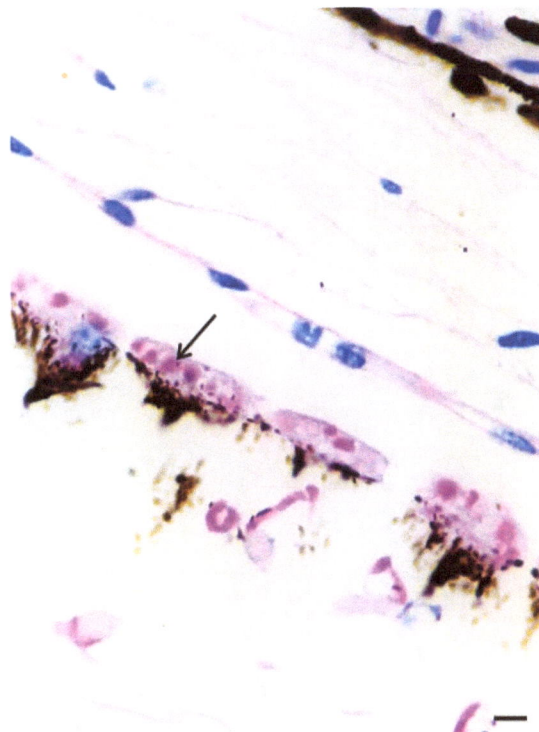

Figure 1.1o. *Periodic acid-schiff/Hematoxylin staining.*

The pigment epithelium of the sturgeon retina shows PAS positive lysosome like structure (arrow) (perhaps ingested phagosome) in the cells. Bar = 50 μm.

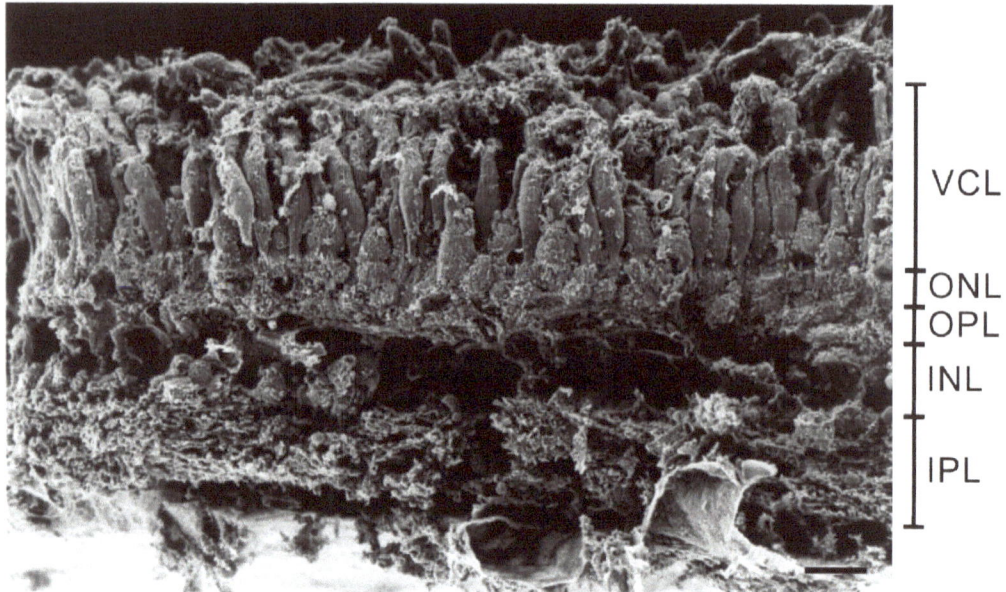

Figure 1.1p.

This figure shows the scanning electron micrograph of the anterior retina of the sturgeon. Note the size of the photoreceptors in visual cell layer (VCL). They are shorter and smaller than those seen in the central part as in figure 1.1q. Bar = 10 μm.

(INL - Inner nuclear layer; IPL - Inner plexiform layer; ONL - Outer nuclear layer; OPL - Outer plexiform layer; VCL - Visual cell layer).

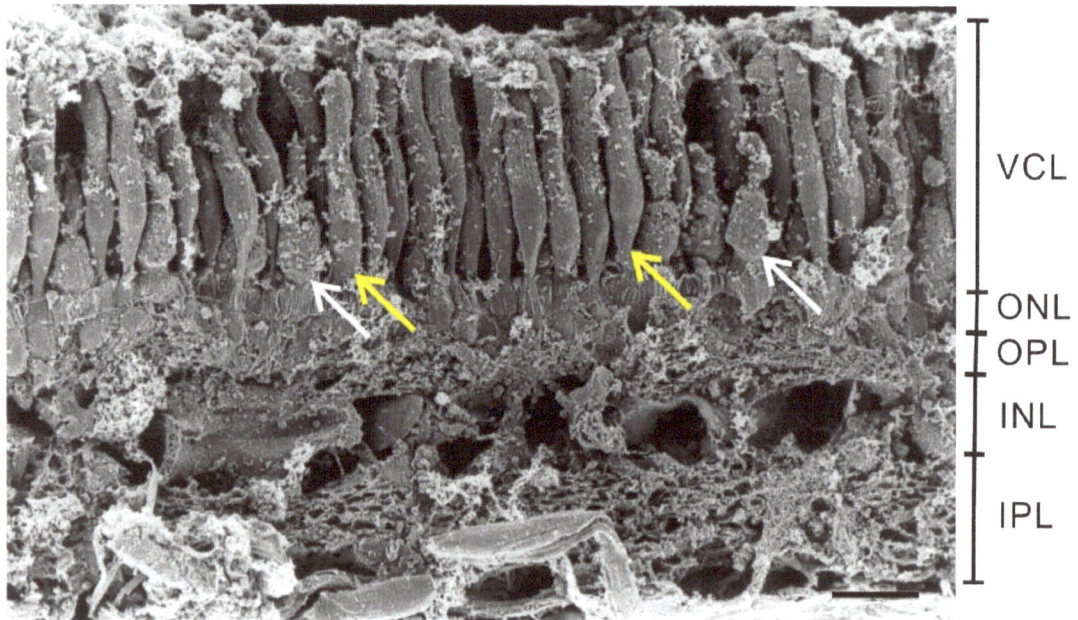

Figure 1.1q.

The visual cells in the central region are taller. There are various kinds of cone cells. Some appear as short and flask-like (white arrows), others are tall and cylindrical in shape (yellow arrows). Bar = 10 μm.

(INL - Inner nuclear layer; IPL - Inner plexiform layer; ONL - Outer nuclear layer; OPL - Outer plexiform layer; VCL - Visual cell layer).

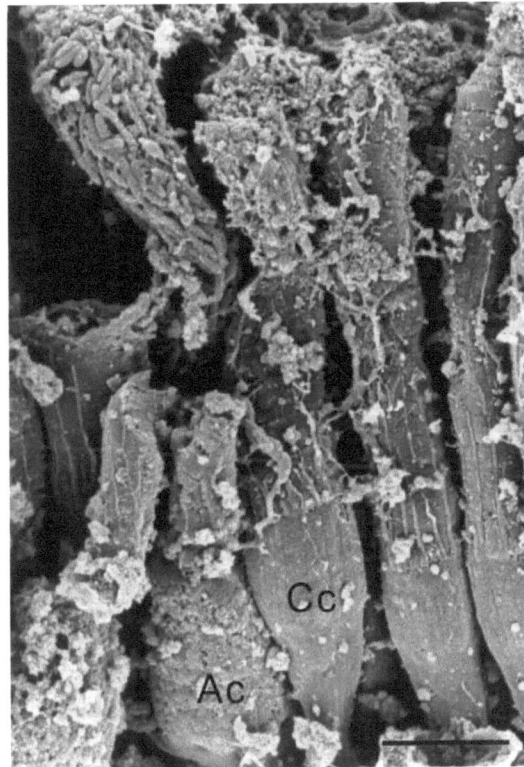

Figure 1.1r.

A double cone is displayed. The cell with the pear shaped inner segment is the accessory cone (Ac). The chief cone (Cc) appears to be taller and has a thinner proximal inner segment. Bar = 5 μm.

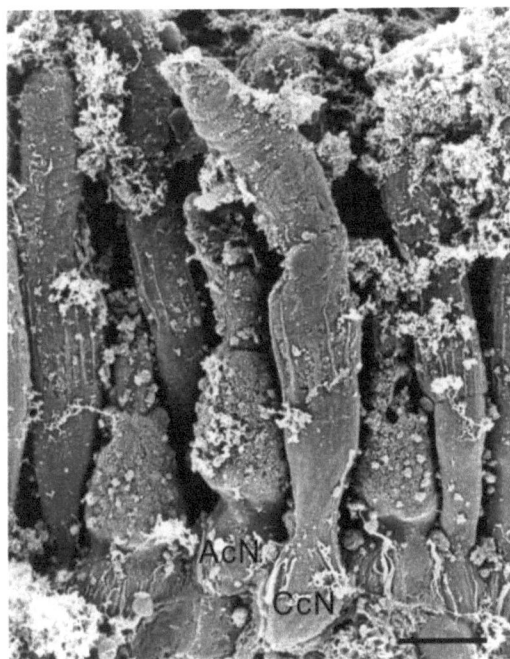

Figure 1.1s.

Another double cone seen in the peripheral retina. Note the positional difference of the chief (CcN) and accessory (AcN) cell nuclei. The accessory cone nucleus is always located superior to the chief cone nucleus. Bar = 5 μm.

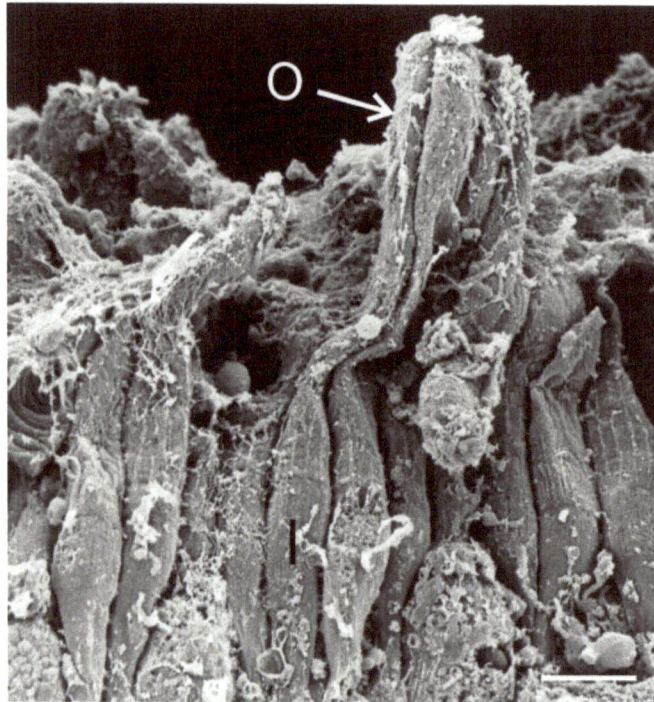

Figure 1.1t.

Note the very long outer segments (O) of the visual cells in area near the centre. They are about 3 times longer than the inner segments (I). Bar = 5 μm.

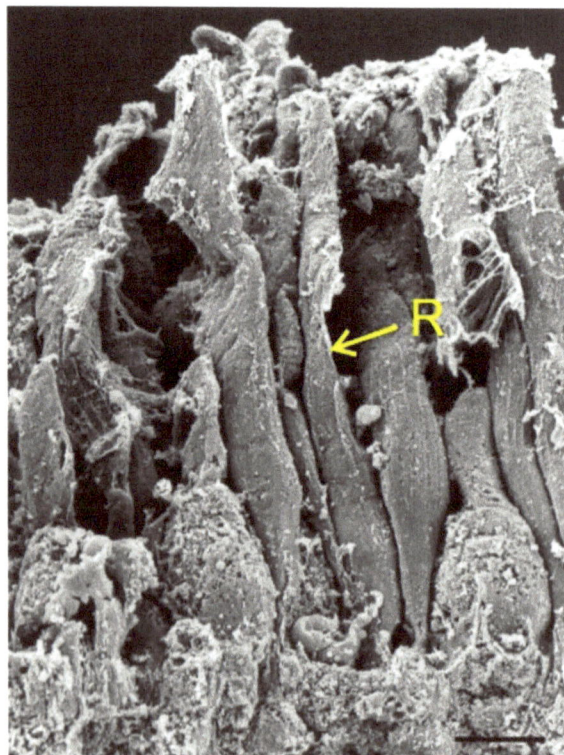

Figure 1.1u.

Among the various cone cells, a rod (R) is noted. Bar = 5 μm.

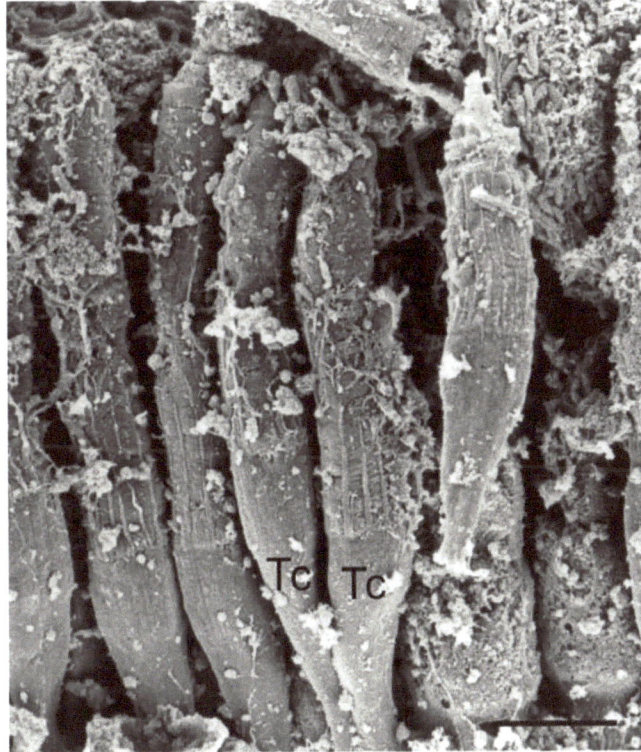

Figure 1.1v.

This figure indicates a twin cone (Tc) of equal height in the sturgeon. The proximal parts of the two components are adhered together. Bar = 5 μm.

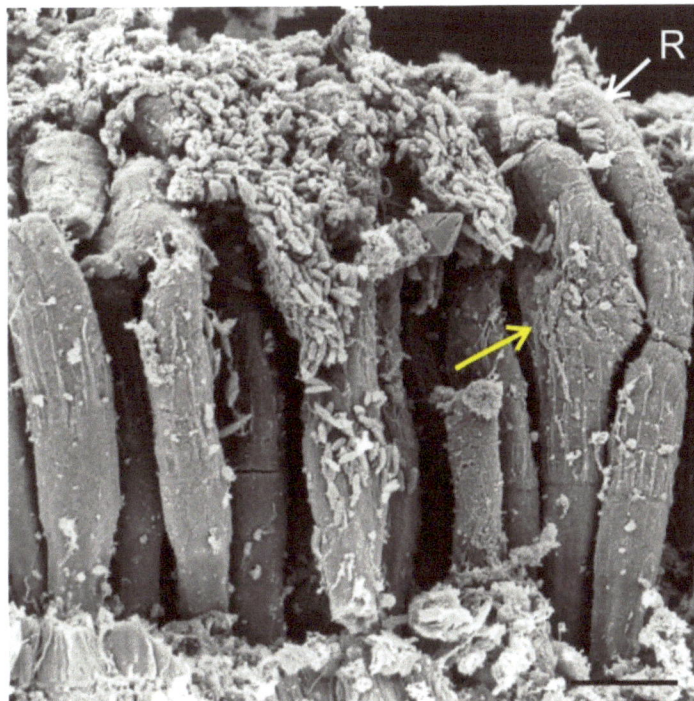

Figure 1.1w.

A cone cell with double outer segments is indicated by a yellow arrow. At its side is a rod cell (R). Bar = 5 μm.

2. EEL

The eels which inhabit both ocean and freshwater streams during their life-cycle have a retina with a thick outer nuclear layer highly packed with cell bodies of visual cells. The inner nuclear layer, on the other hand, has fewer and spaced out cells which form a great contrast to the outer nuclear layer. The ganglion cells, though not few in number, are small in size. The visual cells of this animal are numerous and closely packed. They have distinctive tall outer segments but short inner segments.

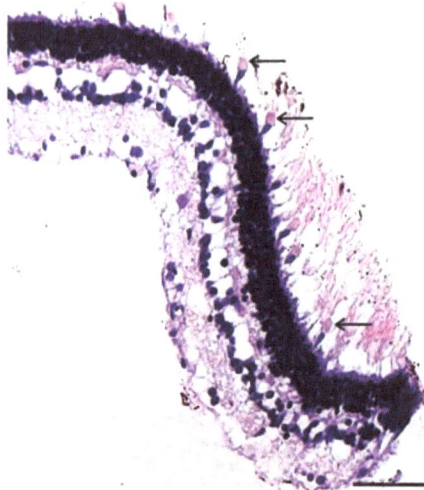

Figure 1.2a. *Anterior retina.*

There are only a few number of visual cells (arrows) present in the anterior retina of the Japanese eel. Bar = 30 μm.

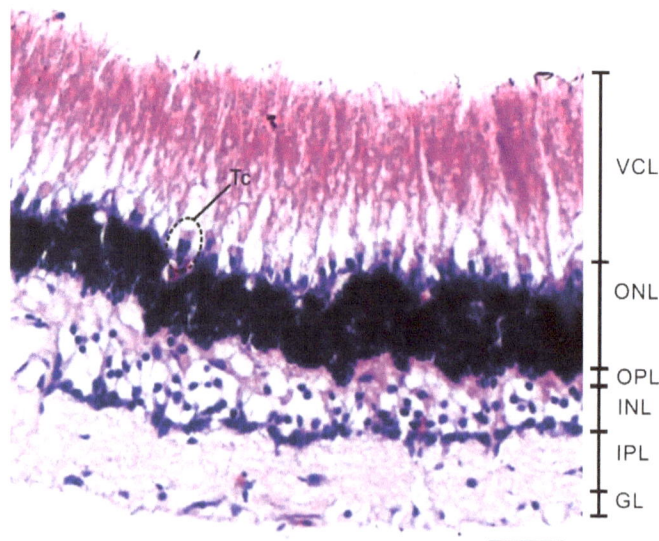

Figure 1.2b. *Peripheral retina.*

Retinal layers are identified. The Japanese eel has a very thick pigment epithelial layer (PE) as compared with the visual cell layer (VCL). Moreover, the outer nuclear layer (ONL) is also multilayered and highly occupied by various cell nuclei. Visual cells in this region are sparsely distributed. A possible twin cone (Tc; circle) is noted in this figure. Bar =30 μm.

(GL - Ganglion cell layer; INL - Inner nuclear layer; IPL - Inner plexiform layer; ONL - Outer nuclear layer; OPL - Outer plexiform; VCL - Visual cell layer).

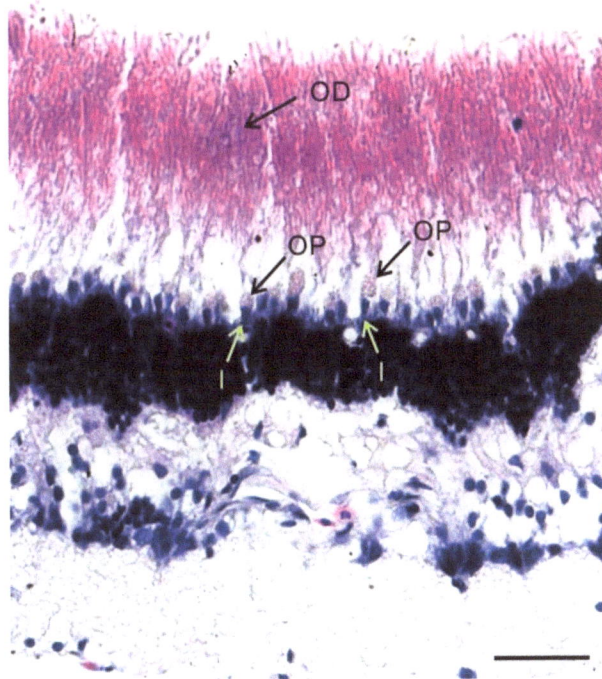

Figure 1.2c. *Peripheral retina.*

Visual cell outer and inner segments of the Japanese eel are identified. The outer segments of this animal are distinctively long, almost 4 times longer than the inner segments. They are divided into an oval shaped proximal part (OP) and an elongated distal part (OD). The inner segments (I), on the other hand, are short and appear as inverted triangles. Bar = 30 µm.

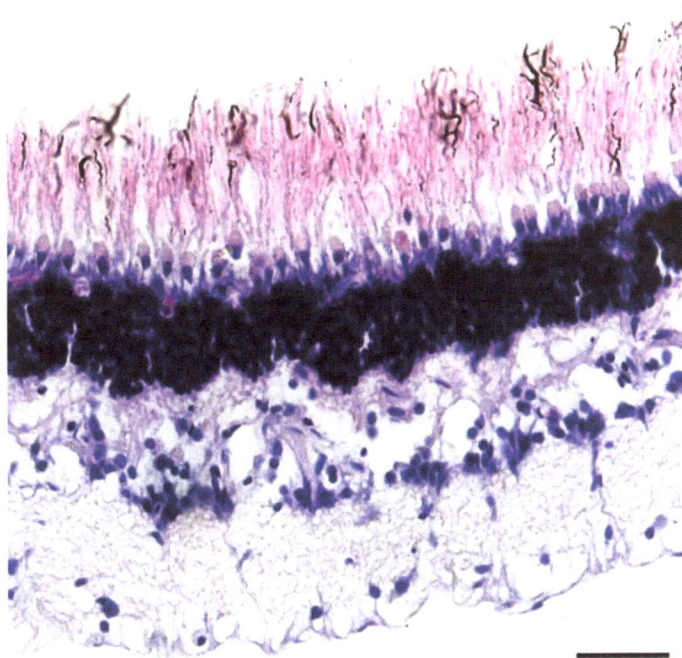

Figure 1.2d. *Central retina.*

This figure shows the retina in the central region near the fovea. As in the peripheral region (figures 1.2b and 1.2c), the density of the visual cells is not high. Bar = 30 µm.

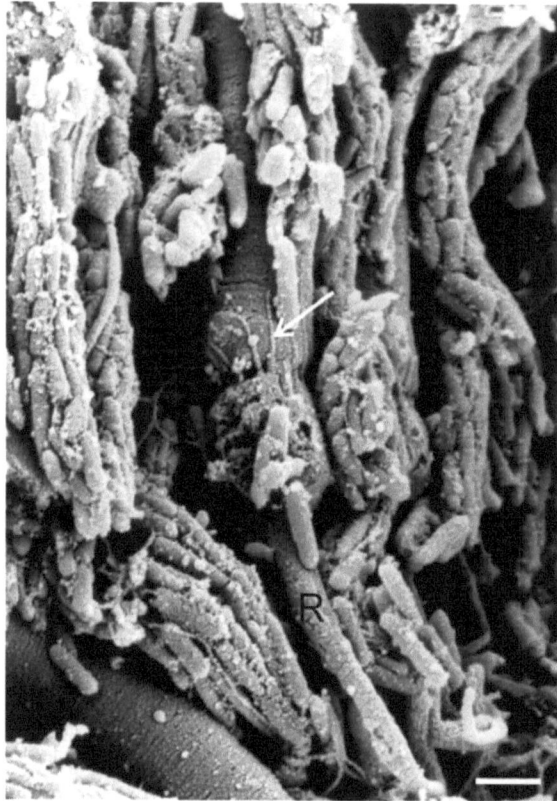

Figure 1.2e.

The visual cells identified as rod cells under light microscopy are confirmed with scanning electron microscopy. In this figure, a rod (R) is shown. Note its slender inner segment with a dilated distal part. The typical microvilli (white arrow) that surround the beginning of the outer segment are also present in this animal. Bar = 1 μm.

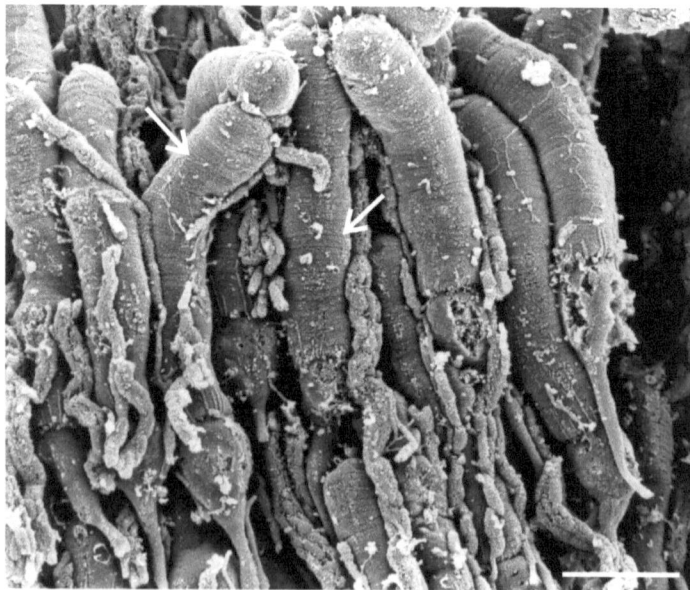

Figure 1.2f.

This figure shows a few rods with their outer segments. The characteristic "stacked membranes" of the outer segments are seen (white arrows). Bar = 3 μm.

3. GOLDFISH

The goldfish's natural habitat is the freshwater streams and ponds. The retina of this animal has a comparatively thin outer nuclear layer composed of two layers of tightly packed visual cells bodies. The inner nuclear layer is thicker but with widely spaced small cells. The ganglion cells are also small and relatively few in this animal. The visual cells are not as closely packed as seen in some freshwater fish like the garpike. Both the typical twin cones which are common in fish and the double cones are noted in the goldfish.

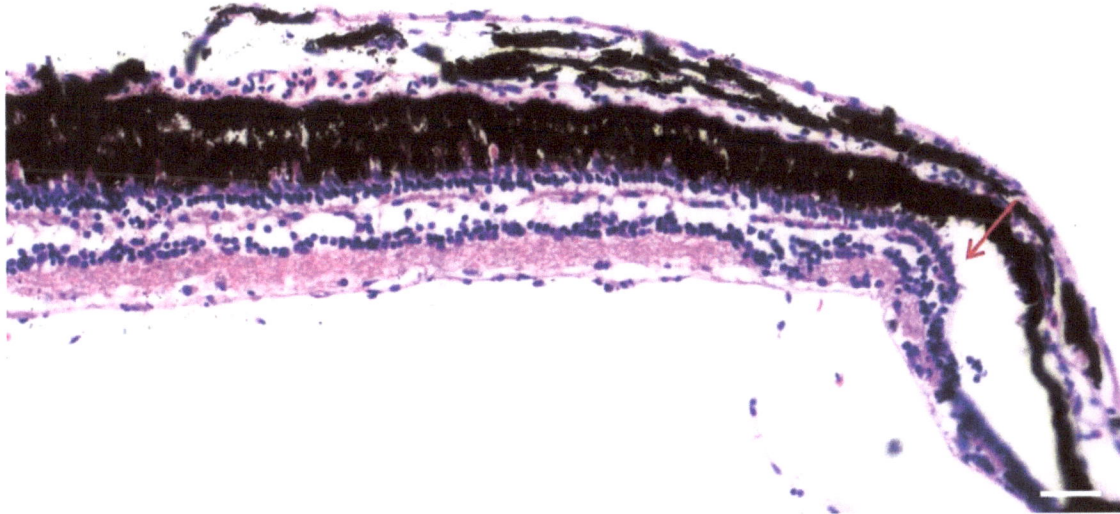

Figure 1.3a. *Anterior retina, near ora serrata.*

This figure shows the anterior region of the retina in goldfish. The visual cell layer is tighly attached to the pigment epithelium, which is almost as thick as the retina itself. Although the visual cells are not clearly seen as they are mostly covered near the transitional zone between the retina and ora serrata (red arrow), the number of visual cells obviously decreases when approaching the ora serrata. Bar = 30 μm.

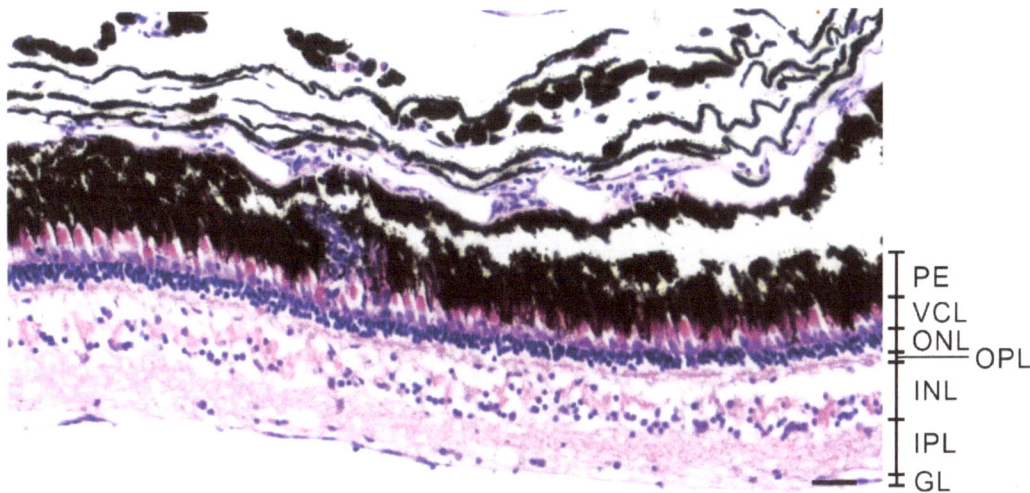

Figure 1.3b. *Peripheral retina.*

The retinal layers of the goldfish are identified. Note that the cells in the inner nuclear layers (INL) are relatively scattered in this animal. Bar = 30 μm.

(GL - Ganglion cell layer; PE Pigment epithelium; INL - Inner nuclear layer; IPL - Inner plexiform layer; ONL - Outer nuclear layer; OPL - Outer plexiform layer; VCL - Visual cell layer).

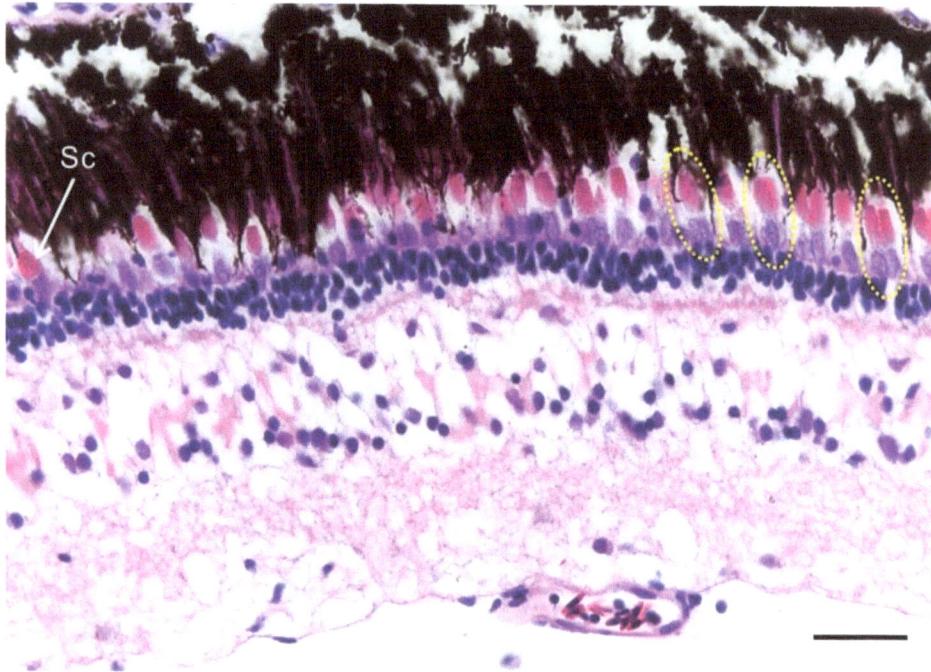

Figure 1.3c. *Central retina.*

In this figure, single cones (Sc) and twin cones (circles) are noted. Members of the twin cones have a similar appearance and are closely adhered to each other. Bar = 30 μm.

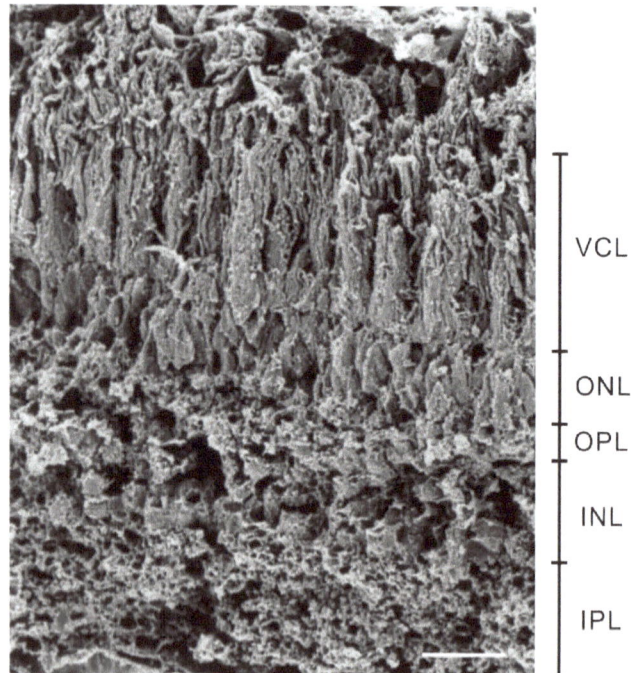

Figure 1.3d.

A scanning electron micrograph showing the different layers of the goldfish retina. Bar = 10 μm.

(INL - Inner nuclear layer; IPL - Inner plexiform layer; ONL - Outer nuclear layer; OPL - Outer plexiform layer; VCL - Visual cell layer).

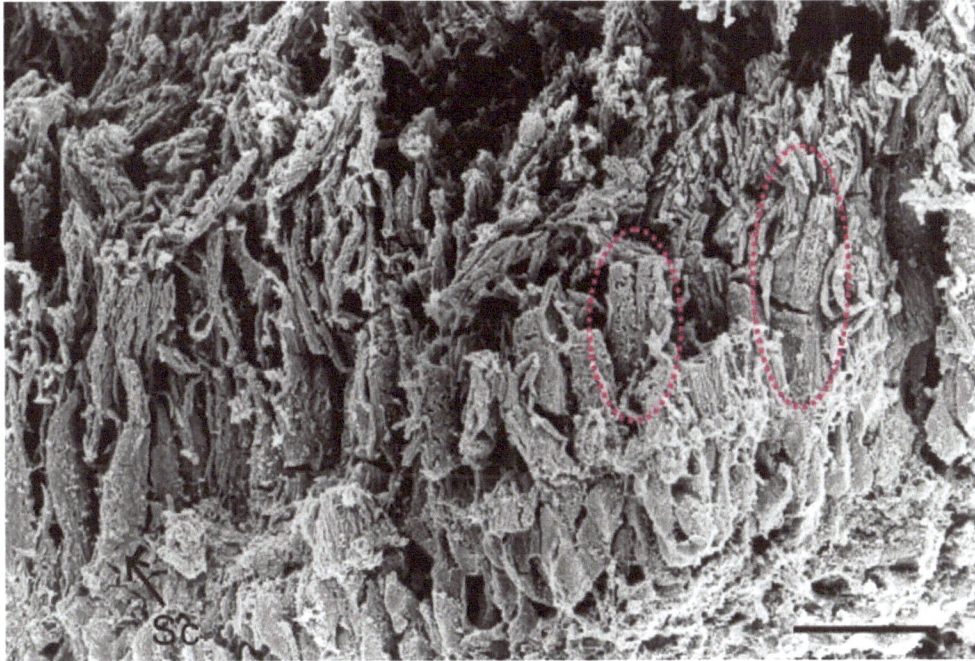

Figure 1.3e.

Among the visual cells shown in this figure, single cones (Sc) and twin cones (circles) are noted. Although the structures of the twin cones are not completely shown, their identities can be deduced from the adherence of the two morphologically identical and much adhered inner segments and their similarity in appearances. Bar = 10 μm.

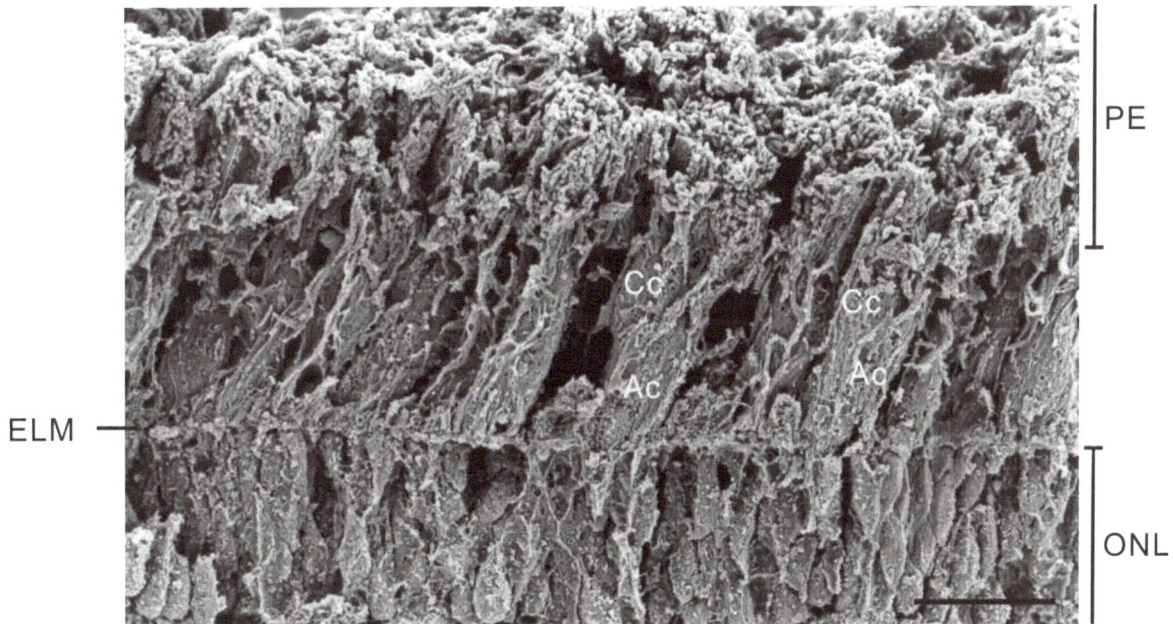

Figure 1.3f.

Typical double cones with short accessory cone (Ac) and tall chief cone (Cc) are shown in this figure. As the pigment epithelium (PE) is still highly attached to the visual cells, most of the outer segments of the visual cells are covered. The microvilli of the pigment epithelium that extend into the visual cell layer are not obvious in the goldfish. The outer nuclear layer (ONL) of this animal is multilayered, having about 3 to 4 layers of cell nuclei. Bar = 10 μm.

(ELM - External limiting membrane).

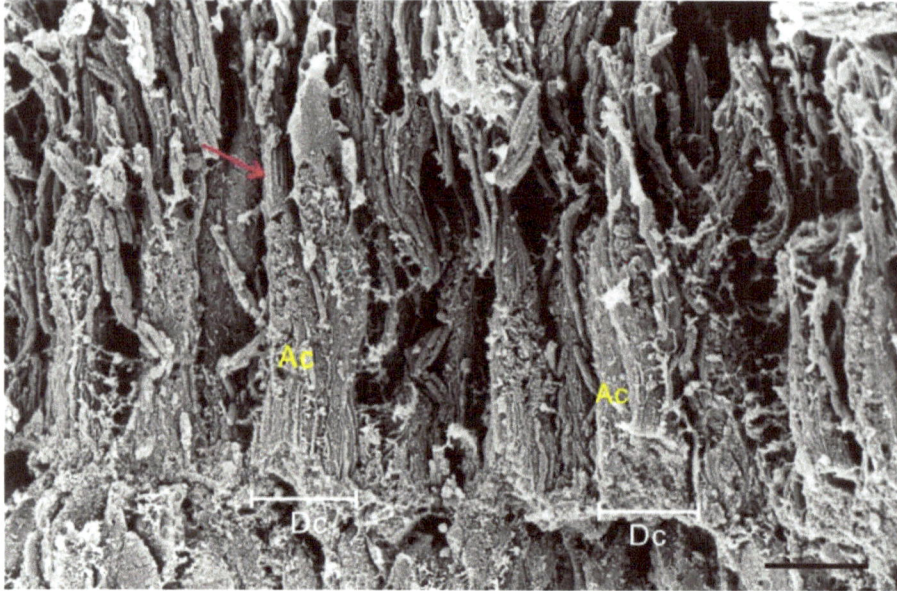

Figure 1.3g.

Double cones (Dc) with longer accessory cones (Ac) are also noted in this animal. A red arrow indicates a ring of microvilli from the inner segment surrounding the surface of the outer segment. Bar = 5 μm.

4. LIP SHARK

The lip shark is a distinct branch of fish (elasmobranchii) which has a thicker outer nuclear layer with elongated cell bodies in its retina. A lot of rods and some twin rods are seen as well. Again, the inner nuclear layer is formed by sparsely spaced cells, as in the sturgeon. The horizontal cells in this animal are large in size. A few ganglion cells are present.

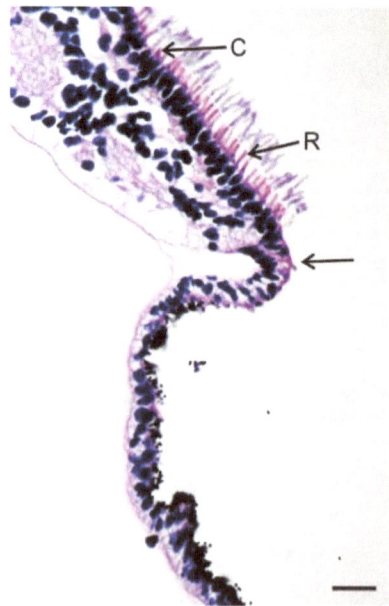

Figure 1.4a. *Anterior retina near ora serrata.*

Both cones (C) and rods (R) are present in the anterior retina of the shark; however, there are more rods than cones. Beyond the anterior retina is the ora serrata (arrow) where there are no visual cells. Bar = 50 μm.

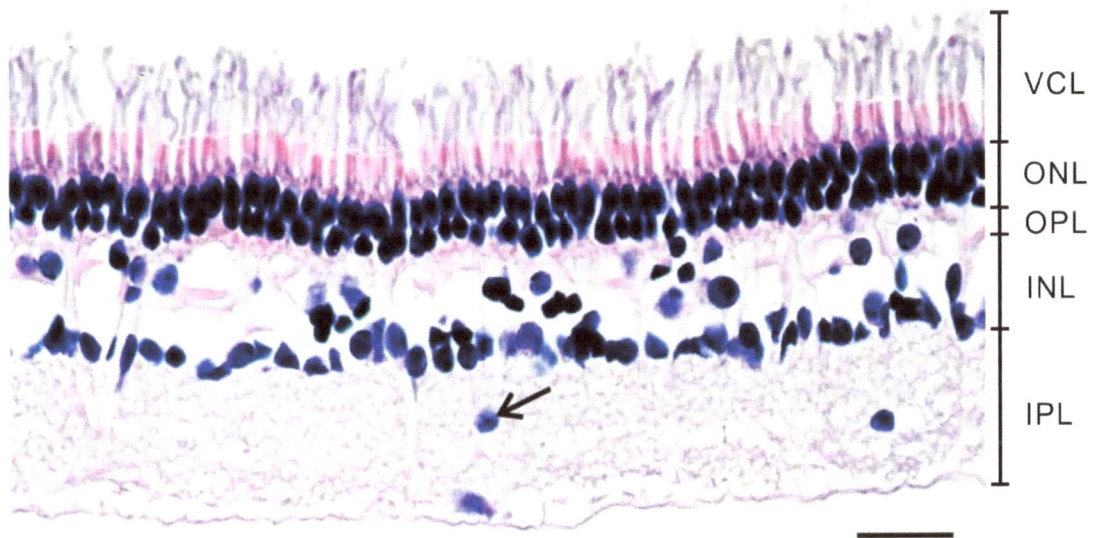

Figure 1.4b. *Anterior retina.*

Layers of the retina are shown. The outer nuclear layer (ONL) consists of nuclei of the visual cells. The external boundary of the inner nuclear layer (INL) of this animal is not discrete, some cells are scattered in the outer plexiform layer (OPL). Even in the inner plexiform layer (IPL), some displaced cells (arrow) are seen. Bar = 50 μm.

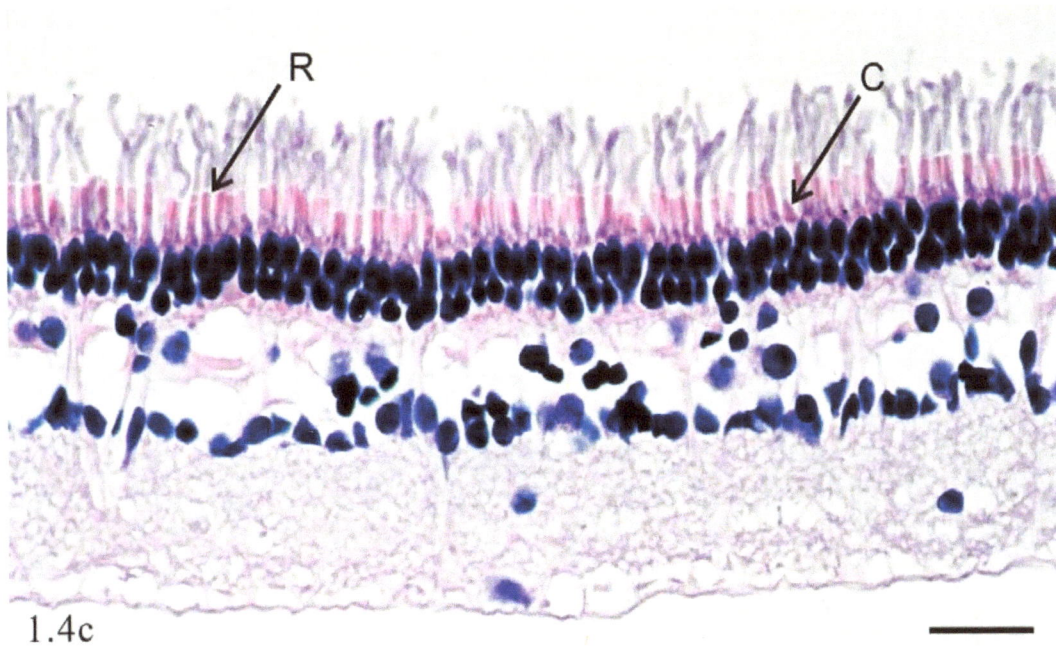

Figure 1.4c. *Anterior retina.*

Further away from the ora serrata, there are still many rods (R) but a few cones (C) are also noted. Bar = 50 μm.

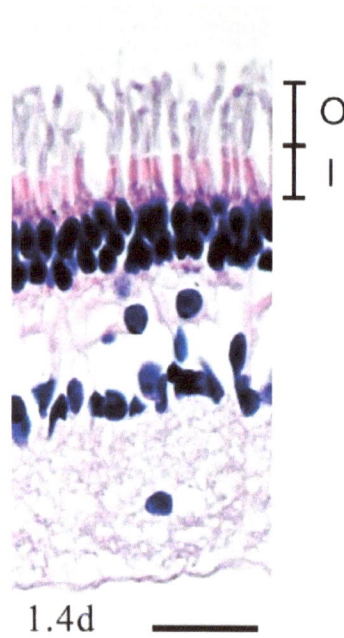

Figure 1.4d. *Visual cell.*

Outer (O) and inner (I) segments of the visual cells are identified. Bar = 50 μm.

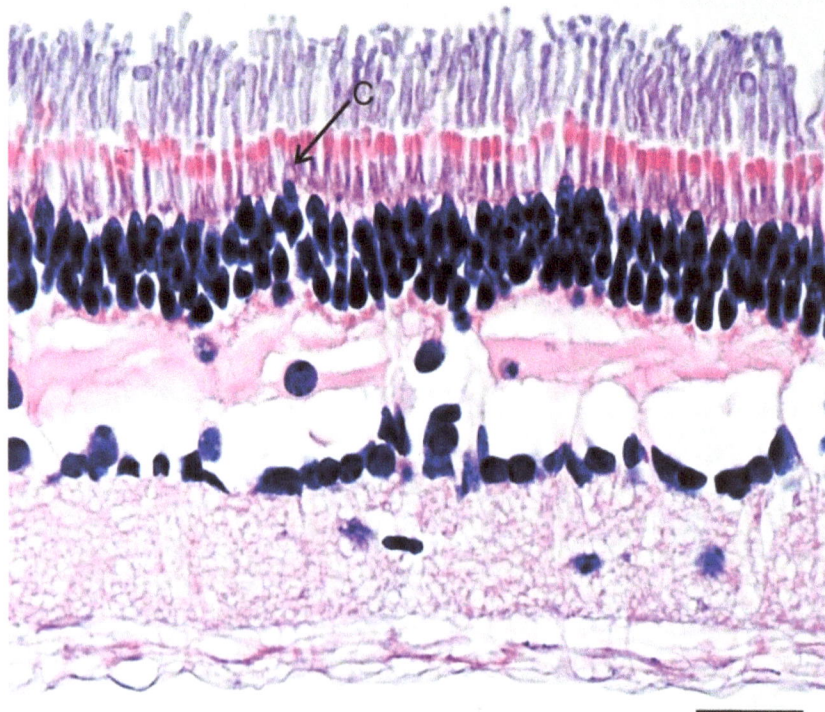

Figure 1.4e. *Peripheral retina.*

Rod cells dominate the peripheral retina of the shark. A cone with flask-like inner segment (C) is noted among the rod cells. Bar = 50 μm.

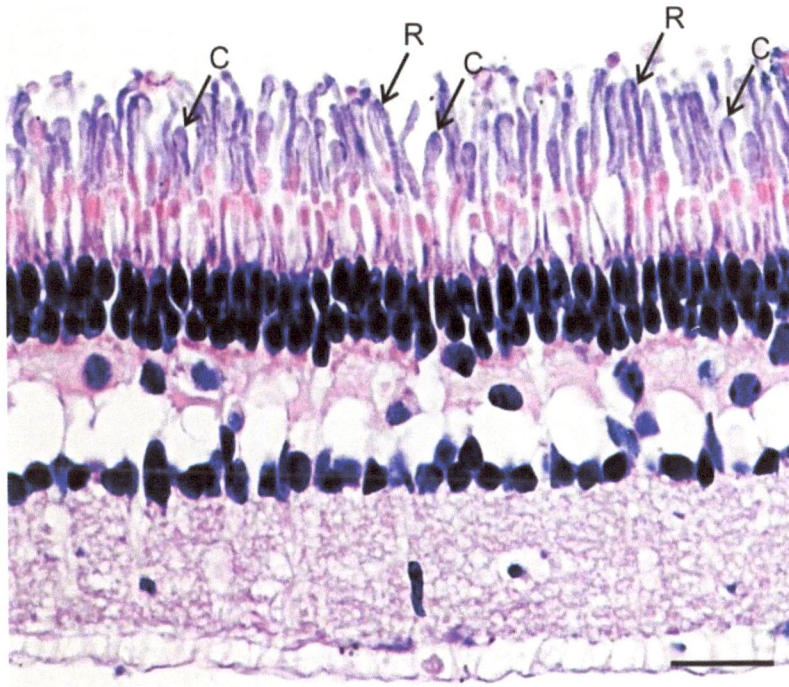

Figure 1.4f. *Mid-peripheral retina.*

The mid-peripheral retina is also full of rods (R) and a few cones (C) with thicker and round outer segments are seen. Bar = 50 μm.

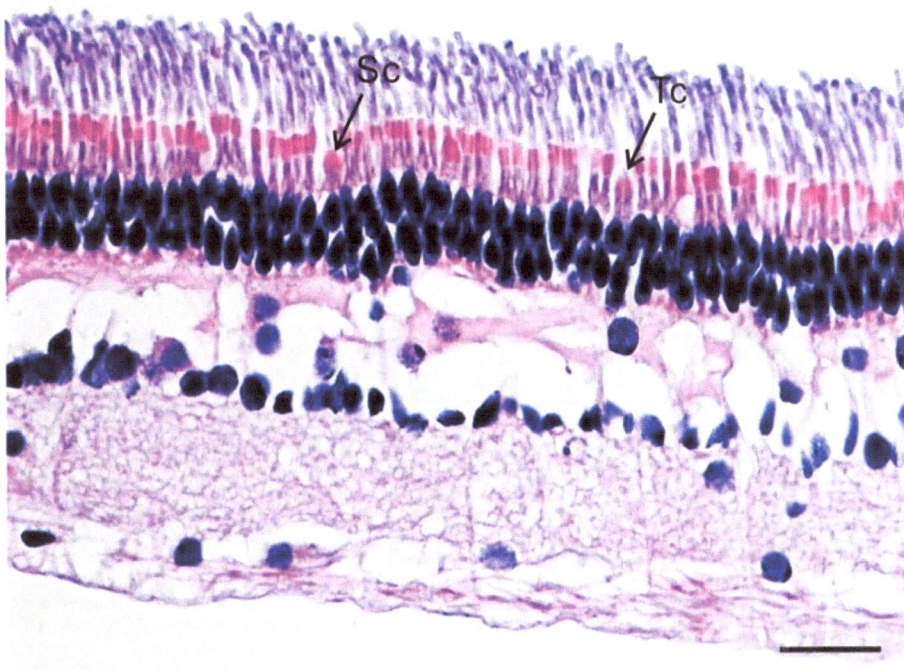

Figure 1.4g. *Mid-peripheral retina.*

In the middle portion of the peripheral retina, there are single cone cells (Sc) and possibly twin cone cells (Tc). Bar = 50 μm.

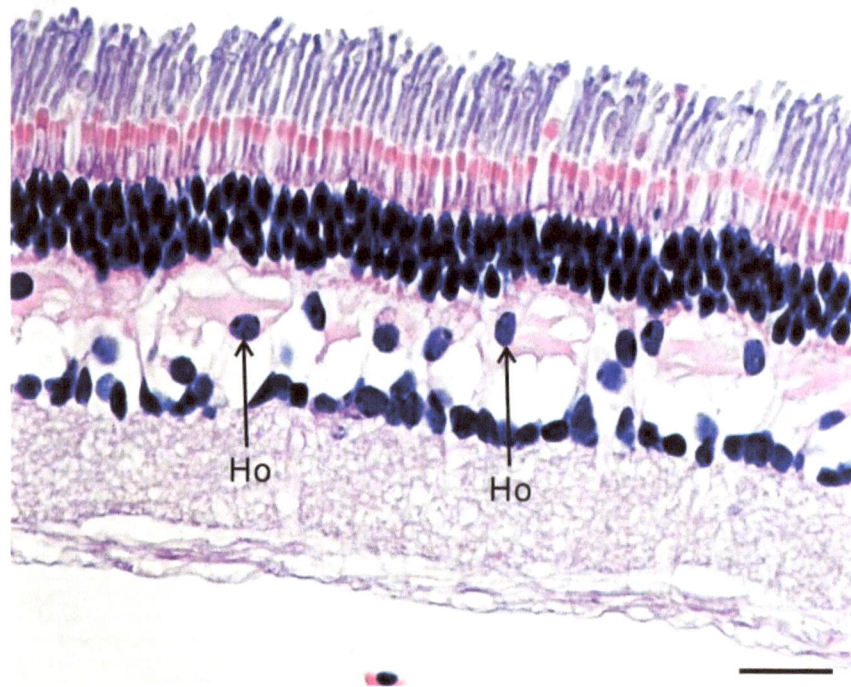

Figure 1.4h. *Mid-peripheral retina.*

Large horizontal cells (Ho) are located near the thin outer plexiform layer. Bar = 50 μm.

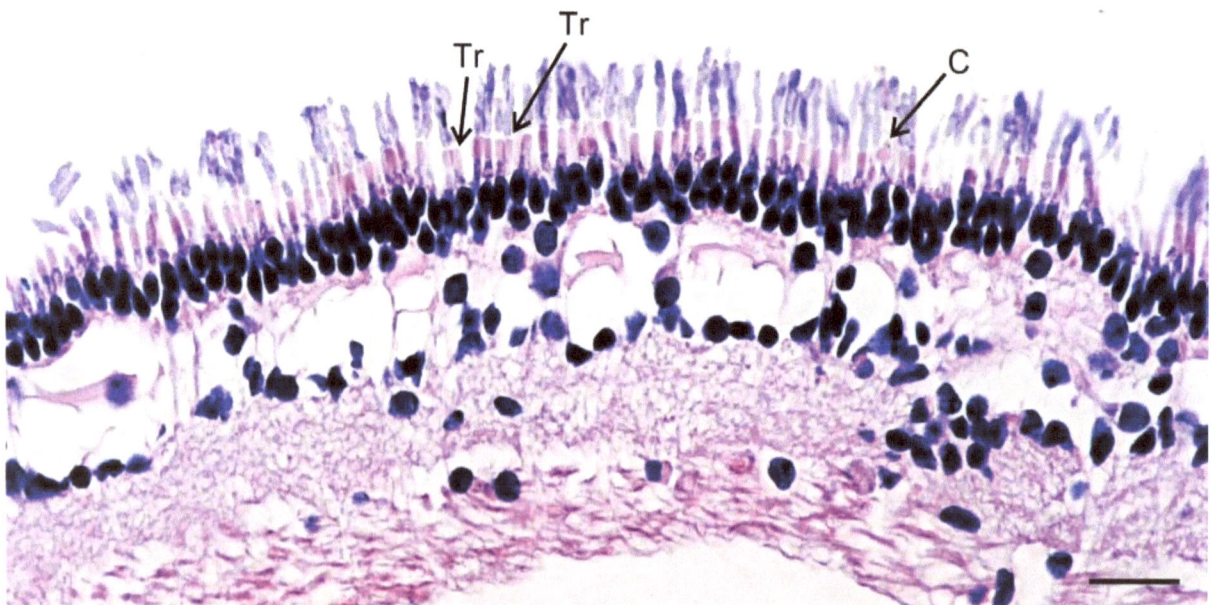

Figure 1.4i. *Central retina.*

Cone cells (C) are not numerous in the central retina. However, different types of visual cells can be seen including twin rods (Tr). Bar = 50 μm.

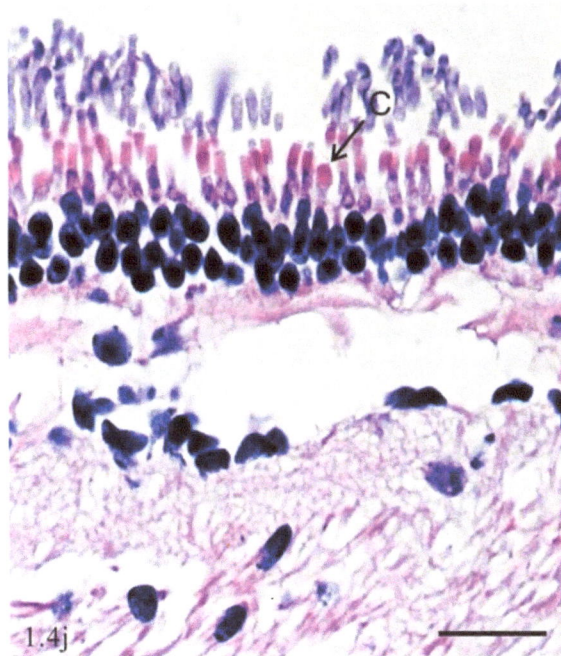

Figures 1.4j and 1.4k. *Near fovea.*

Near the fovea, the visual cells become shorter in statue. Standard cone cells (C), however, are not numerous. Bar = 50 µm.

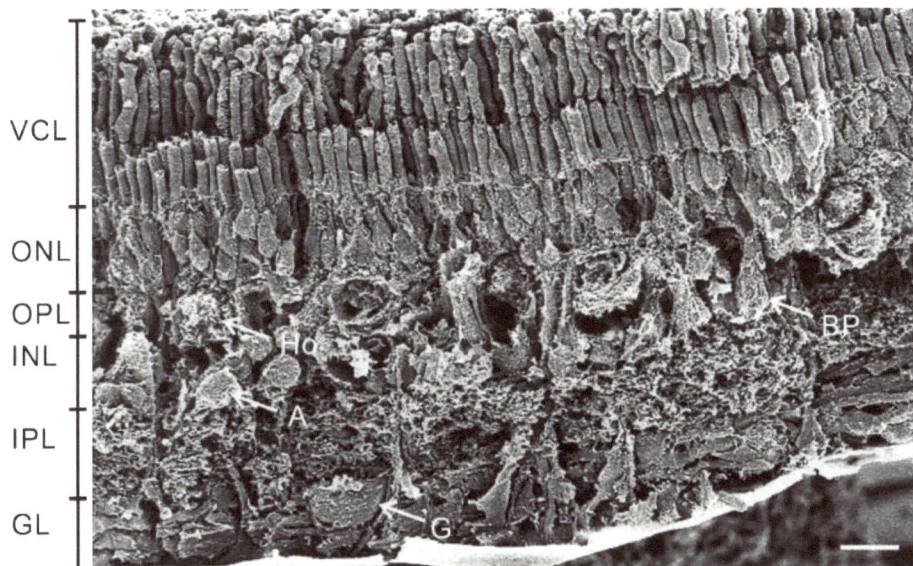

Figure 1.4l.

Scanning electron micrograph showing the retina of the shark. A row of visual cells is seen, forming the visual cell layer (VCL). The outer nuclear layer (ONL) and the inner nuclear layer (INL) are of about the same thickness. The outer plexiform layer (OPL) is thin whereas the inner plexiform layer (IPL) is thick. Large ganglion cells (G) are noted. "Ho" stands for horizontal cells and "BP" stands for bipolar cells. "A" stands for amacrine cells. Bar = 10 µm.

(GL - Ganglion cell layer; INL - Inner nuclear layer; IPL - Inner plexiform layer; ONL - Outer nuclear layer; OPL - Outer plexiform layer; VCL - Visual cell layer).

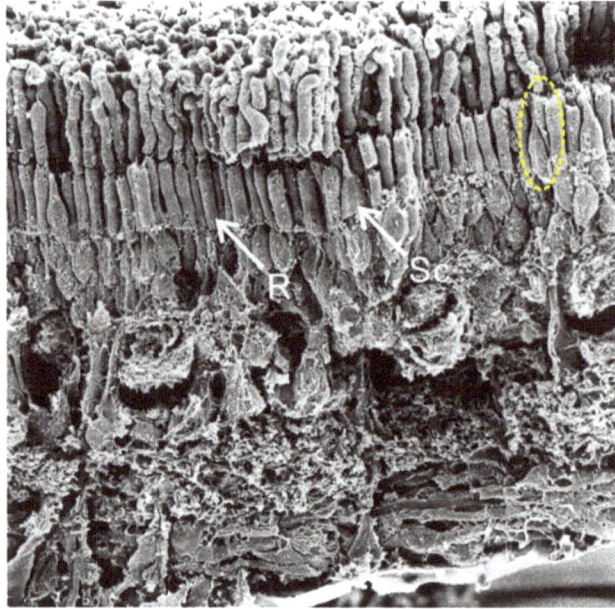

Figure 1.4m.

There are many rods (R) in the shark. A possible double cone (circle) with an accessory cone and chief cone components are noted. "Sc" is a single cone. Bar = 10 μm.

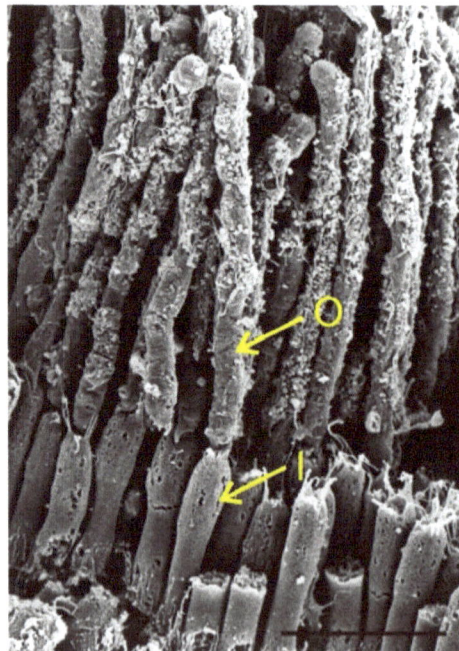

Figure 1.4n.

The long outer segment (O) and inner segment (I) of the rods are shown. Bar = 10 μm.

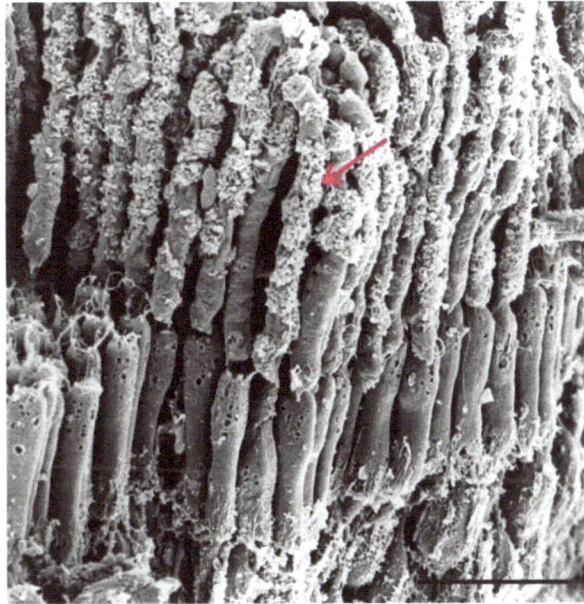

Figure 1.4o.

The outer segments are covered by mucopolysaccharides (red arrow) mixed with pigment granules. Bar = 10 μm.

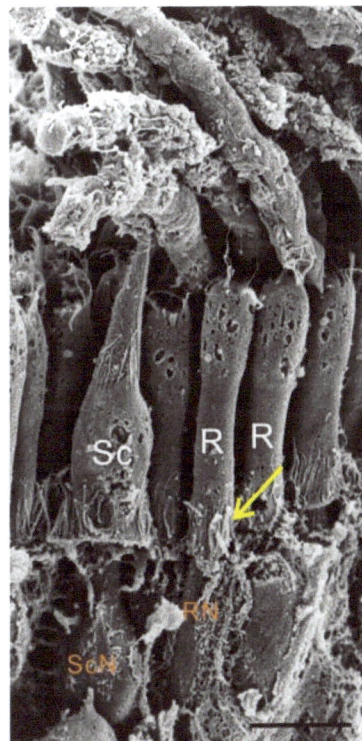

Figure 1.4p.

A pear shaped single cone (Sc) with its nucleus (ScN) is shown. On the side of the single cone are many rods (R). Their nuclei are also noted (RN). Surrounding the base of the visual cells are many Müller cell processes (yellow arrow). Bar = 5 μm.

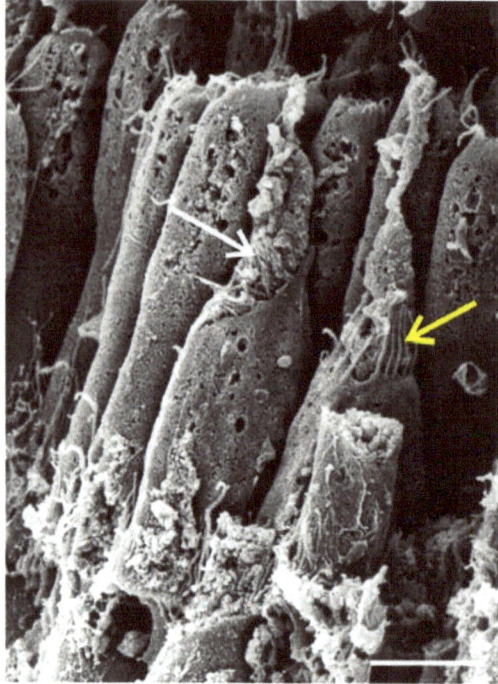

Figure 1.4q.

This figure displays two cones in the lip shark retina. The white arrow indicates the stack of membranes inside the outer segment of one cone; and the yellow arrow shows the microvilli surrounding the proximal outer segment of another cone. These arise from the inner segment. Bar = 3 μm.

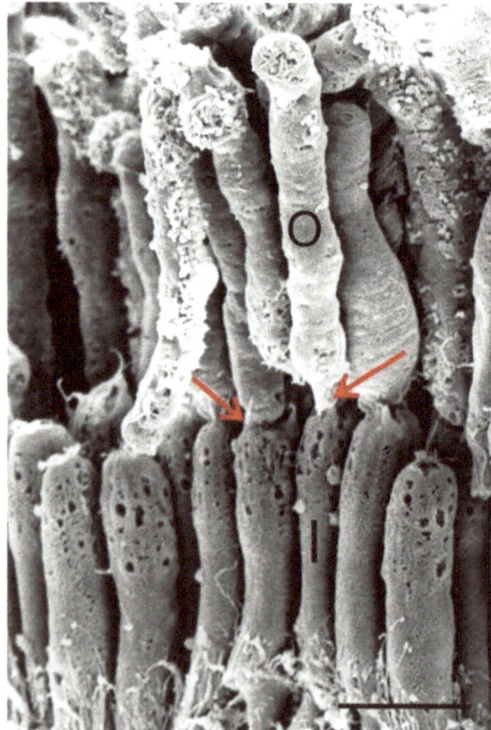

Figure 1.4r.

Arrows point to the cilia of the visual cells leading to the outer segment (O) from the inner segment (I). Bar = 5 μm.

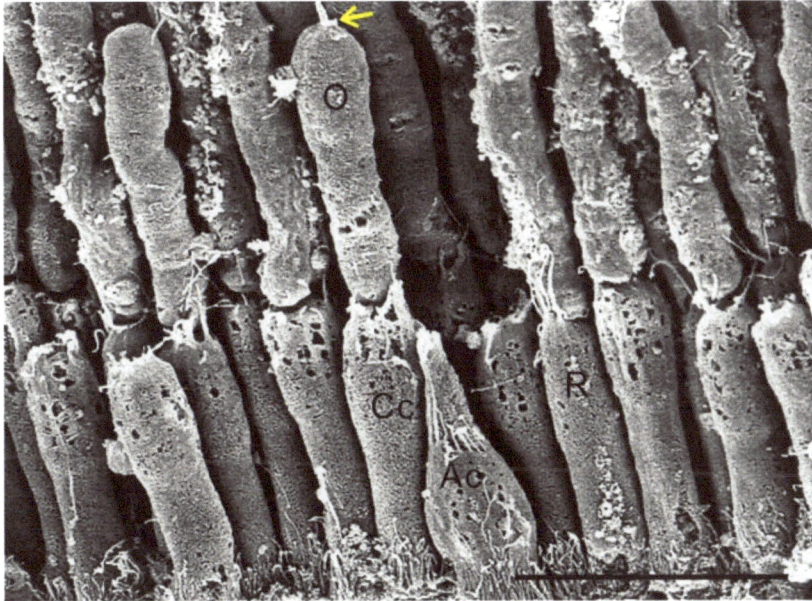

Figure 1.4s.

A possible chief cone (Cc) and accessory cone (Ac) of a double cone are shown. A rod (R) is also visible. Note the pointed end (yellow arrow) of the outer segment (O) of the chief cone. Bar = 10 μm.

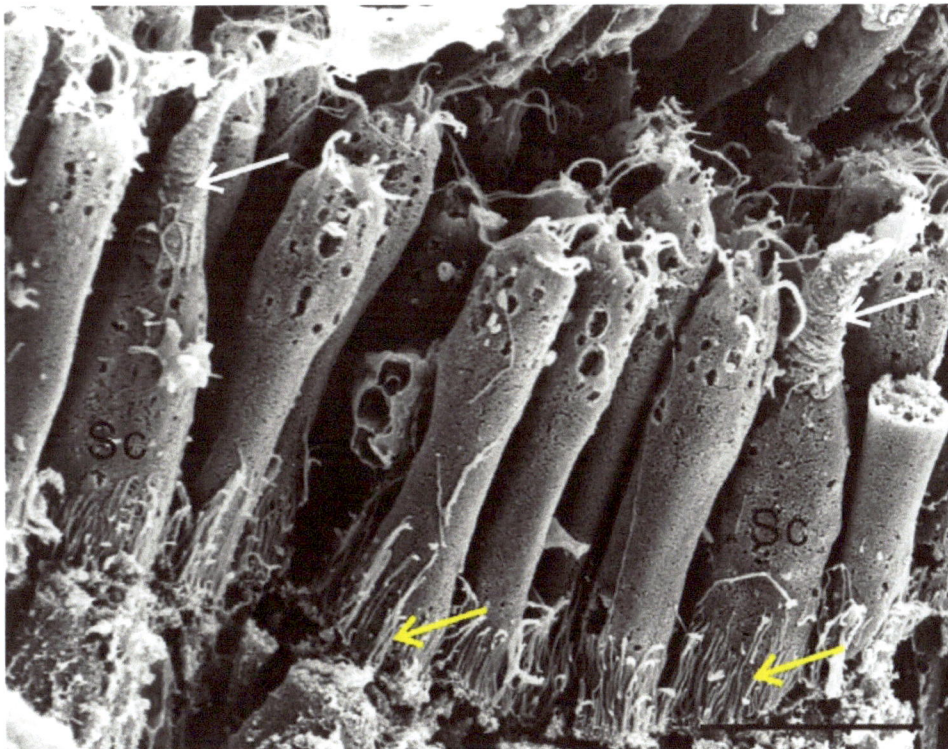

Figure 1.4t.

Single cones (Sc) with short and conical shaped outer segments (white arrows) are shown. Microvilli from the external limiting membrane are indicated by yellow arrows. Bar = 5 μm.

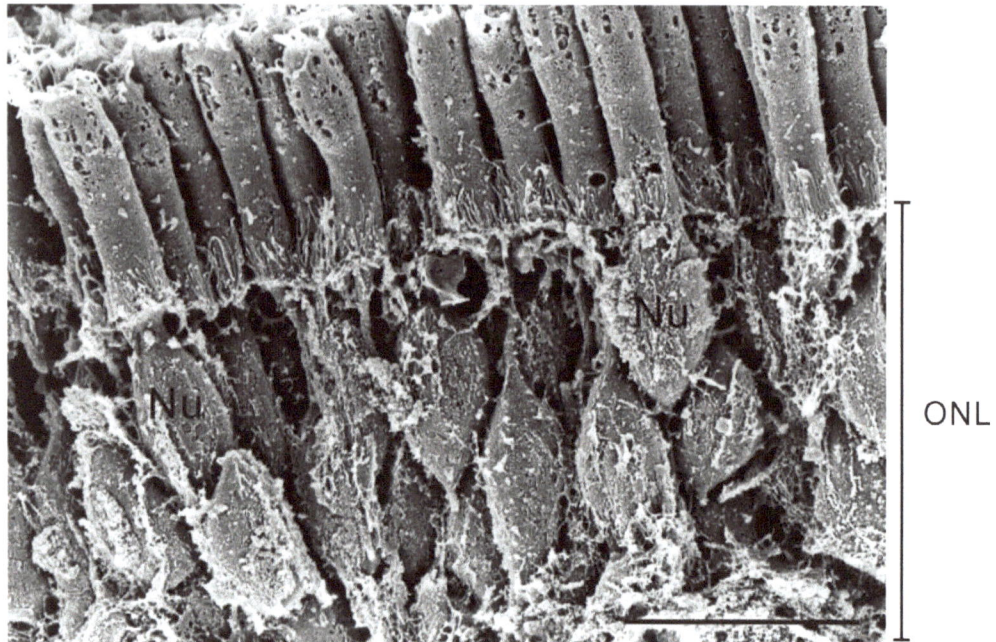

Figure 1.4u.

The outer nuclear layer (ONL) of the lip shark's retina is normally not more than three layers thick. Note the relatively large size of the visual cell nuclei (Nu). Bar = 10 μm.

5. ORIENTAL WEATHER FISH

The oriental weather fish has a retina with a thin outer nuclear layer with two well stratified layers and a much thicker inner nuclear layer. The ganglion cells are also more plentiful in this fish.

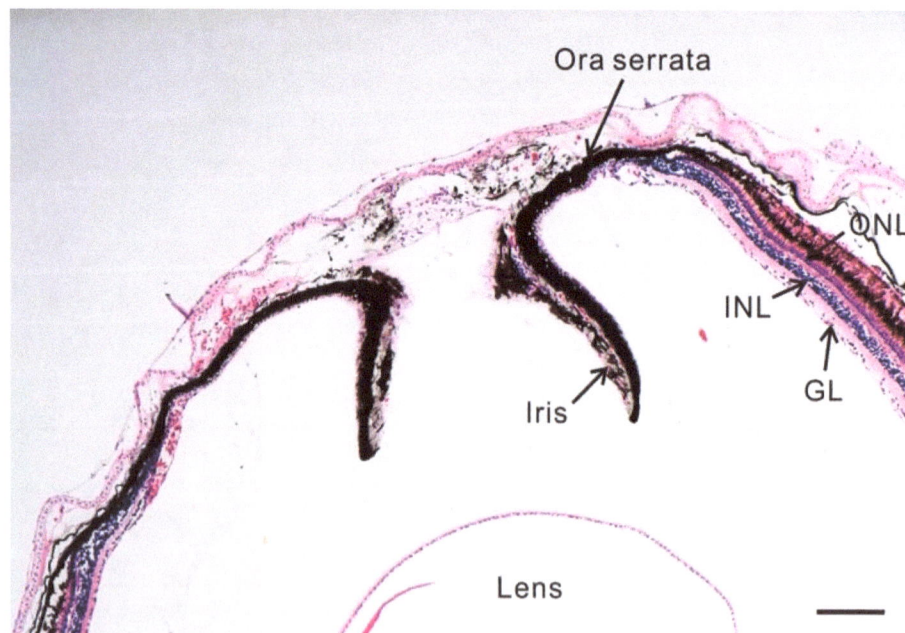

Figure 1.5a. *Anterior eye.*

This figure shows the anterior region of the eye in an oriental weather fish. Bar = 100 μm.

(GL - Ganglion cell layer; INL - Inner nuclear layer; ONL - Outer nuclear layer).

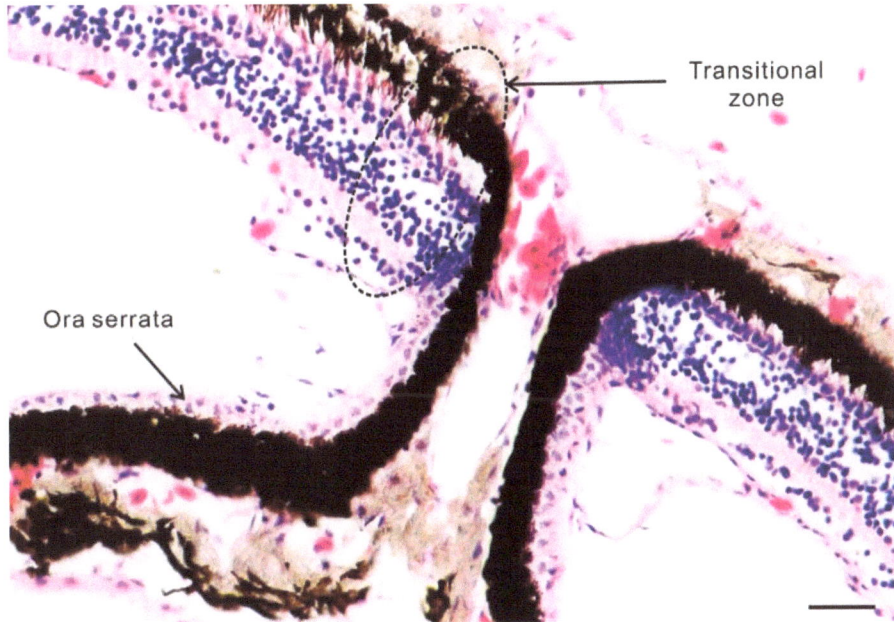

Figure 1.5b. *Ora serrata and anterior retina.*

Note the absence of visual cells in the ora serrata. Bar = 50 μm.

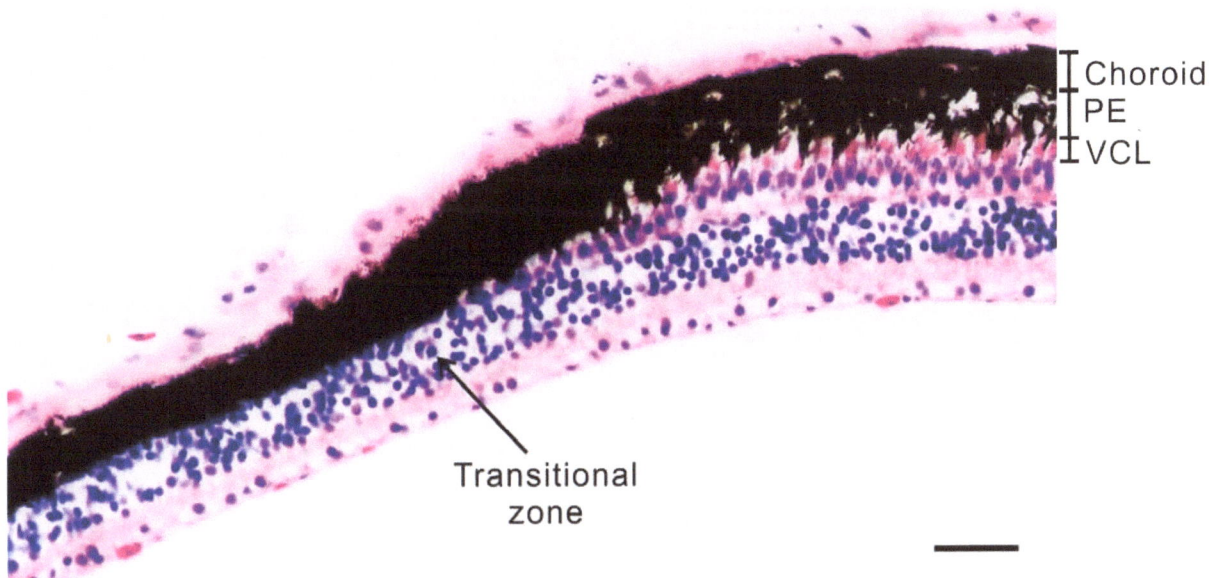

Figure 1.5c. *Ora serrata and anterior retina.*

This figure displays the transitional zone into ora serrata. On the right, a layer of visual cells (VCL) is still present. The black layer represents the choroid and pigment epithelium (PE) combined. Bar = 50 μm.

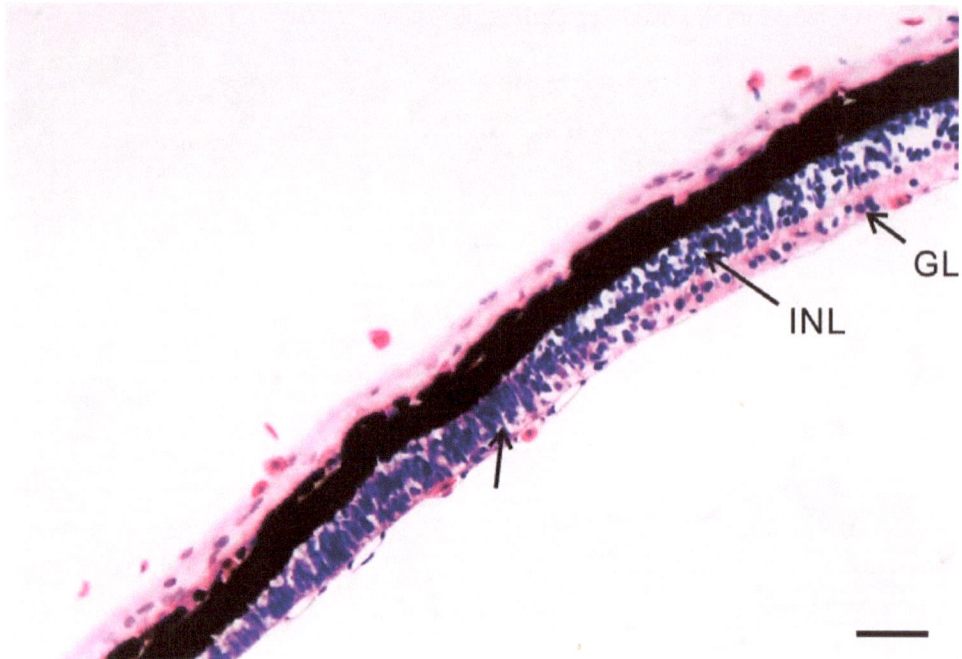

Figure 1.5d. *Ora serrata and anterior retina.*

The anterior retina finally becomes more layered posteriorly. An inner nuclear layer (INL) and a ganglion cell layer (GL) can be identified. In the more anterior region, the inner nuclear layer develops into a palisade layer of elongated cells (arrow). Bar = 50 μm.

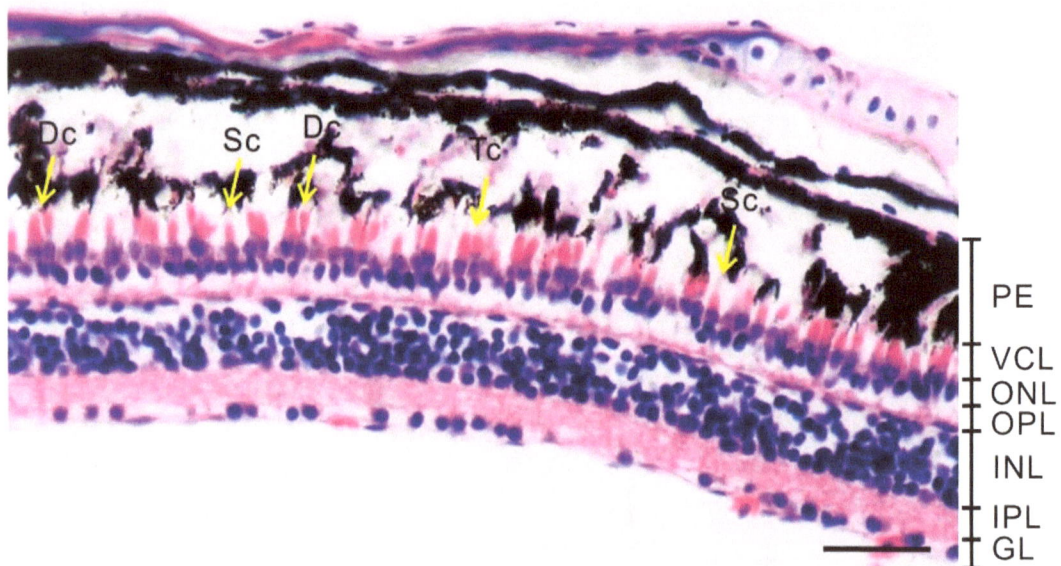

Figure 1.5e. *Peripheral retina.*

The peripheral retina of this fish still contains a lot of cones; a double cone (Dc) with a tall chief cone and a short accessory cone is shown. The nuclei of these cones are situated in the uppermost layer of the outer nuclear layer (ONL), as are the single cone (Sc) nuclei. The two cones of equal height and size are possibly twin cones (Tc). Bar = 50 μm.

(GL - Ganglion cell layer; INL - Inner nuclear layer; IPL - Inner plexiform layer; ONL - Outer nuclear layer; OPL - Outer plexiform layer; PE - Pigment epithelium; VCL - Visucal cell layer).

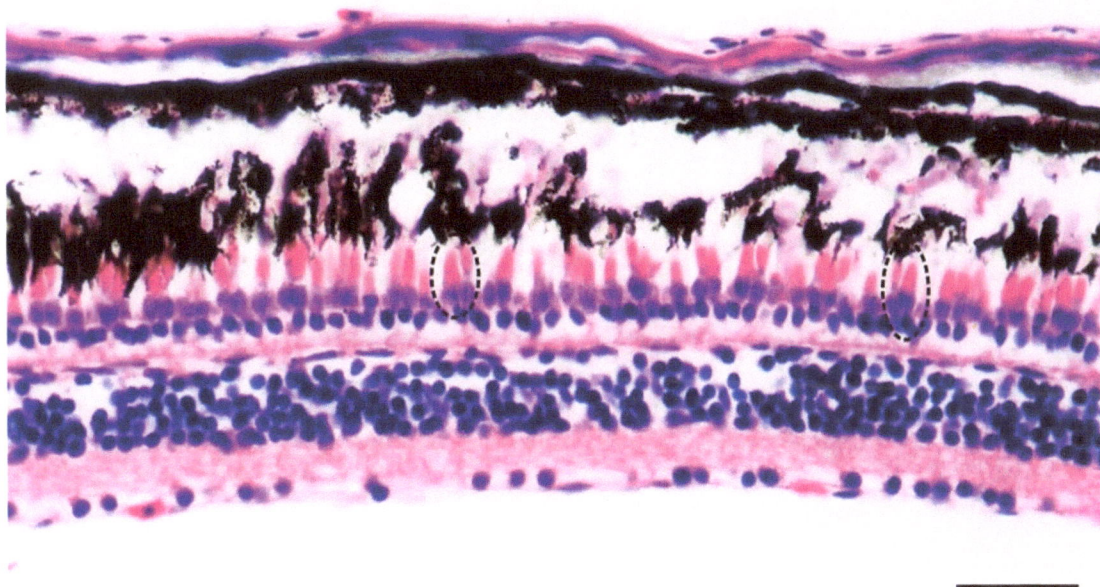

Figure 1.5f. *Peripheral retina.*

The visual cells in this region of the retina are few and sparsely distributed. The circles indicate the double cones. Bar = 50 μm.

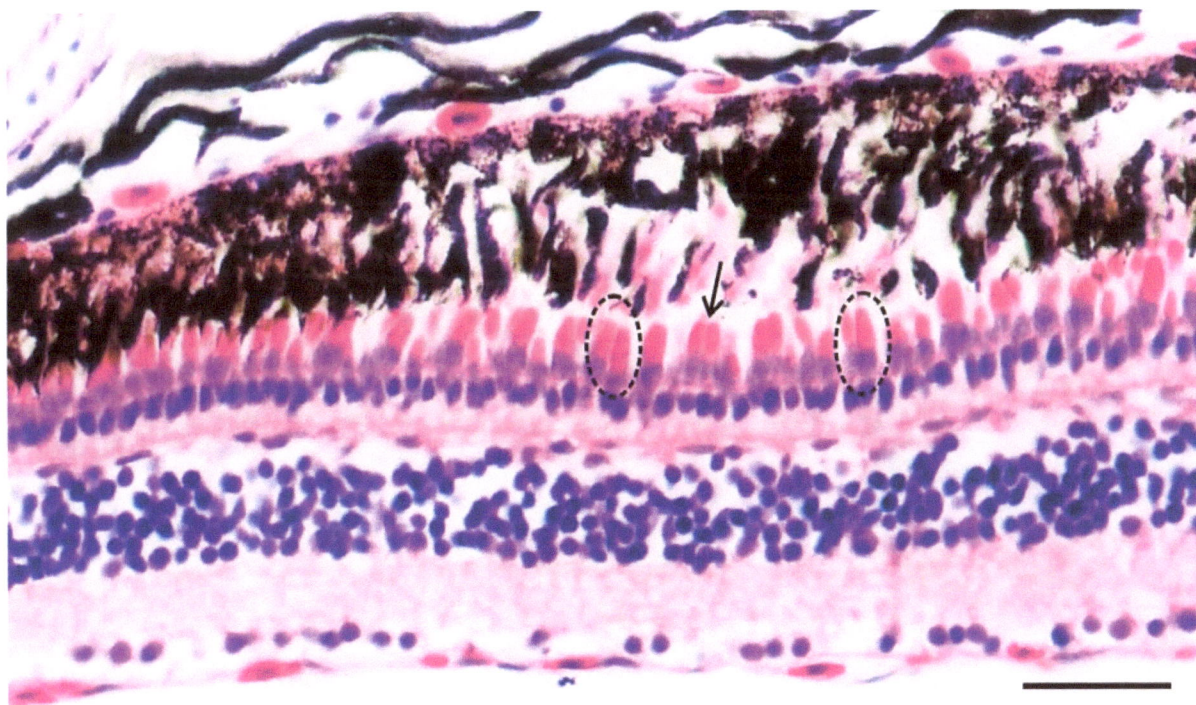

Figure 1.5g. *Peripheral retina.*

Again, this figure shows the double cones (circles) and twin cones (arrow) in the peripheral retina. Note that the arrangement of their nuclei is different. Twin cones have elongated nuclei. Bar = 50 μm.

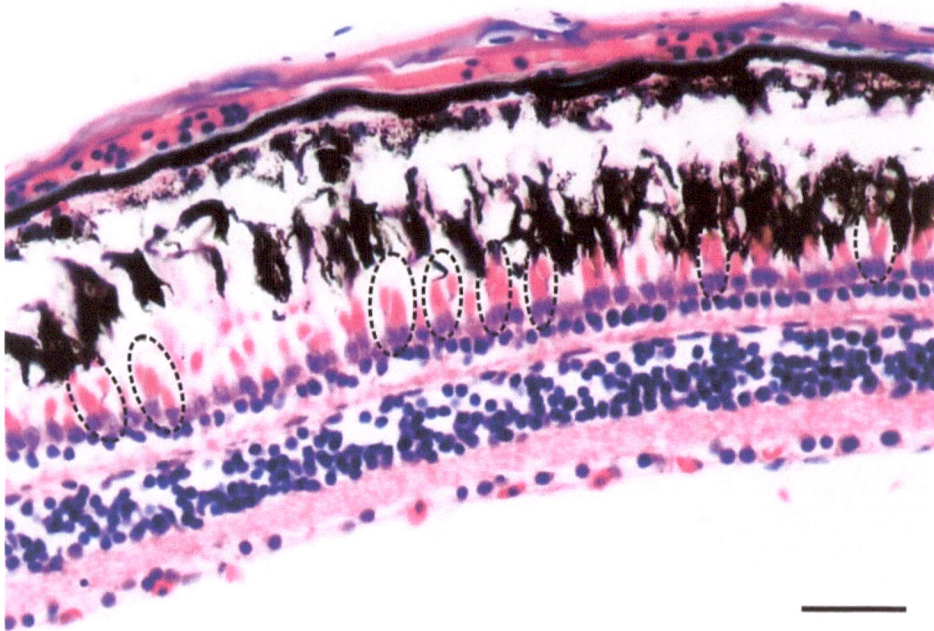

Figure 1.5h. *Mid-peripheral retina.*

In the mid-peripheral region, double cones still dominate the retina (circles). Bar = 50 μm.

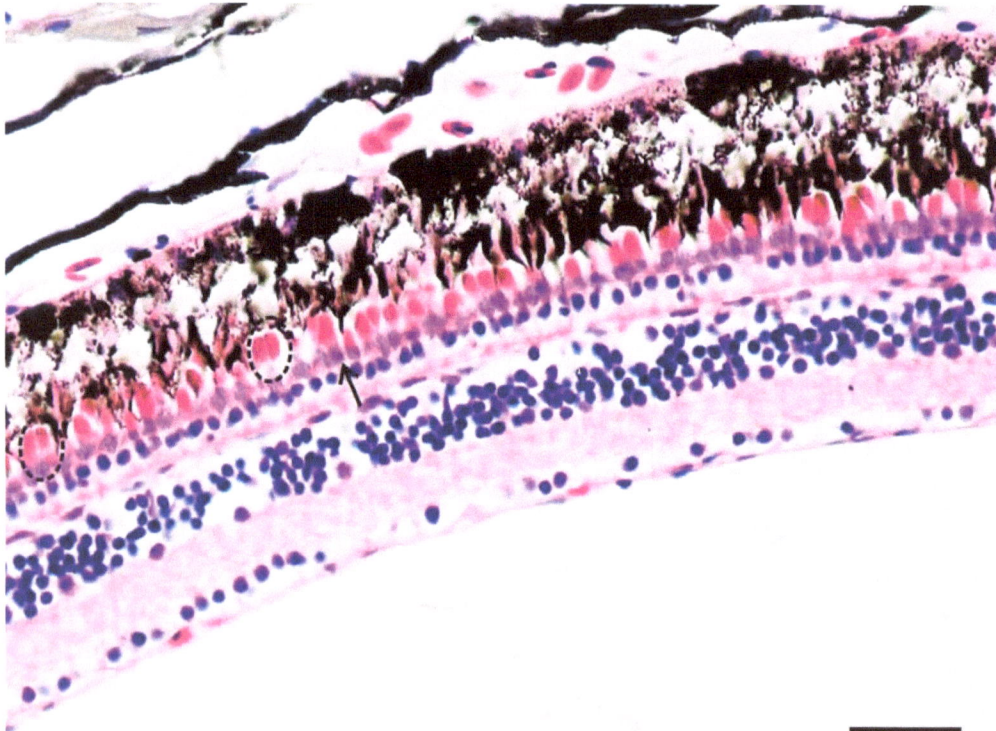

Figure 1.5i. *Mid-peripheral retina.*

Twin cones with inner segments of equal sizes (circles) are observed. These are different from those of the double cones (arrow). Bar = 50 μm.

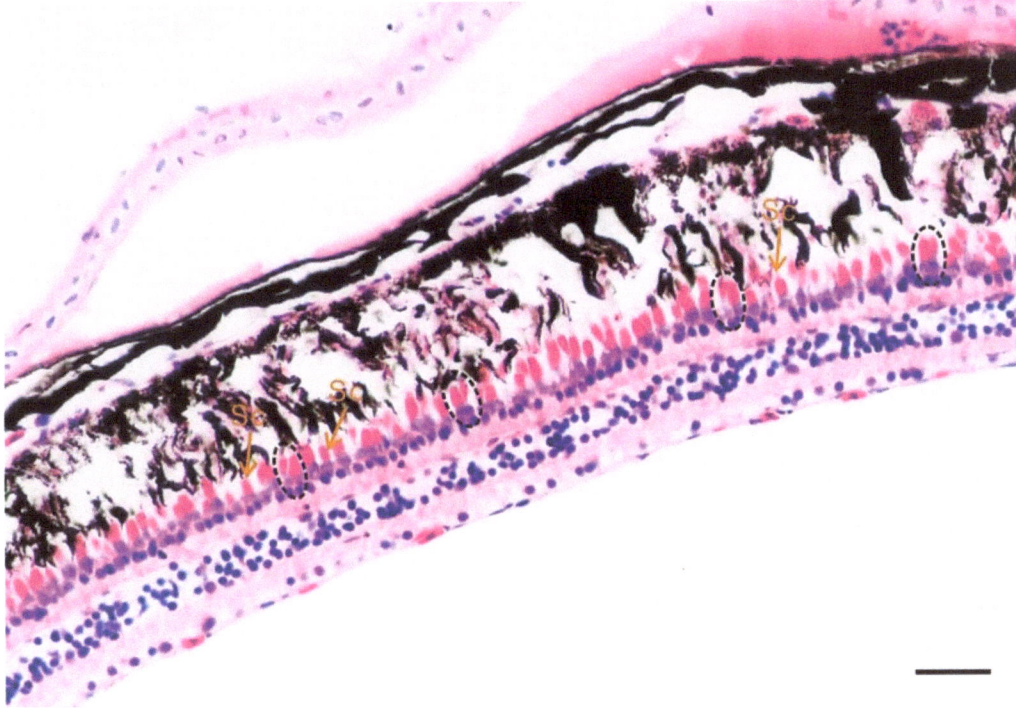

Figure 1.5j. *Central retina.*

In the central retina, visual cells are not highly packed. However, it is still dominated by different types of cones such as double cones (circles) and single cones (Sc). Bar = 50 μm.

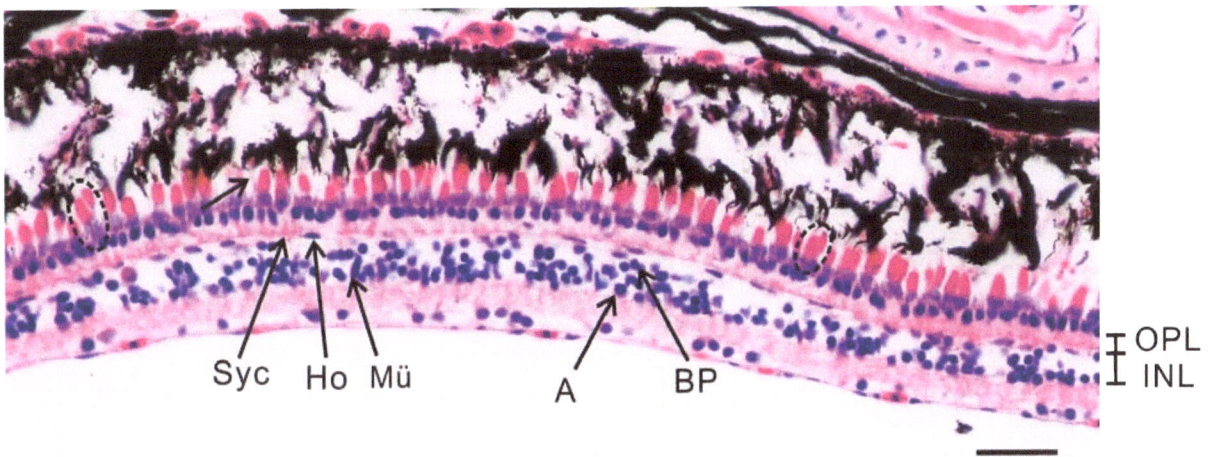

Figure 1.5k. *Central retina.*

Double cones (circles) are seen in the even more central portion of the retina and the rod (arrow) is slender and thin in this species. "I" denotes the synaptic contact with the outer plexiform layer (OPL). Different cell types in the inner nuclear layer (INL) are identified. "A" denotes amacrine cells, "BP" denotes bipolar cells, "Ho" denotes horizontal cells, and "Mü" denotes the Müller cell. Bar = 50 μm.

6. GARPIKE

The garpike is another phylogenetic old fish with much more visual cells especially cones in the retina. There are almost three layers of cells in the outer nuclear layer. The inner nuclear layer of this fish is also thick and houses numerous cells.

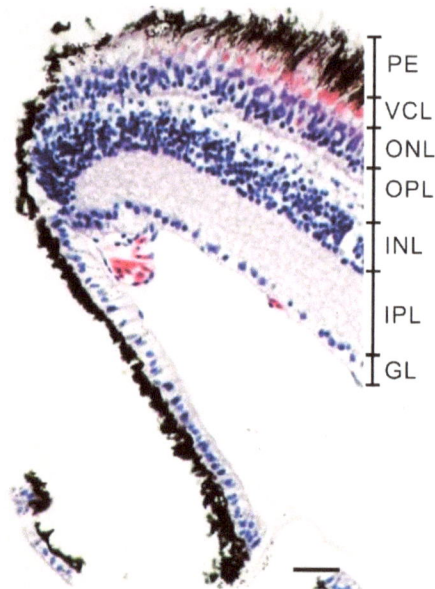

Figure 1.6a. *Ora serrata.*

This figure shows the ora serrata region of the Garpike, a phylogenetically old fish. Layers of the retina are identified. Bar = 50 μm.

(GL - Ganglion cell layer; INL - Inner nuclear layer; IPL - Inner plexiform layer; ONL - Outer nuclear layer; OPL - Outer plexiform layer; PE - Pigment Epithelium;VCL - Visual cell layer).

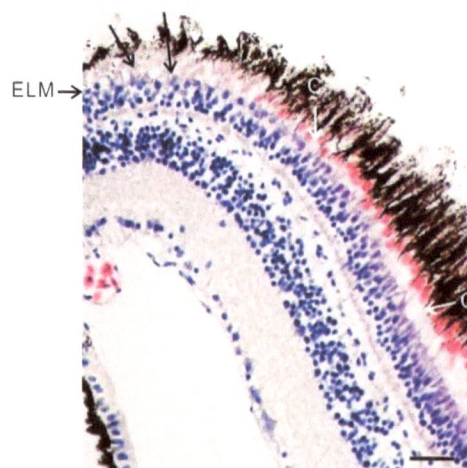

Figure 1.6b. *Ora serrata.*

Around the ora serrata, a lot of nuclei (black arrows) migrate above the external limiting membrane (ELM). The ellipsoid region of the internal segment of the cone cells (C) is highly stained with eosin while the myoid region appears clear. Bar = 50 μm.

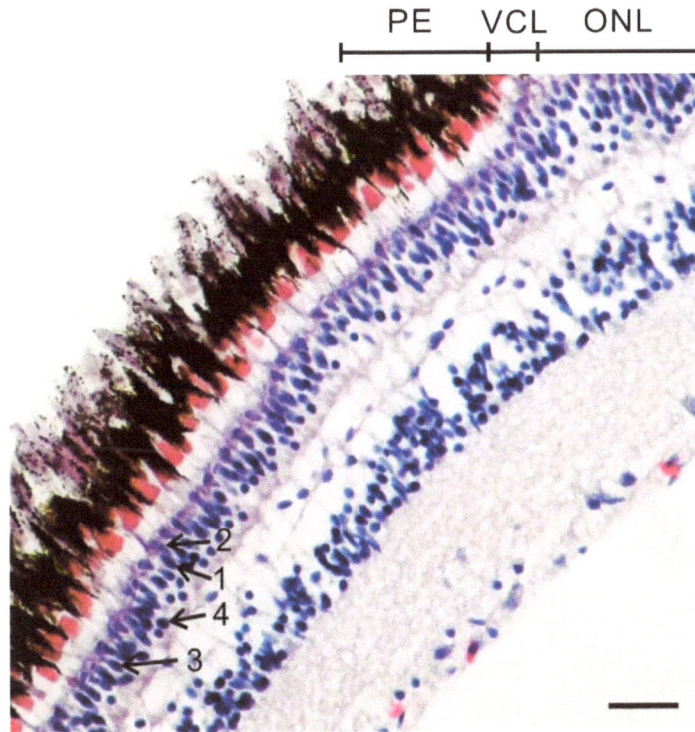

Figure 1.6c. *Peripheral retina.*

The peripheral retina still contains a lot of cones cells. In this figure, the visual cell layer (VCL) is covered by the pigment epithelium (PE). Various cell nuclei in the outer nuclear layer (ONL) can be identified by different location levels. "1" denotes the chief cone nucleus, "2" denotes the accessory cone nucleus, "3" indicates a single cone nucleus, and "4" refers to a rod nucleus. Bar = 50 μm.

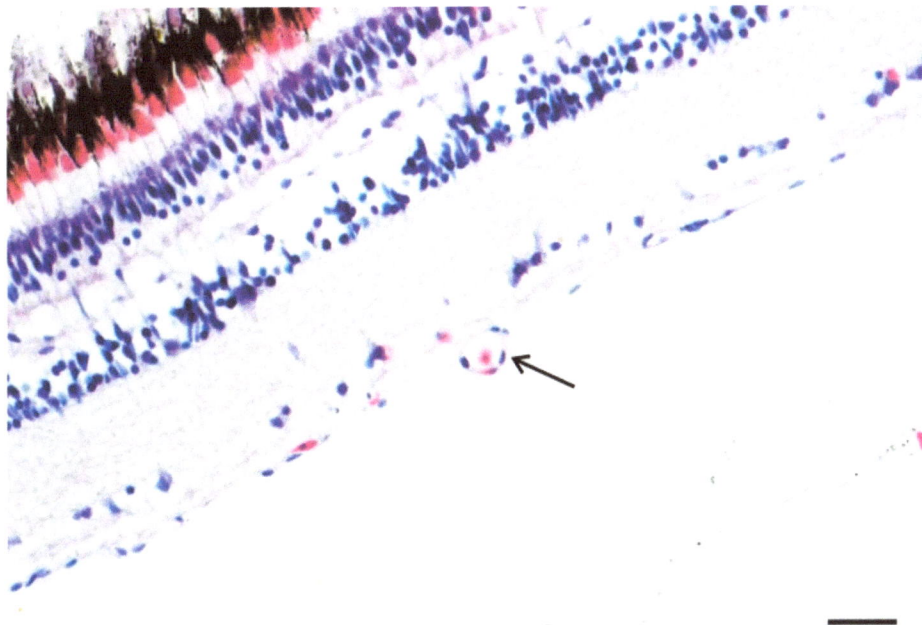

Figure 1.6d. *Epiretinal vessel.*

Epiretinal vessels (arrow) are frequently found on the inner surface of the retina. Bar = 50 μm.

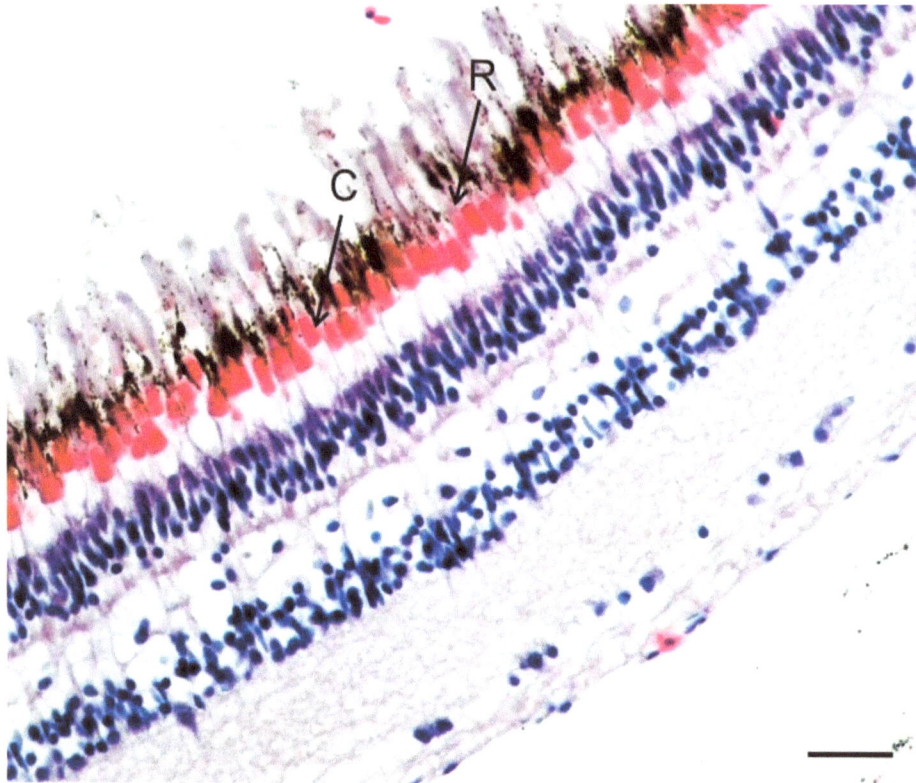

Figure 1.6e. *Central retina.*

In the central retina, cone cells (C) are highly packed. A few rod cells (R) with long and slender inner and outer segments are also noted. Bar = 50 μm.

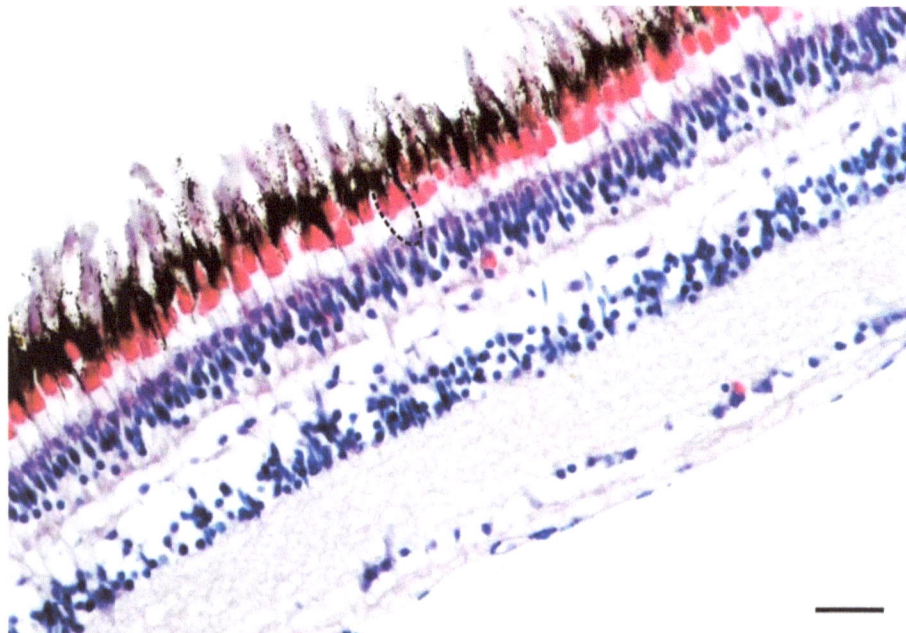

Figure 1.6f. *Cental retina.*

A double cone in the central retina is encircled. A clear separation is seen between the taller chief cone and the shorter accessory cone. Bar = 50 μm.

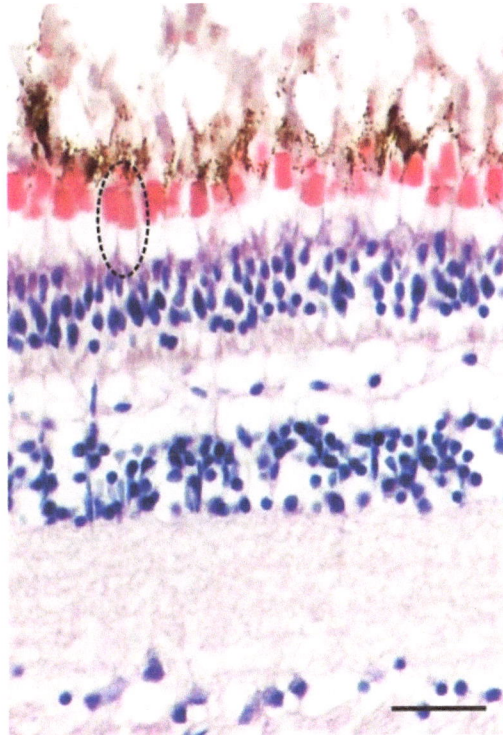

Figure 1.6g. *Central retina.*

A possible twin cone (circle) in the central retina is noted in the retina of the garpike fish (archi-fish). Bar = 50 μm.

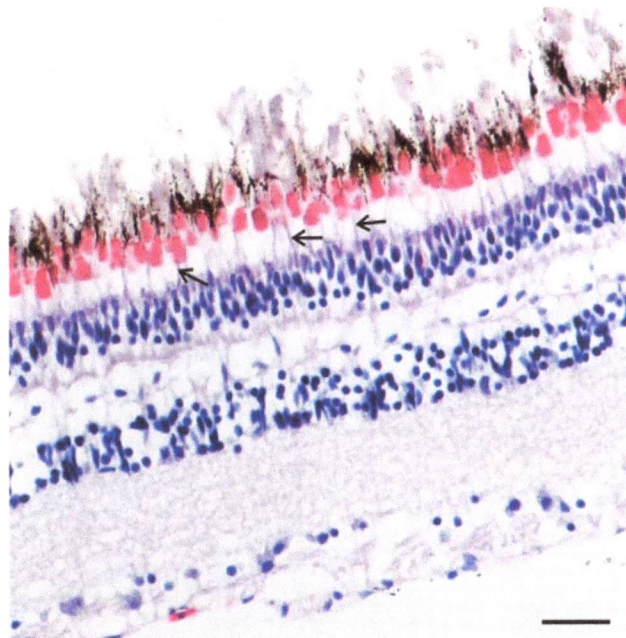

Figure 1.6h. *Central retina.*

Double cones are noted in this haematoxylin and eosin staining eye section. Arrows indicate the chief cones of the double cones. They have characteristically very thin and slender inner segments. Bar = 50 μm.

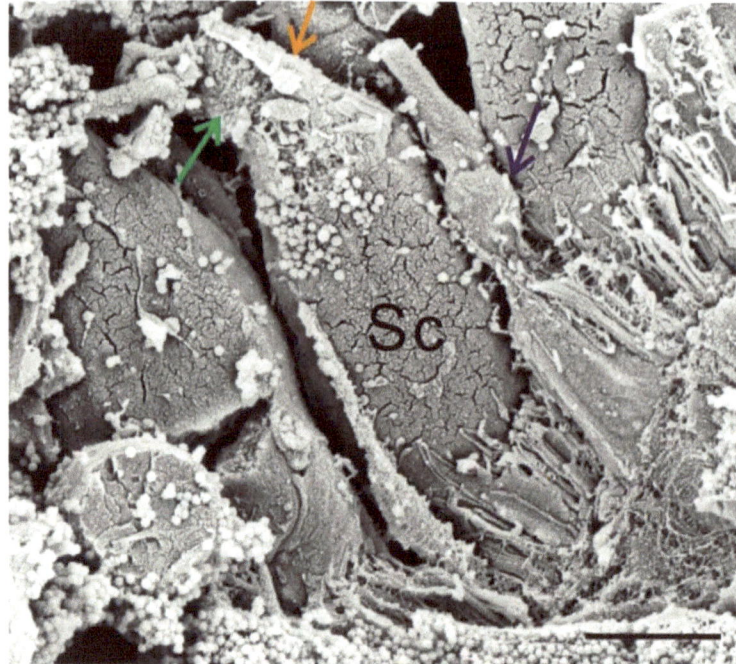

Figure 1.6i.

A single cone with an oval shaped inner segment is shown in this scanning electron micrograph. The green arrow indicates the outer segment of the cone and the orange arrow indicates a cilium. On the side of this cone is another possible smaller cone (purple arrow). Bar = 3 μm.

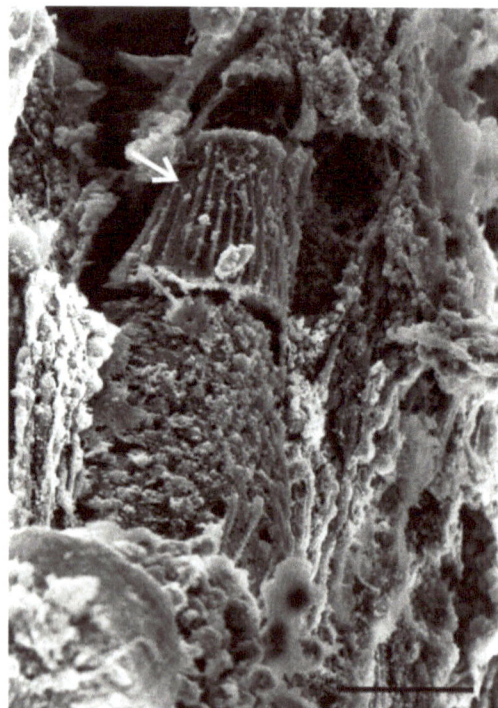

Figure 1.6j.

Another single cone with its plasma membrane of the inner segment ruptured is shown, thus exposing the internal organelles. A white arrow shows the many microvilli surrounding the proximal part of the outer segment. Bar = 3 μm.

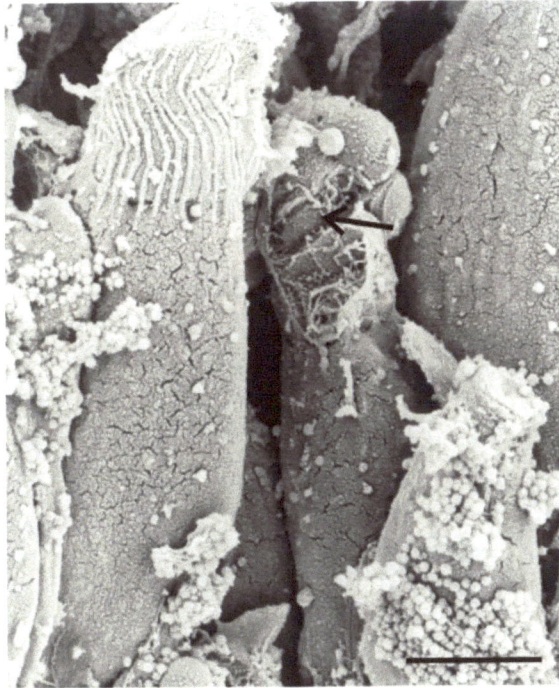

Figure 1.6k.

The stacked membranes (arrow) inside the outer segment of a single cone are exposed. Bar = 3 μm.

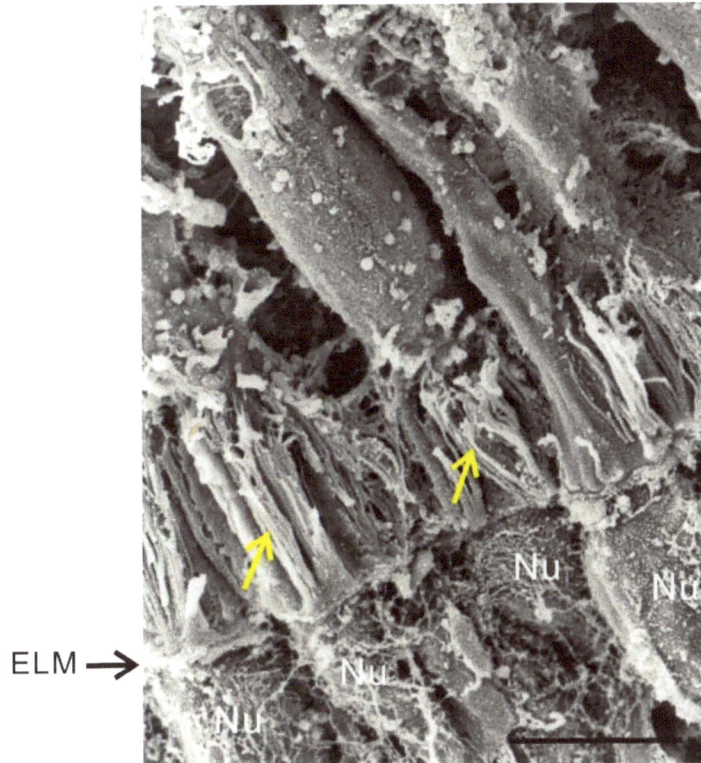

Figure 1.6l.

Numerous microvilli of the Müller cells (yellow arrows) surrounding the basal part of the visual cells are seen. Below the external limiting membrane (ELM) are the nuclei (Nu) of the visual cells. Bar = 3 μm.

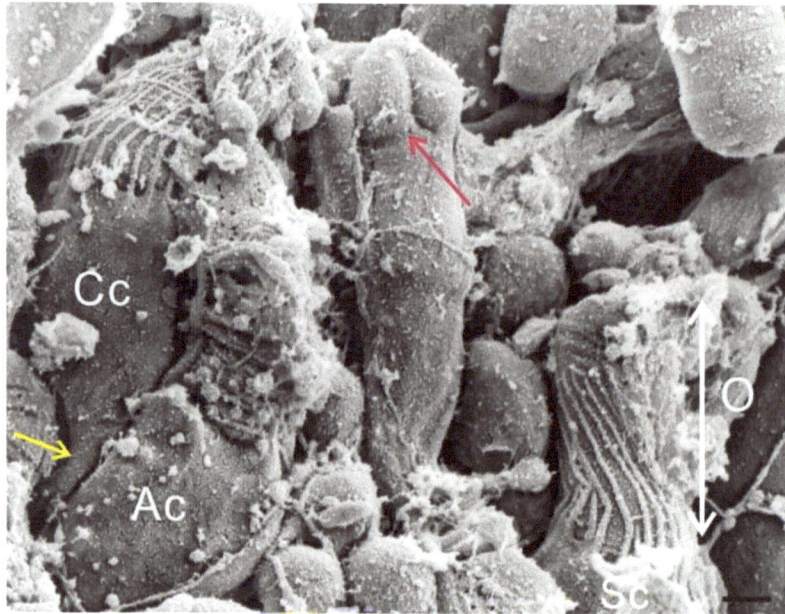

Figure 1.6m.

A double cone with a taller chief cone (Cc) and a shorter accessory cone (Ac) is seen. Note that most part of the inner segment of the chief cone is thin and slender (yellow arrow), except the distal end. The part of the chief cone that is surrounded by many microvilli indicates the origin of the outer segment. The stacked membranes inside the outer segment are displayed in the accessory cone. In the middle of this scanning electron micrograph, a possible twin cone with two developing outer segments is shown (red arrow). A type of single cone (Sc) with many microvilli extending to its outer segment (O) is also noted. Bar = 1 mm.

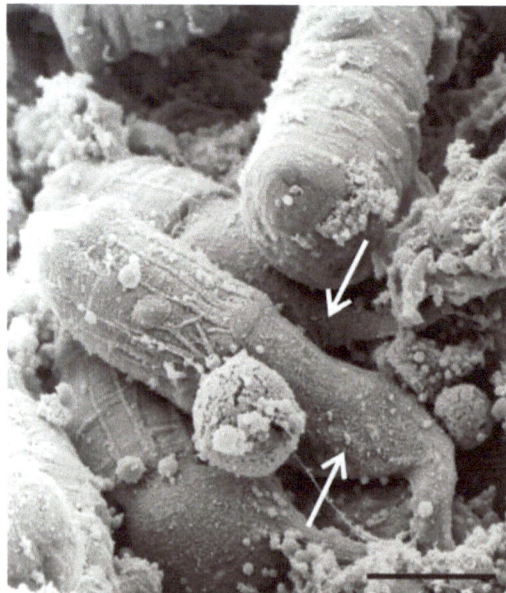

Figure 1.6n.

Two chief cones with reversely tapered shape of inner segments are shown (white arrows). Bar = 3 μm.

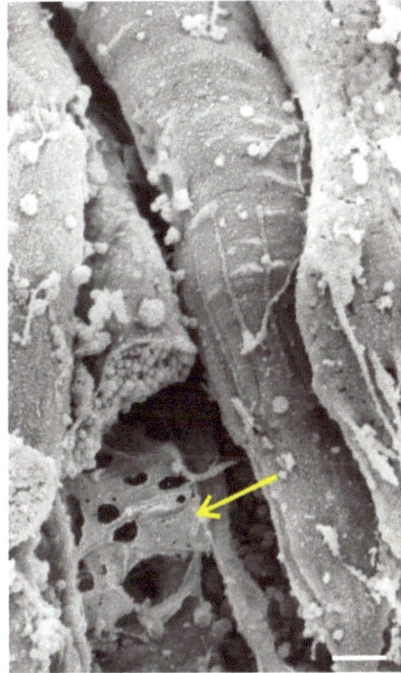

Figure 1.6o.

The yellow arrow indicates the presence of a Müller cell among the proximal portion of the inner segments of visual cells. Extrusion of Müller cell (not microvilli) between visual cells is normally abnormal and indicates degeneration. Bar = 1 μm.

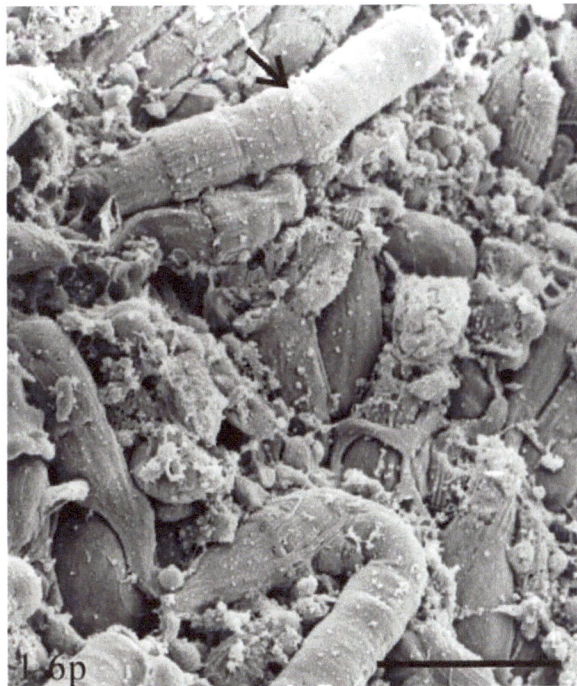

Figure 1.6p.

Long outer segments of the visual cells are indicated (arrow). Bar = 10 μm.

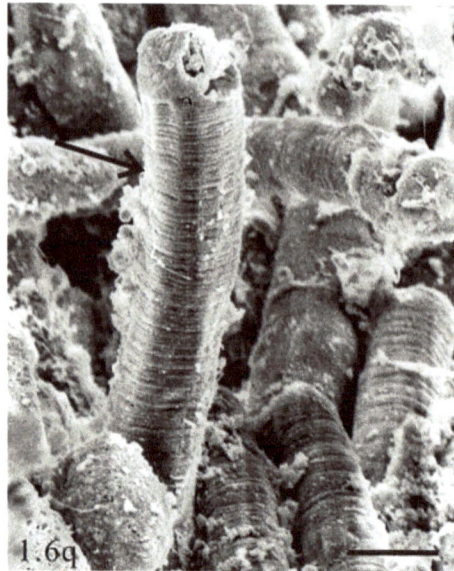

Figure 1.6q.

Regularly spaced membranes are clearly displayed inside the outer segments (arrow). Bar = 3 μm.

7. SOUTHERN FLOUNDER

The southern flounder has eyes on top of its head and the retina has a thick outer nuclear layer with small cell bodies. The cells in the inner nuclear layer are scattered and small in sizes as well.

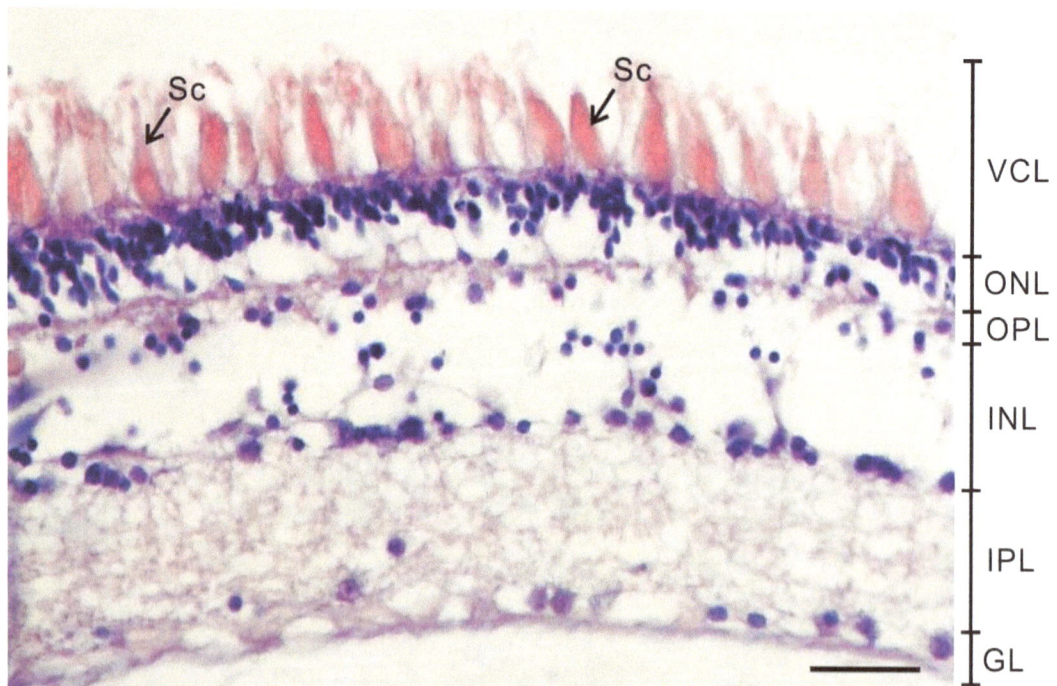

Figure 1.7a. *Anterior retina.*

In the anterior retina near the ora serrata, there are many single cones (Sc) with tall pear shaped inner segments. Bar = 50 μm.

(GL - Ganglion cell layer; INL - Inner nuclear layer; IPL - Inner plexiform layer; ONL - Outer nuclear layer; OPL - Outer plexiform layer; VCL - Visual cell layer).

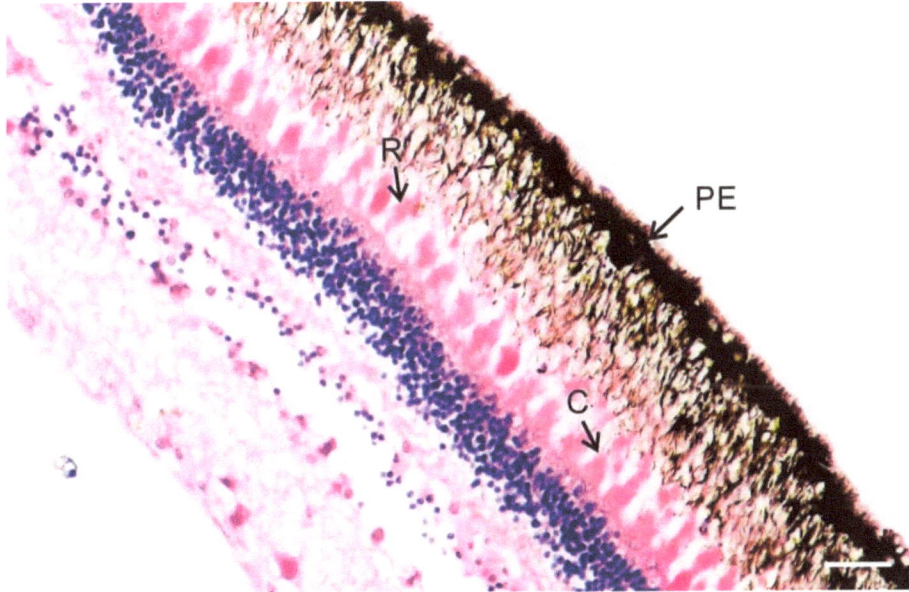

Figure 1.7b. *Peripheral retina.*

Rods (R) are few in number even in the peripheral retina. There are more cones cells (C) present in this region. Bar = 50 μm.

(PE - Pigment epithelium).

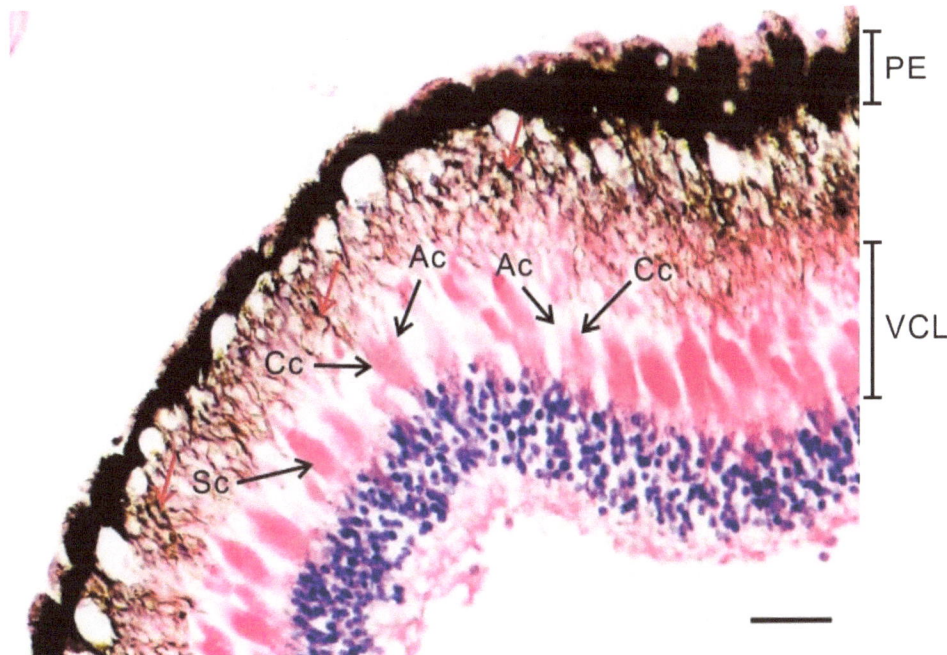

Figure 1.7c. *Central retina.*

The pigment epithelial layer (PE) is still adhered to the visual cell layer (VCL) and their processes are surrounding the outer segments of the visual cells (red arrows). The visual cells in the central retina of this fish include single cones (Sc), double cones with chief cones (Cc) and accessory cones (Ac). Rods are few in the central retina. Bar = 50 μm.

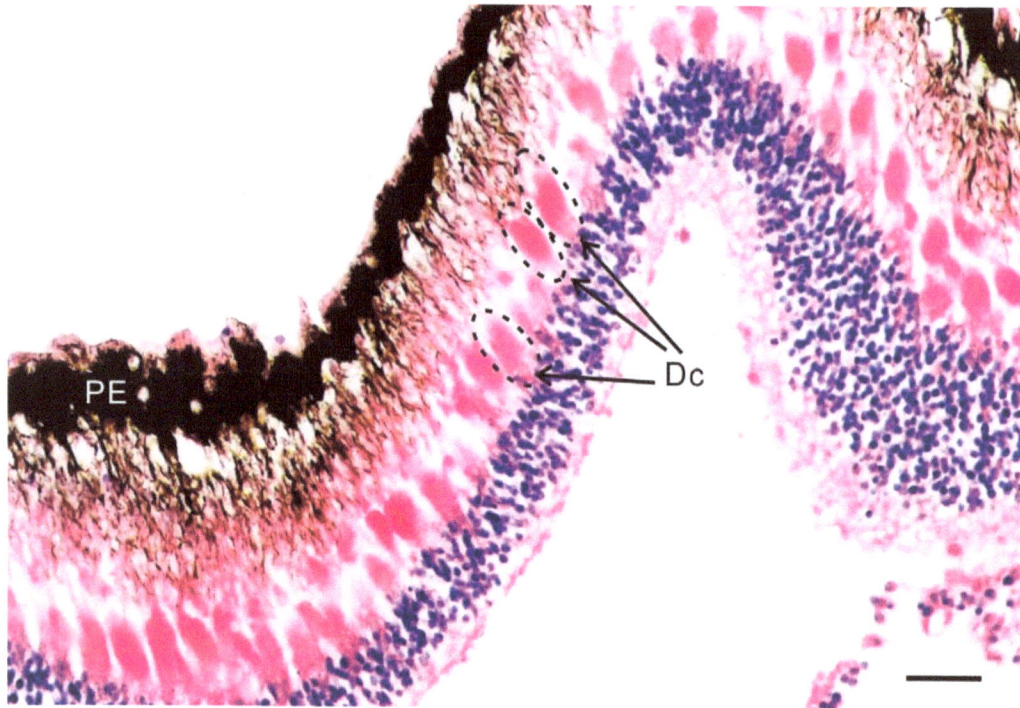

Figure 1.7d. *Central retina.*

More double cones (Dc; circles) with chief and accessory components tightly packed together are shown in other parts of the central region. Bar = 50 μm.

(PE - Pigment epithelium).

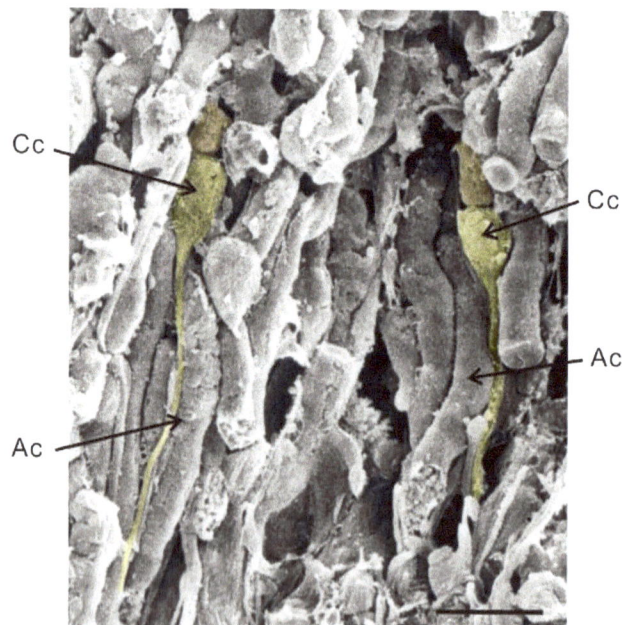

Figure 1.7e.

In this scanning electron micrograph, two double cones are shown. The chief cone (Cc) displays a long and thin proximal part of the inner segment (colored in yellow) whereas the accessory cone (Ac) consists of a thicker and rod-like inner segment. The outer segments of the chief cones are colored in orange. Bar = 5 μm.

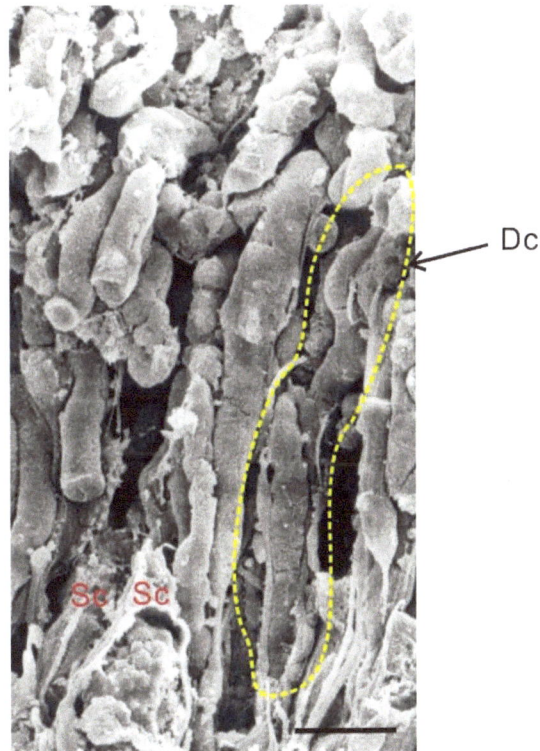

Figure 1.7f.

Another double cone (Dc; circle) is shown in this scanning electron micrograph. A few short and round single cones (Sc) are found. The internal organelles of one of these single cones are displayed. Bar = 5 μm.

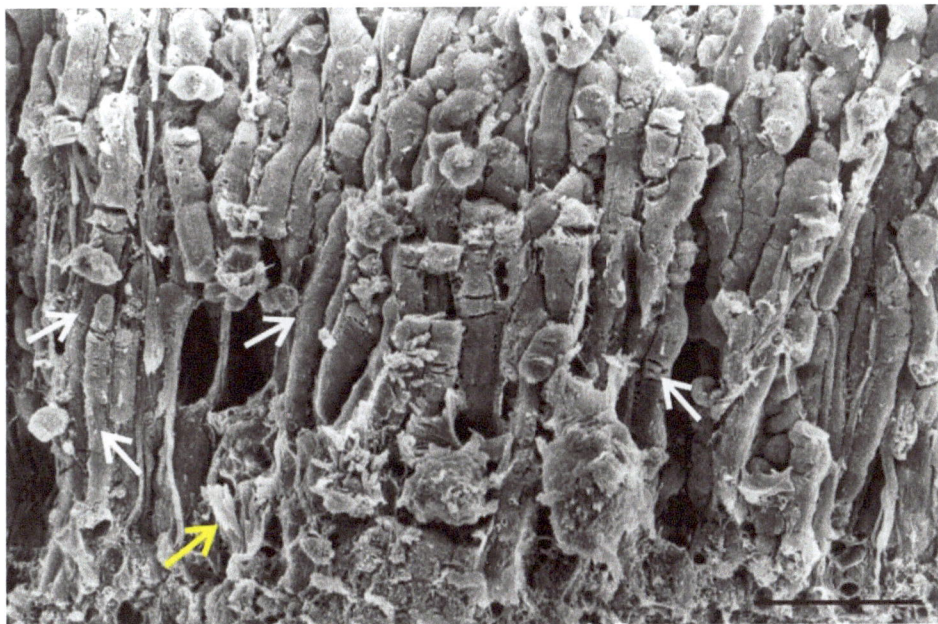

Figure 1.7g.

Among the various types of visual cells, single cones with rod-like inner segments (white arrows) are also seen in this scanning electron micrograph. Microvilli of the Müller cells are indicated by a yellow arrow. Bar = 10 μm.

8. MUDSKIPPER

The mudskipper appears on land at times. The retina of this animal has two well stratified layers of elongated cell bodies in the outer nuclear layer. There is a thickened (8 to 10 layers) inner nuclear layer. Ganglion cells are numerous in this species.

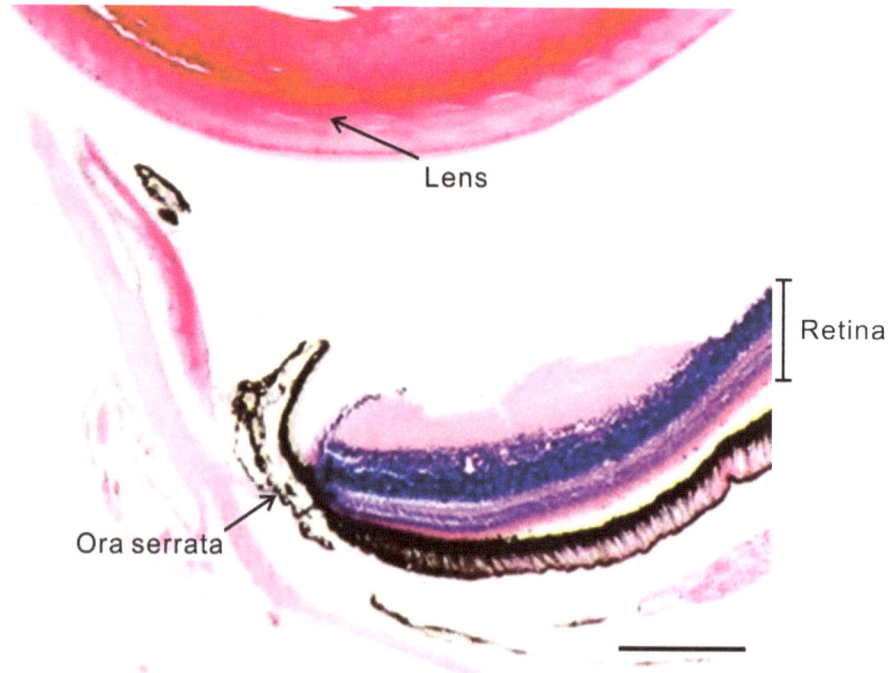

Figure 1.8a. *Ora serrata.*

This figure shows the anterior retina of a mudskipper at the ora serrata region at a low magnification. Bar = 200 μm.

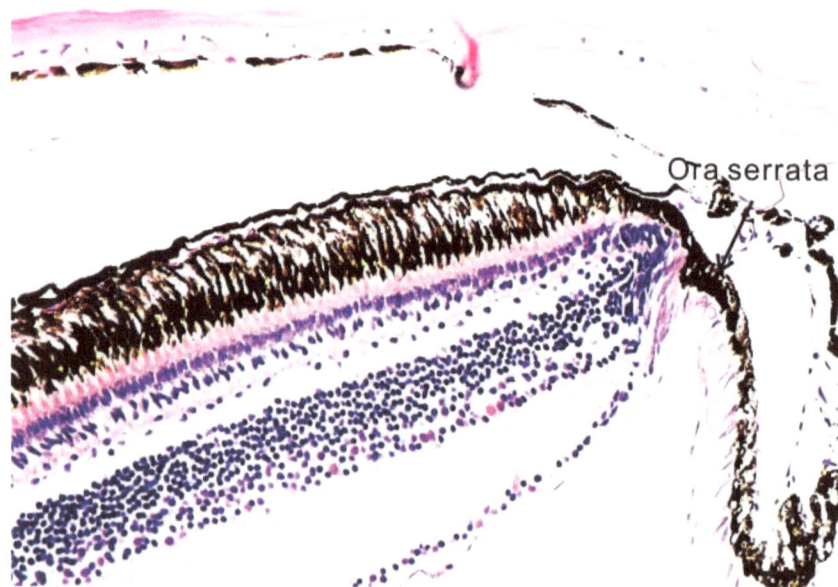

Figure 1.8b. *Ora serrata, Anterior retina.*

The anterior retina and the transition of the ora serrata is shown in higher magnification. A gradual reduction of the thickness is seen in the retina towards the ora serrata. Bar = 50 μm.

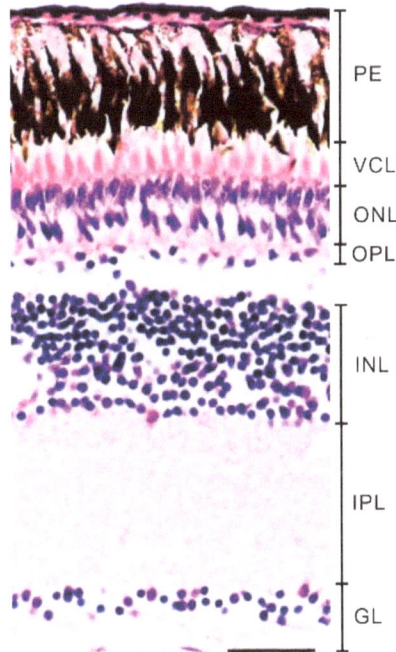

Figure 1.8c. *Peripheral retina.*

Different retinal layers of the mudskipper are shown. Visual cells, which are mostly cone cells, are arranged in a regular pattern below the pigment epithelium (PE). Bar = 50 μm.

(GL - Ganglion cell layer; INL - Inner nuclear layer; IPL - Inner plexiform layer; ONL - Outer nuclear layer; OPL - Outer plexiform layer; PE - Pigment epithelium; VCL - Visual cell layer).

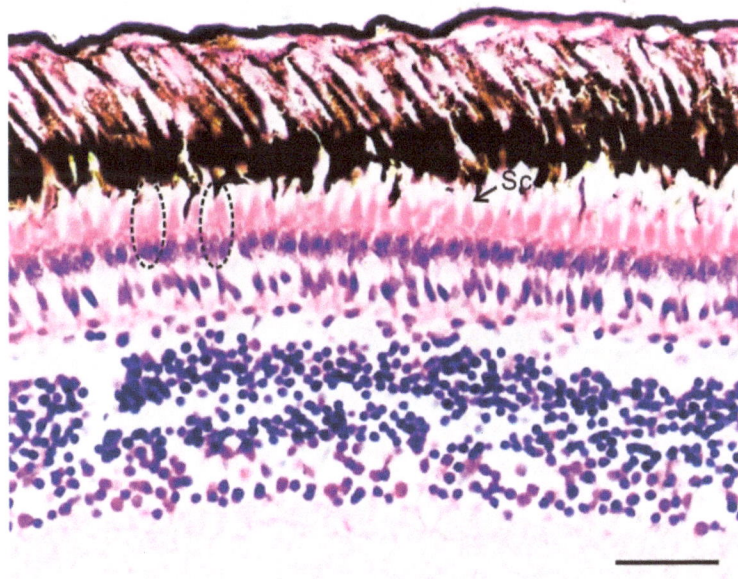

Figure 1.8d. *Peripheral retina.*

Single cones (Sc) and double cones (circles) are noted among the different visual cells. Bar = 50 μm.

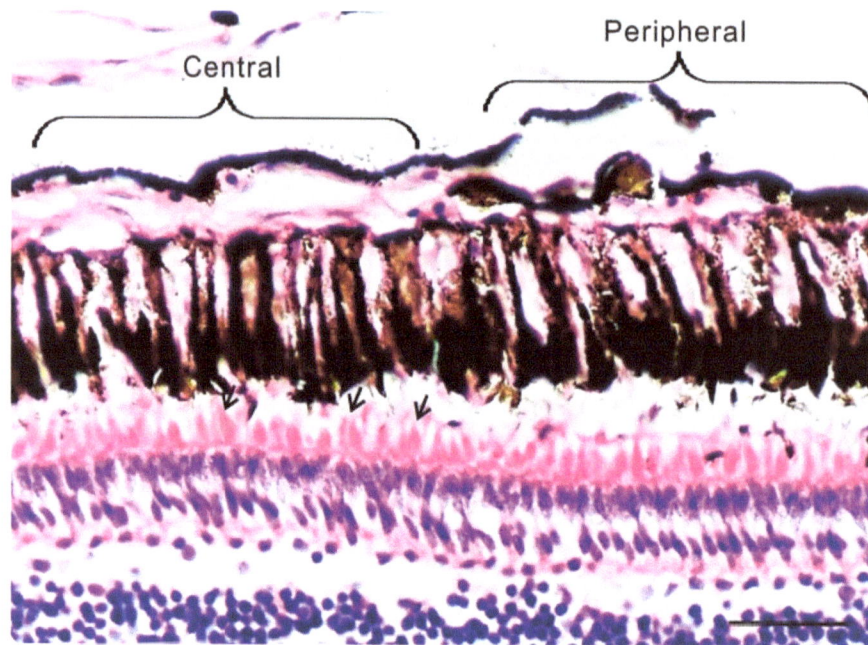

Figure 1.8e. *A transition between peripheral and central retina.*

The transitonal zone between the central and peripheral retina. There appears to be more double cones (arrows) in the central region. Bar = 50 μm.

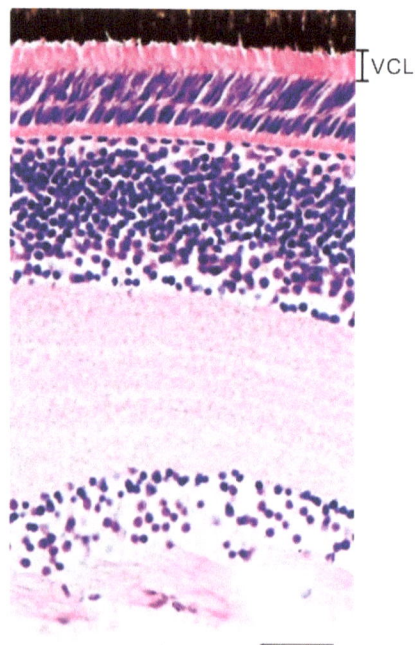

Figure 1.8f. *Central retina.*

The visual cells are highly packed in the central region. Bar = 50 μm.

(VCL - Visual cell layer).

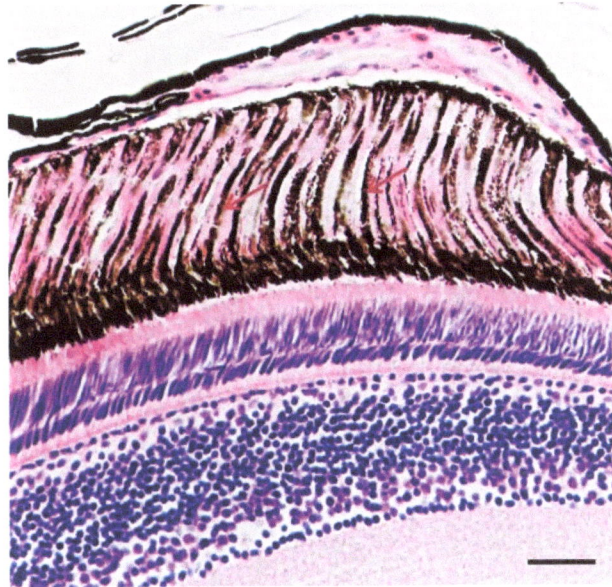

Figure 1.8g. *Central retina.*

The processes of the pigment cells (red arrows) in the mudskipper are longer along the entire retina in general. Bar = 50 μm.

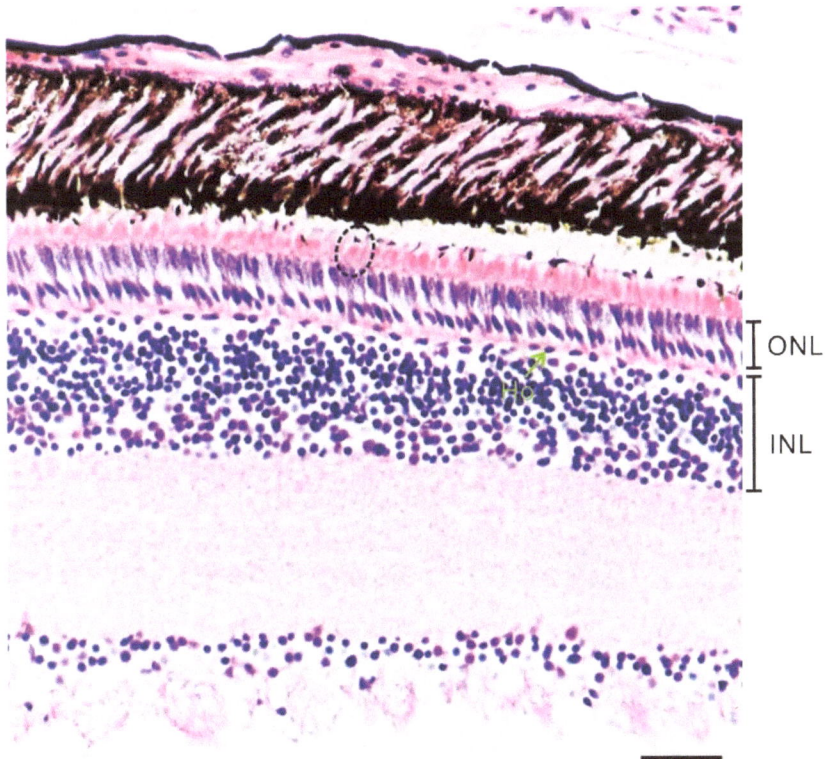

Figure 1.8h. *Central retina.*

The central retina has a lot of double cones (circle) with a rounder chief cone and a more slender accessory cone. The outer nuclear layer (ONL) is formed by a row of dark and elongated basal nuclei. The inner nuclear layer (INL) is thick and the superior layer is possibly formed by a row of horizontal cells (Ho). Bar = 50 μm.

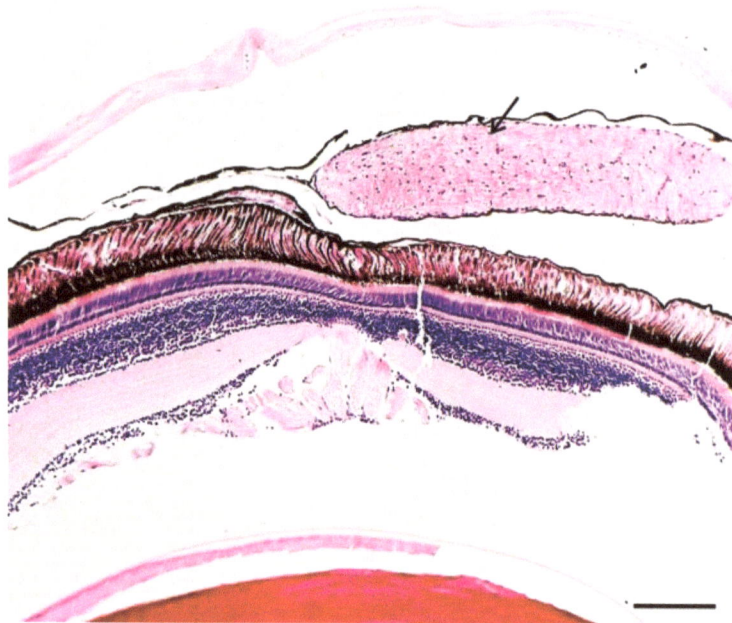

Figure 1.8i. *Optic nerve.*

The fovea of the mudskipper. The optic nerve (arrow) is also shown. Bar = 200 μm.

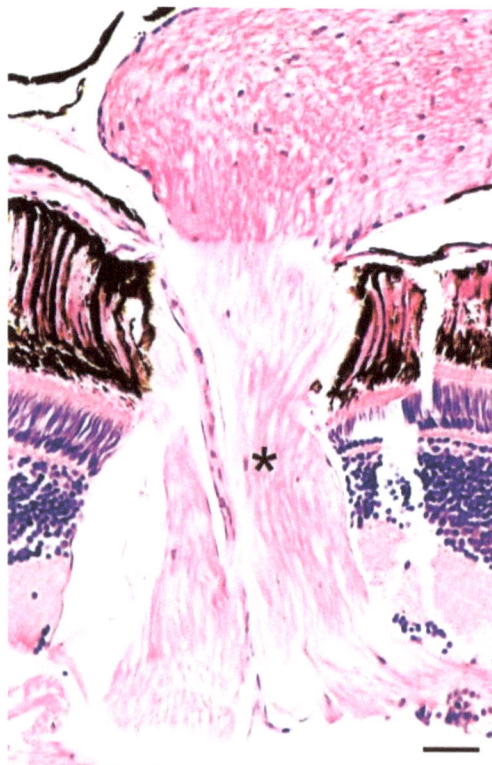

Figure 1.8j. *Optic nerve.*

Observation under a higher power reveals that there are less glial components in the stalk (asterisk) of the optic nerve. Bar = 50 μm.

9. LUNGFISH

The spotted African lungfish is another old but phylogenetically important fish, having many retinal features similar to the sturgeon. The outer nuclear layer of this fish is thin but contains large cell bodies. Proximal parts of the inner segments of the cone cells are very much dilated. Moreover, the nuclei of the pigment epithelial cells are particularly large in this species.

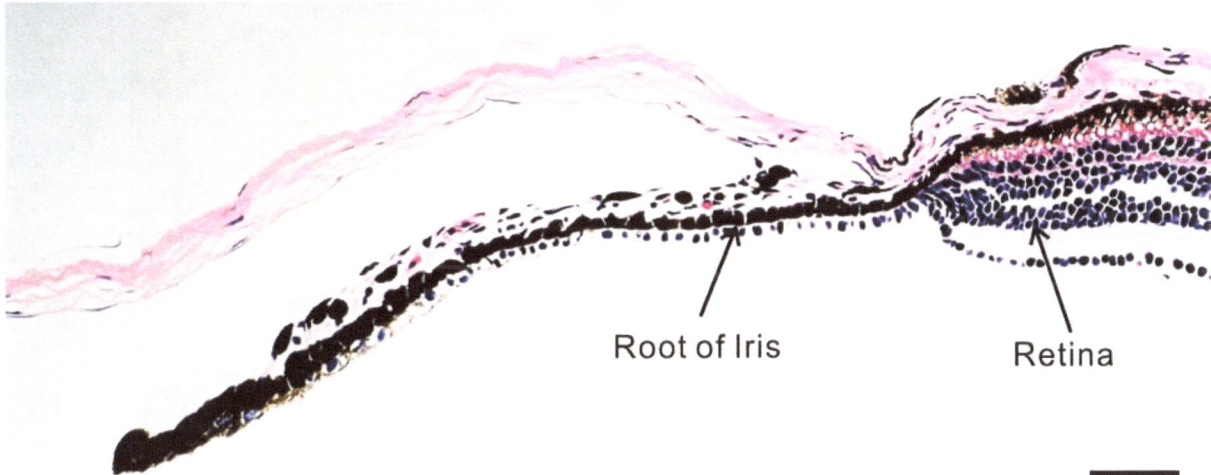

Figure 1.9a. *Ora serrata.*

This figure shows the junction between the retina and iris of the lungfish. Bar = 100 μm.

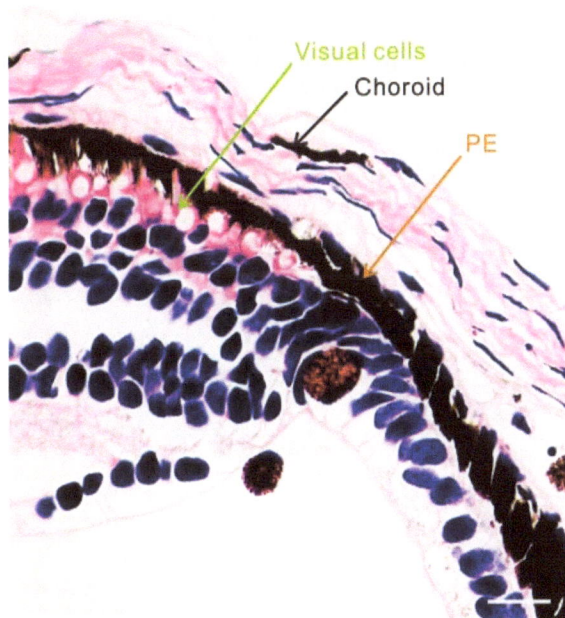

Figure 1.9b. *Ora serrata.*

A magnified photo of figure1.9a, showing the depletion of visual cells anteriorly. Some retinal layers are missing at this region. Bar = 50 μm.

(PE - Pigment epithelium).

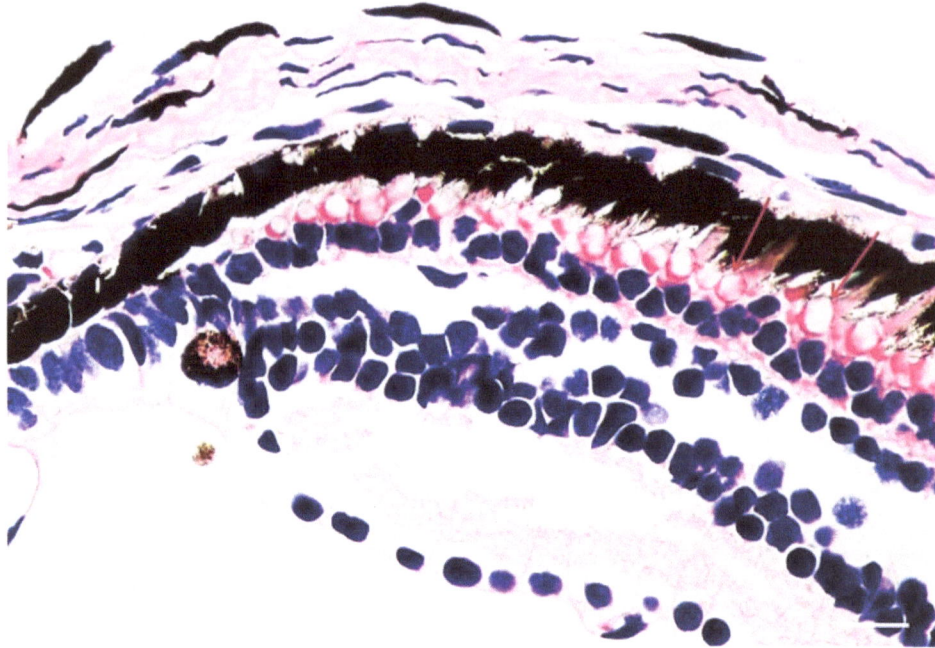

Figure 1.9c. *Anterior retina, near ora serrata.*

Large number of cone cells (red arrows) in the anterior segment of the retina near the ora serrata. Bar = 50 μm.

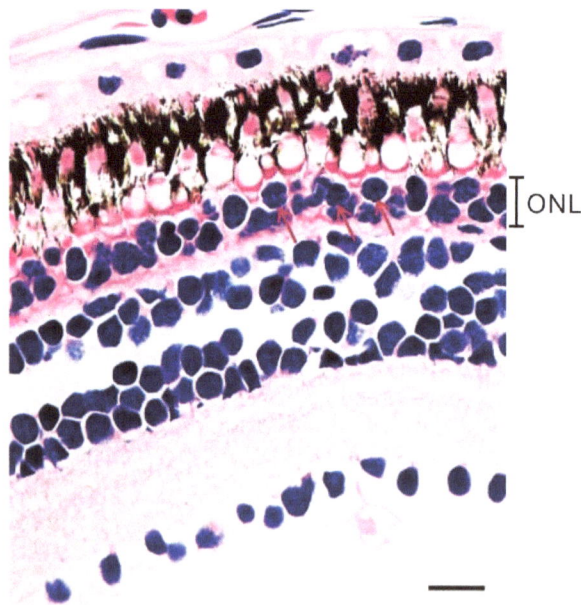

Figure 1.9d. *Peripheral retina.*

The retinal layers of the spotted African lungfish are shown and identified. A layer of cartilage is located exterior to the choroid of this fish. Moreover, a layer of pigment epithelial cells (arrows) which are large and rectangular in shape are apparently evident. Bar = 50 μm.

(ELM - External limiting membrane; GL - Ganglion cell layer; INL - Inner nuclear layer; IPL - Inner plexiform layer; ONL - Outer nuclear layer; OPL - Outer plexiform layer; PE - Pigment epithelium; VCL - Visual cell layer).

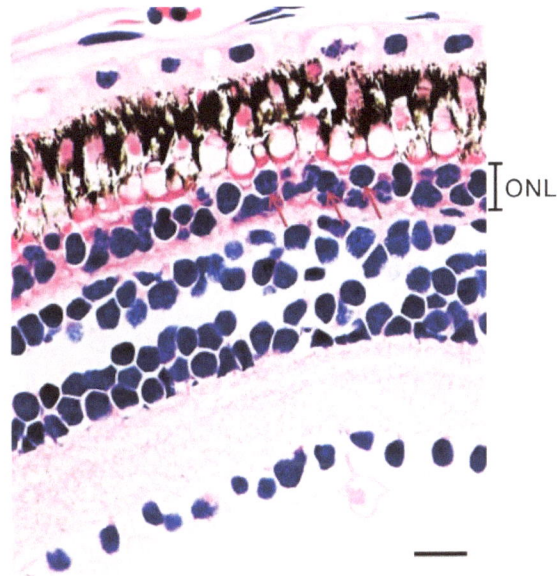

Figure 1.9e. *Peripheral retina.*

In the peripheral retina, numerous cone cells with round inner segments are observed. Smaller cone cells which are possibly the accessory components of the double cones are shown to have nuclei (red arrows) positioned in the upper border of outer nuclear layer (ONL). Bar = 50 μm.

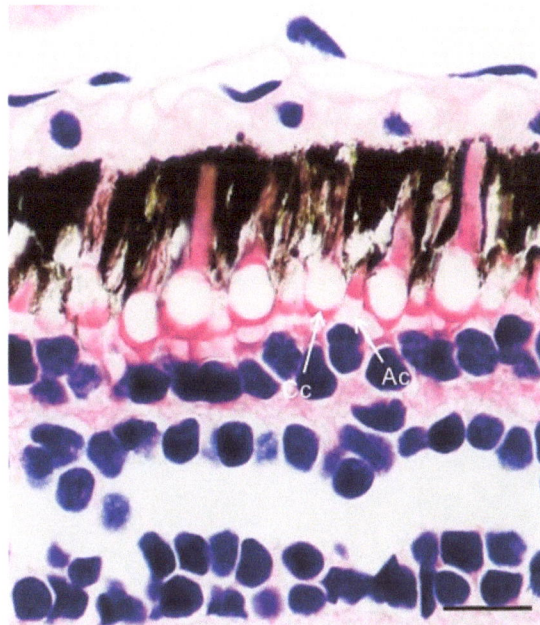

Figure 1.9f. *Peripheral retina.*

A possible double cone is shown. The chief cone is indicated as "Cc" while the accessory cone is labeled as "Ac". Their nuclei are located at different levels. The one which belongs to the accessory cone is more superior than that of the chief cone. Bar = 50 μm.

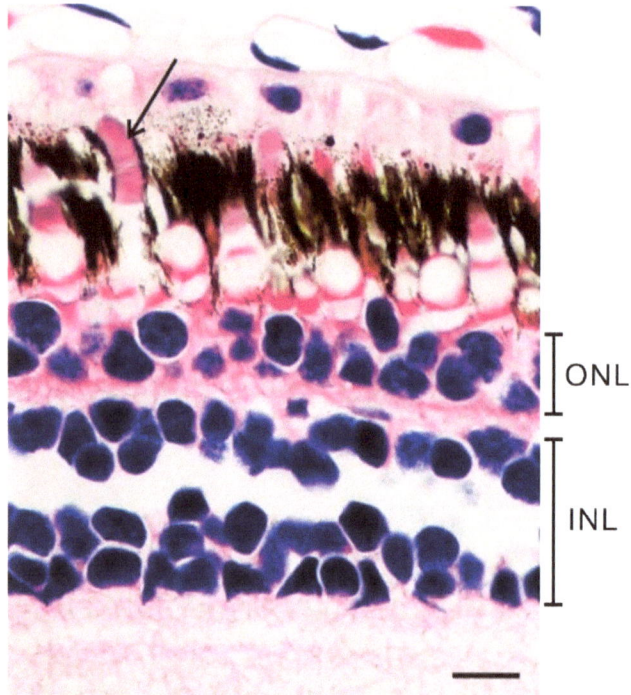

Figure 1.9g. *Transition between central and peripheral retina.*

An arrow shows a rod in the peripheral retina of the spotted African lungfish. Note that the outer nuclear layer (ONL) is thin and the inner nuclear layer (INL) is thick in this animal. Bar = 50 μm.

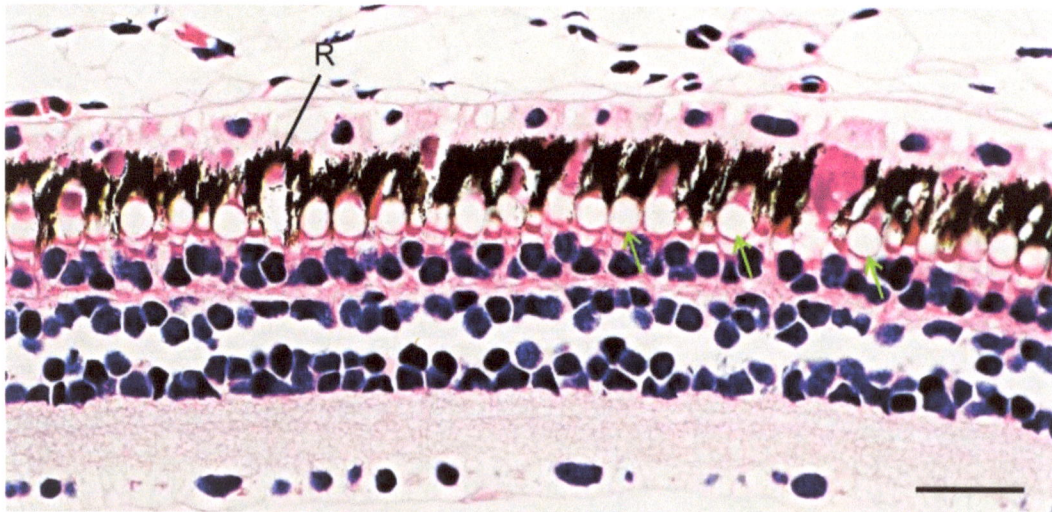

Figure 1.9h. *Central retina.*

The density of the cone cells in the central region is similar to that in the peripheral region. In terms of cell types, more cones are observed in the central region. However, an occasional rod (R) is seen on the left of this figure. The rod is shorter and thicker than those of other fish species. The round proximal ends of the inner segments which appear empty in the cones (green arrows) which are actually consisted of a large amount of glycogen. Bar = 100 μm.

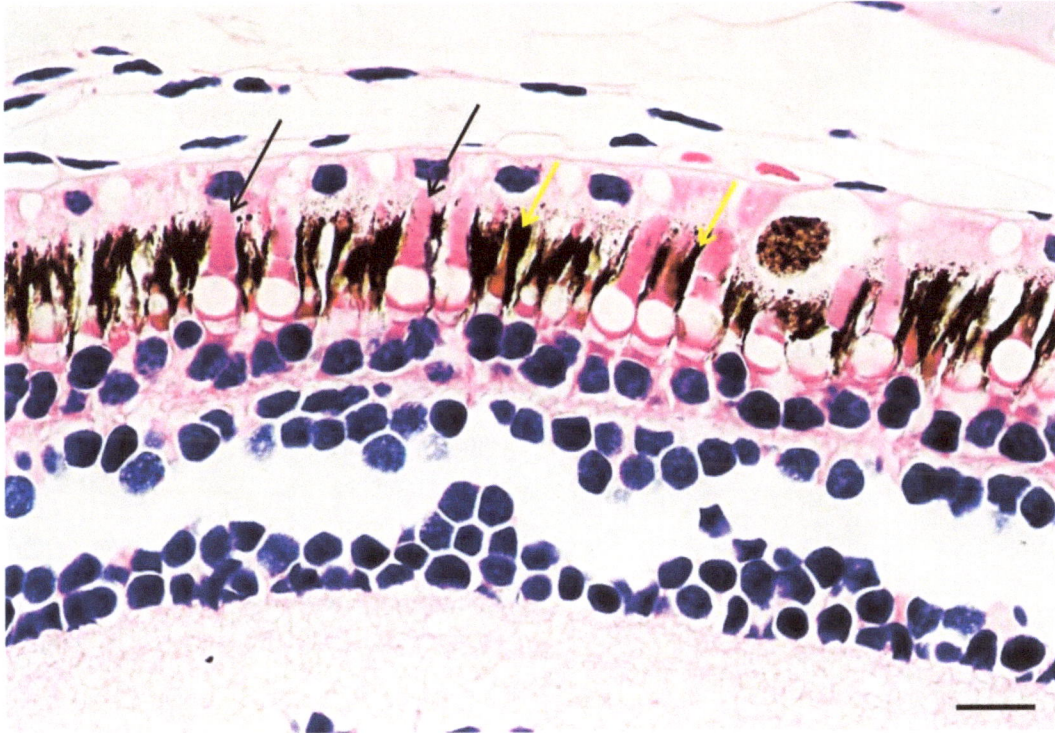

Figure 1.9i. *Central retina.*

The pointed outer segments (black arrows) of the visual cells are clearly shown among the processes of the pigment epithelium (yellow arrows). Bar = 50 μm.

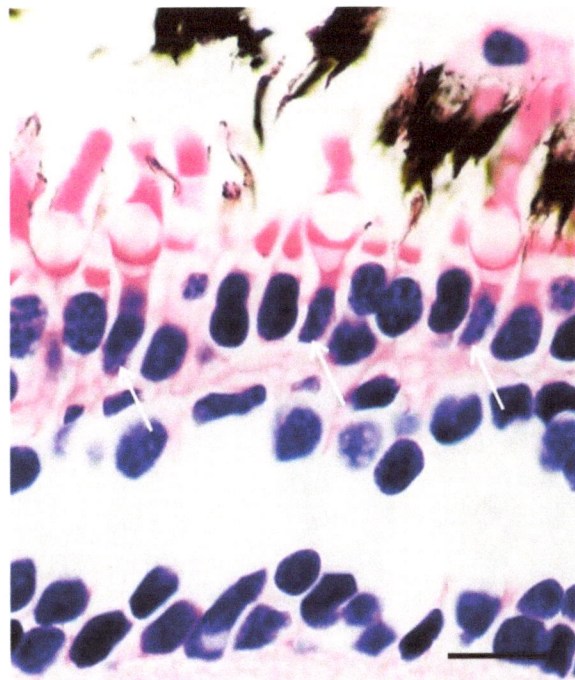

Figure 1.9j. *Central retina.*

The nuclei of the chief cones appear elongated (green arrows). Bar = 50 mm.

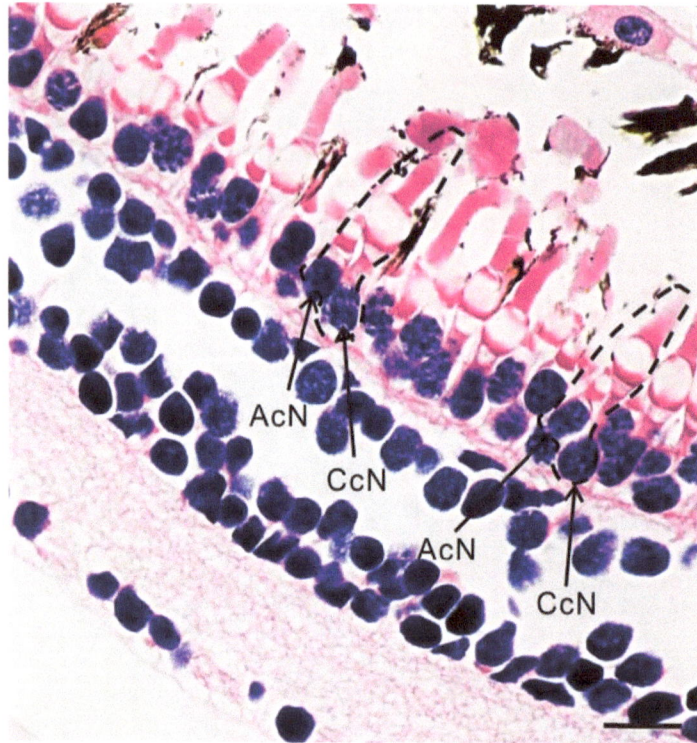

Figure 1.9k. *Central retina.*

Double cones (circles) are clearly shown in this figure. The nuclei of the two components are denoted as "CcN" for the chief cones and "AcN" for the accessory cones respectively. Bar = 50 μm.

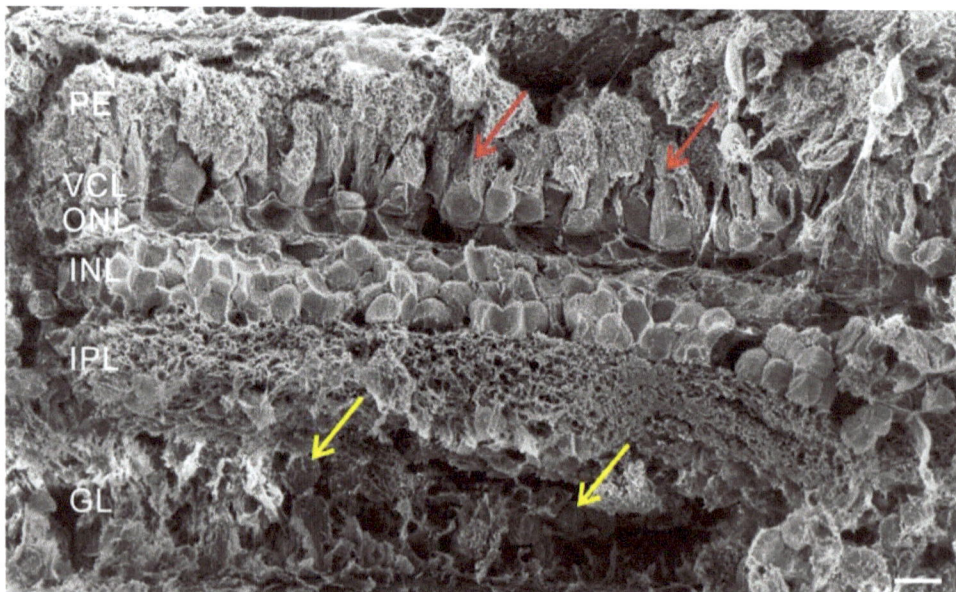

Figure 1.9l.

This electron scanning micrograph shows the retinal layers of the spotted African lungfish. The visual cell layer (VCL) and the pigment epithelium (PE) are closely attached. The outer part of the visual cells (red arrows) are interdigitated by the processes of the epithelial layer. Some spherical cells (yellow arrows) located in the innermost layer are ganglion cells. Bar = 10 μm.

(GL - Ganglion cell layer; INL - Inner nuclear layer; IPL - Inner plexiform layer; ONL - Outer nuclear layer; PE - Pigment epithelium; VCL - Visual cell layer).

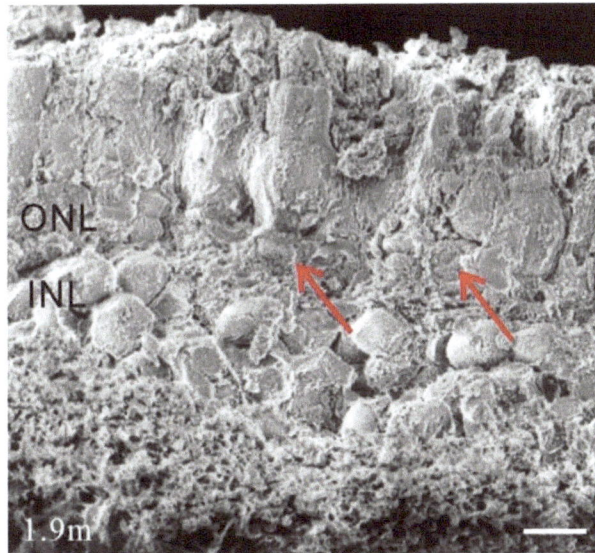

Figures 1.9m and 1.9n.

This electron micrograph indicates the different thickness of the two nuclear layers in the lungfish. The outer nuclear layer (ONL) of this fish is relatively thin and composed of a fewer number of visual cell bodies (red arrows). Bar = 10 μm.

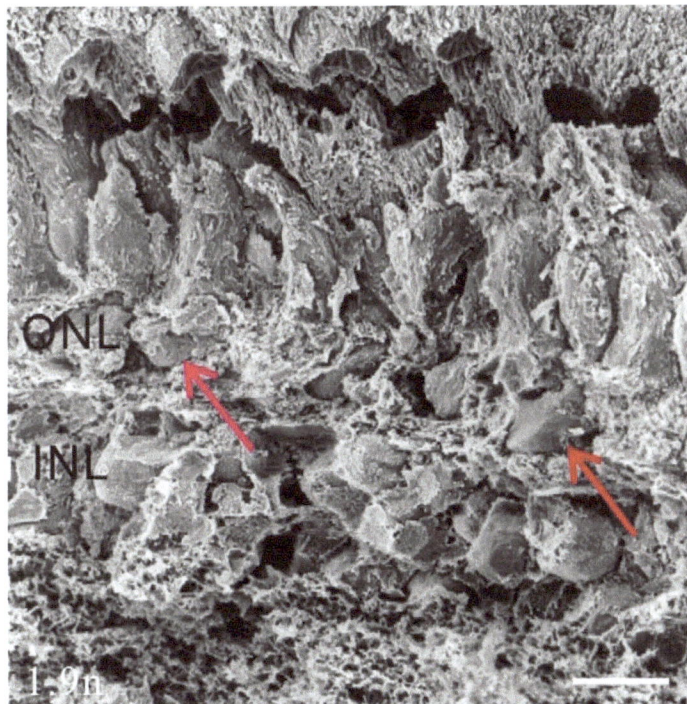

Figure 1.9o.

A continuous row of double cones is seen in this figure. A layer of synaptic contacts between different retinal cells, known as the outer plexiform layer (OPL) is also identified. Bar = 10 μm.

(Ac - Accessory cone; Cc - Chief cone).

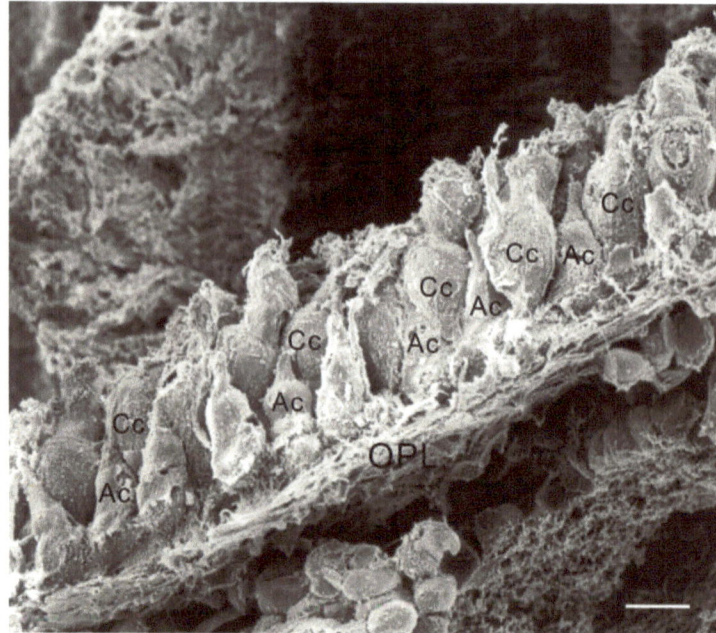

Figure 1.9p.

Cone cells (C) in the outer nuclear layer (ONL) have wide synaptic contacts (i.e. pedicles) (yellow dotted outline) with cells of the inner nuclear layer (INL) while the rod cell (R) has a smaller area of contacts (i.e. spherule) (red solid outline) with inner nuclear cells. Bar = 10 μm.

(IPL - Inner plexiform layer).

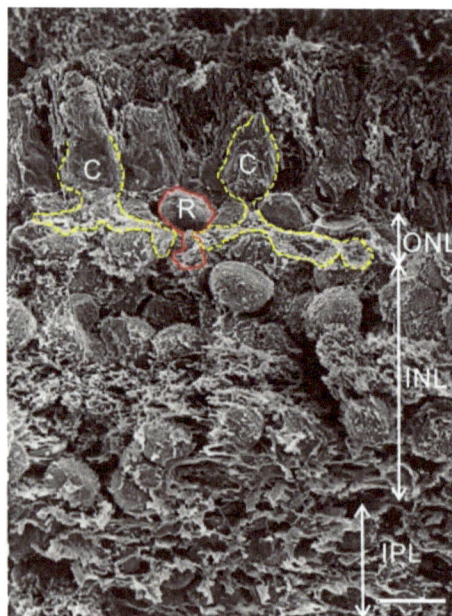

Figure 1.9q.

This scanning electron micrograph shows chief cones (Cc) and accessory cones (Ac) in the lungfish retina. The chief cones are larger and taller than the accessory cones. In between the outer segments of the cones lie the pigment epithelial processes (red arrows). The nuclei of the accessory cones (AcN) are also noted in this figure. On the right, the outer (O) and inner (I) segments of a chief cone are indicated. Bar = 10 μm.

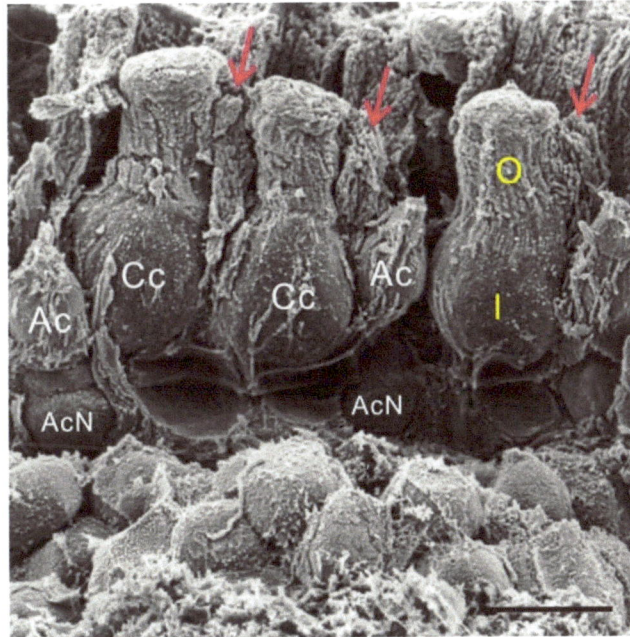

Figure 1.9r.

A magnified chief cone (Cc) with its blunt outer segment (O) is shown. Bar = 5 μm.

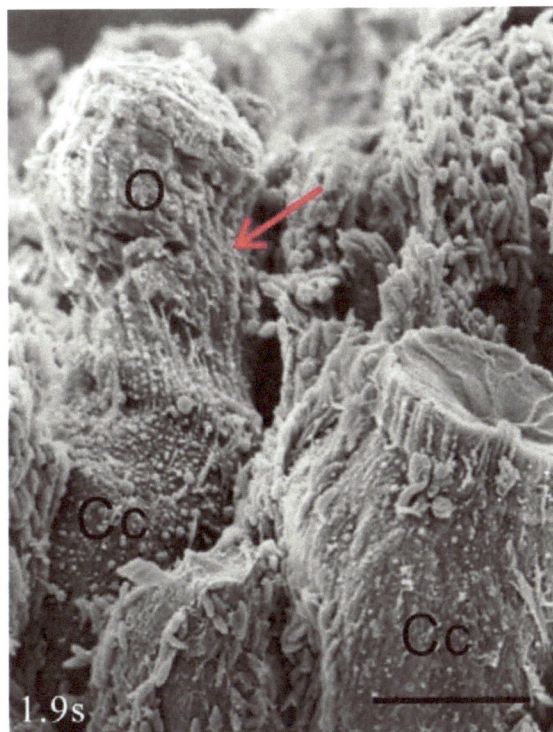

Figure 1.9s.

There are many microvilli (red arrow) on the surface of the chief cone outer segments (O). Bar = 5 μm.

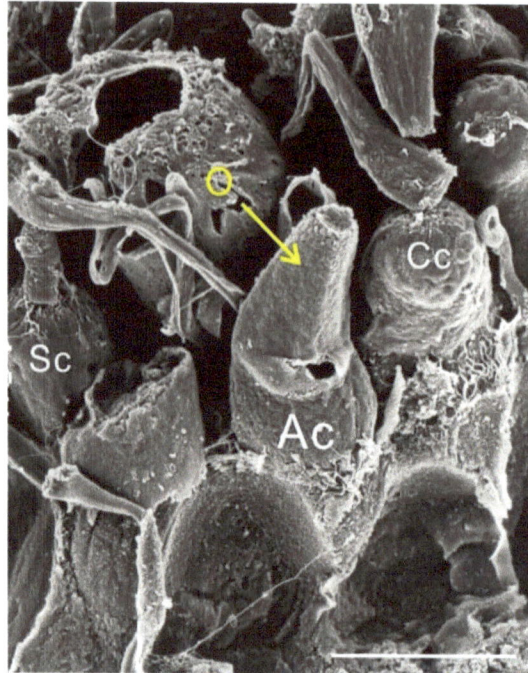

Figure 1.9t.

A chief cone (Cc) and an accessory cone (Ac) with taper outer segment (O) are shown. In addition, an elongated outer segment of a single cone (S) is also noted on the left. Bar = 10 μm.

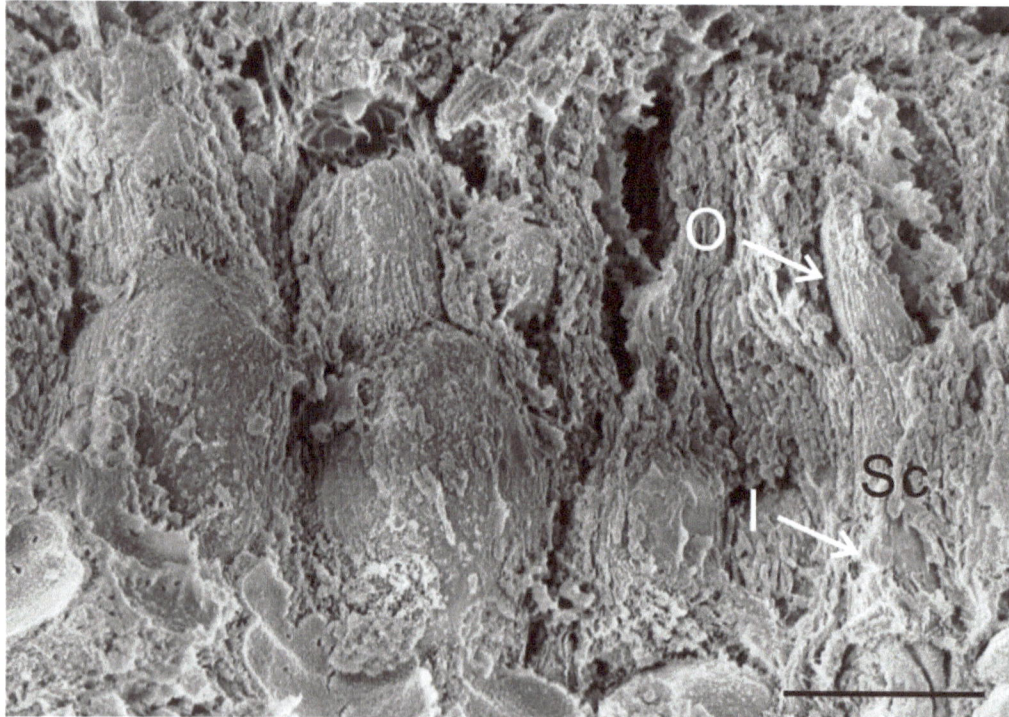

Figure 1.9u.

Another single cone (Sc) with its nucleus is shown. "I" denotes its short and column-like inner segment and "O" denotes its long and tapered outer segment. Bar = 10 μm.

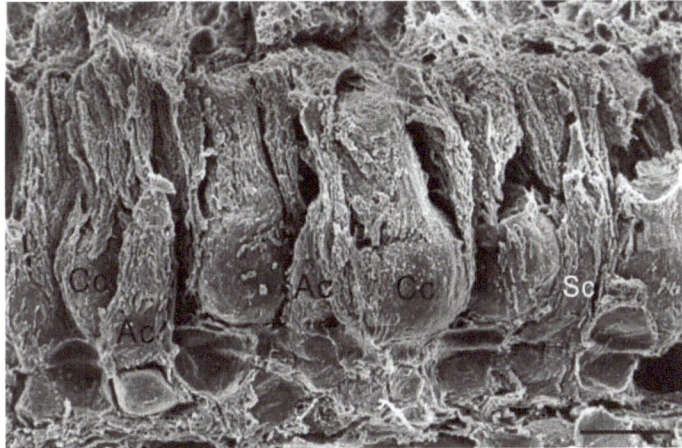

Figure 1.9v.

In this figure another slender single cone (Sc) with a tapered outer segment is seen. In addition, a few double cones are also noted. The outer segments of the chief cones (Cc) appear wide whereas the outer segments of the accessory cones (Ac) are short and tapered in shape. Bar = 10 μm.

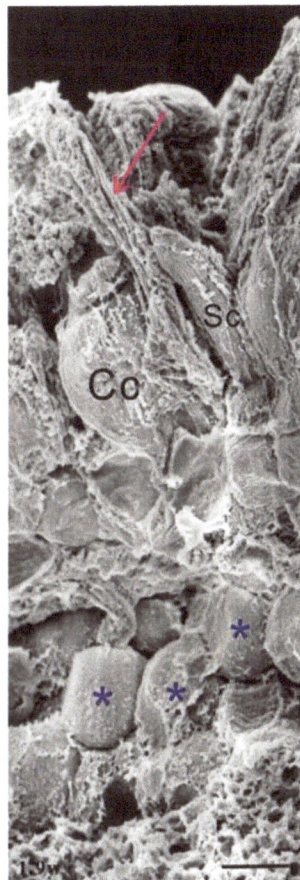

Figure 1.9w.

In this figure, a short single cone (Sc), probably another type of single cone, is separated from the neighboring round chief cone by a microvillus with pigment epithelial granules (red arrow). The round cells indicated by asterisks are examples of other retinal cells inside the inner nuclear layer (INL). Bar = 5 μm.

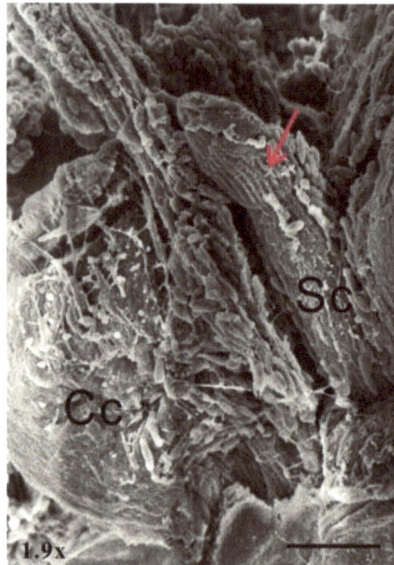

Figure 1.9x.

A higher magnification of figure 1.9w is shown. The beginning of the outer segment of a single cone is illustrated with a circumference of evenly spaced microvilli (red arrow) from the crown between the outer and inner segments. The outer segment of the chief cone is missing. Bar = 3 μm.

10. JAPANESE FIRE BELLY NEWT

The retina of the Japanese Fire Belly newt (salamander) is formed by large cells. The outer nuclear layer is only two layers thick while the inner nuclear layer is about six layers thick. The ganglion cell layer is more than one layer thick and is usually about three layers thick at least. The visual cells have no oil droplets. Twin cones which were originally a feature in fish are constantly observable in this animal. Double cones are also seen.

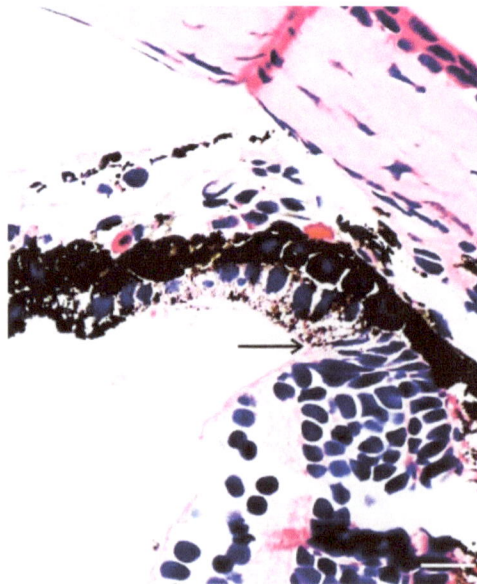

Figure 1.10a. *Anterior retina, near ora serrata.*

This figure shows the abrupt transition (arrow) from the anterior retina into the ora serrata. Note the absence of visual cells in the ora serrata. Bar = 50 μm.

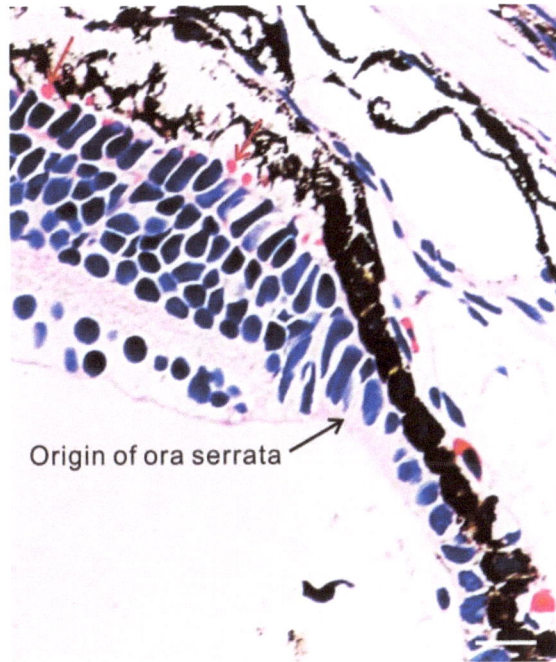

Figure 1.10b. *Ora serrata.*

The eosin stained cells are visual cells (red arrows) in the anterior retina. More anteriorly is the ora serrata, where there is a depletion of visual cells and a decrease of retinal layers. Bar = 50 μm.

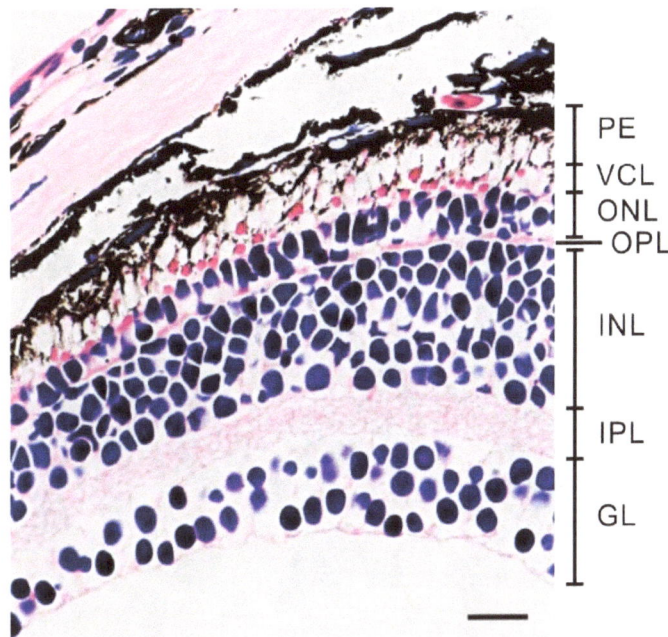

Figure 1.10c. *Anterior retina.*

The different layers of the retina in the salamander are identified. This amphibian shows a characteristically large number of retinal cells in the inner nuclear layer (INL) and ganglion cell layer (GL). Bar = 50 μm.

(GL - Ganglion cell layer; INL - Inner nuclear layer; IPL - Inner plexiform layer; ONL - Outer nuclear layer; OPL - Outer plexiform layer; PE - Pigment epithelium; VCL - Visual cell layer).

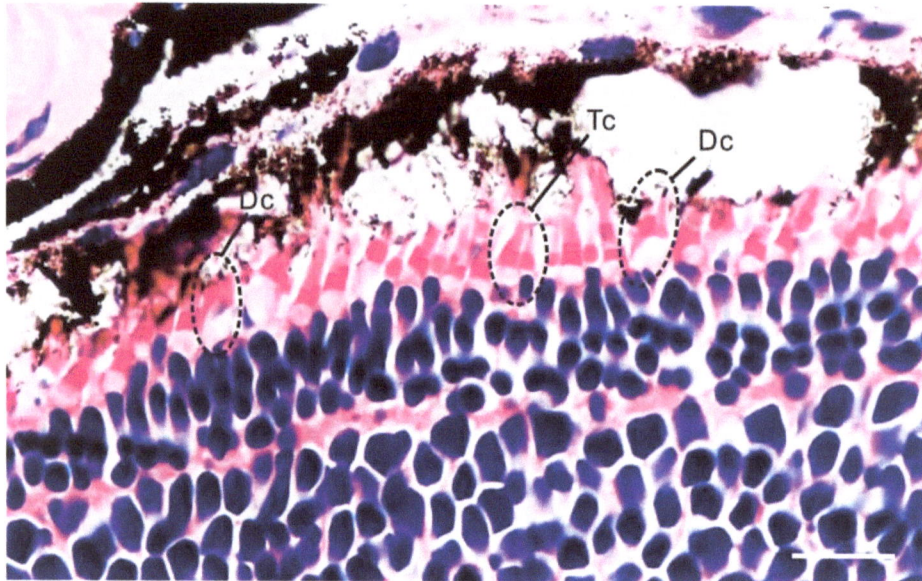

Figure 1.10d. *Peripheral retina.*

Numerous cones are noted in this figure. Among the cones are a few pairs of double cones (Dc) and twin cones (Tc). Rods are not prominent in this region of the retina. Bar = 50 μm.

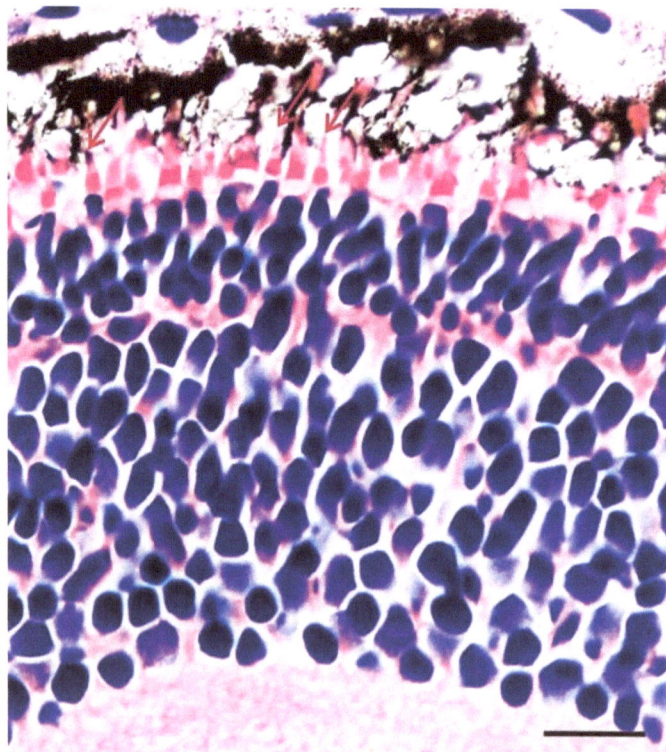

Figure 1.10e. *Peripheral retina.*

This figure shows the single cones (red arrows) with taper outer segments in the peripheral region. Bar = 50 μm.

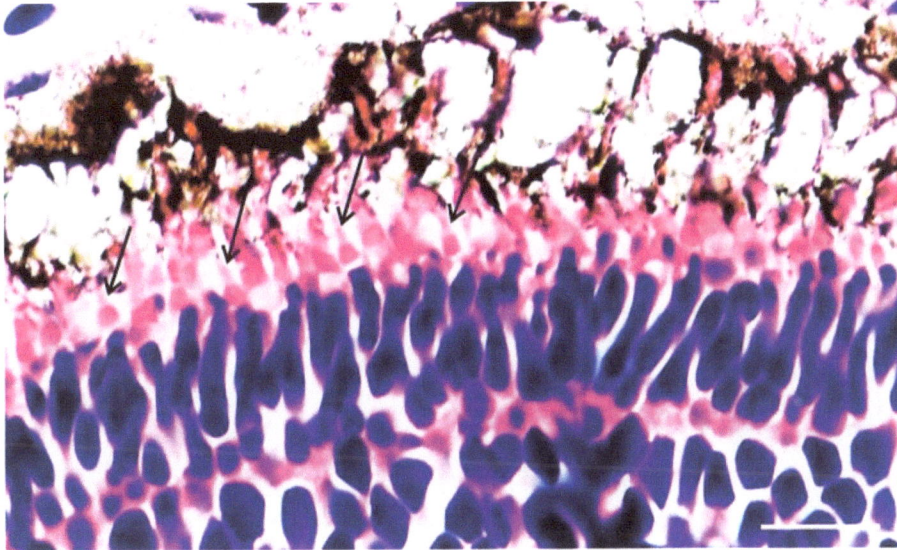

Figure 1.10f. *Central retina.*

The central retina also has a fair number of single cones (arrows) with appearance similar to that seen in the peripheral region. Bar = 50 μm.

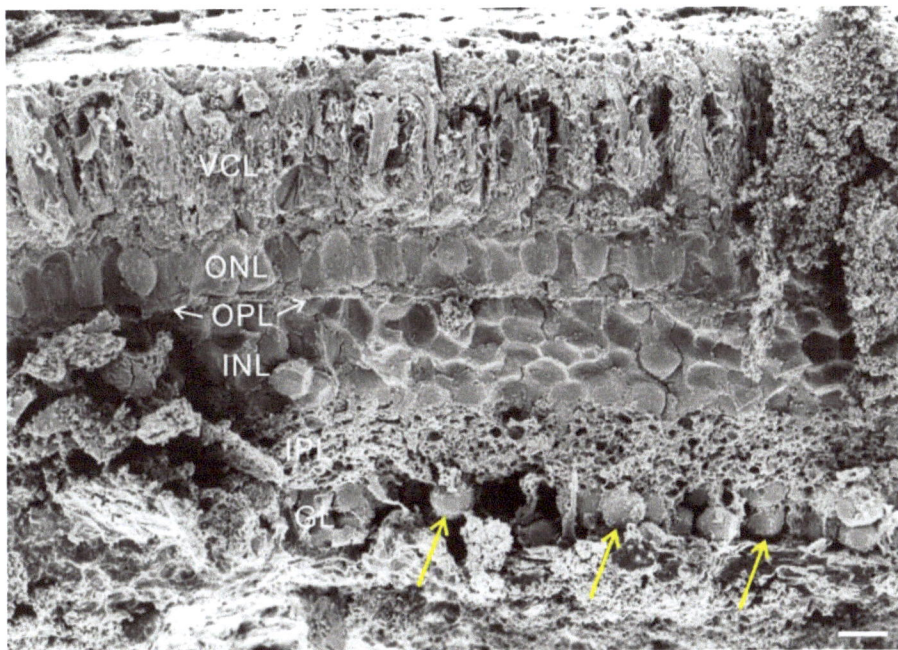

Figure 1.10g.

View under scanning electron microscopy showing the various layers of retina in salamander. The outer nuclear layer (ONL) is made up of 1 to 2 layers of cell nuclei whereas the inner nuclear layer is multilayered with 4 to 5 layers of cells. Spherical ganglion cells (yellow arrows) are noted in the innermost layer. Bar = 10 μm.

(INL - Inner nuclear layer; IPL - Inner plexiform layer; PE - Pigment epithelium; ONL - Outer nuclear layer; OPL - Outer plexiform layer; VCL - Visual cell layer).

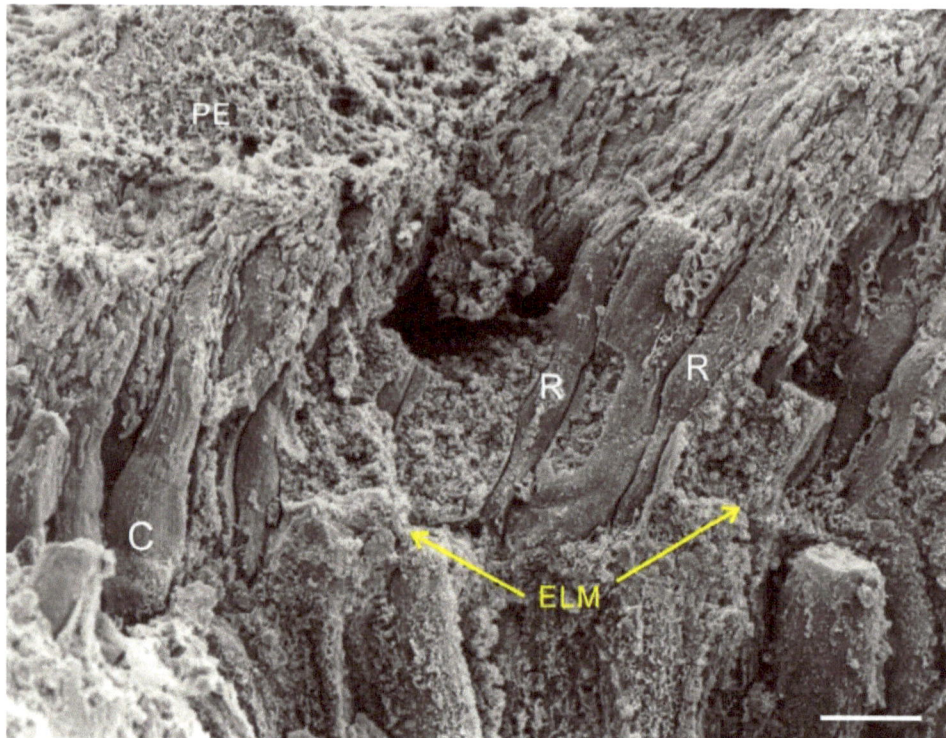

Figure 1.10h.

This figure shows the morphology of both rods (R) and cones (C) in the salamander. Bar = 5 μm.

(ELM - External limiting membrane; PE - Pigment epithelium).

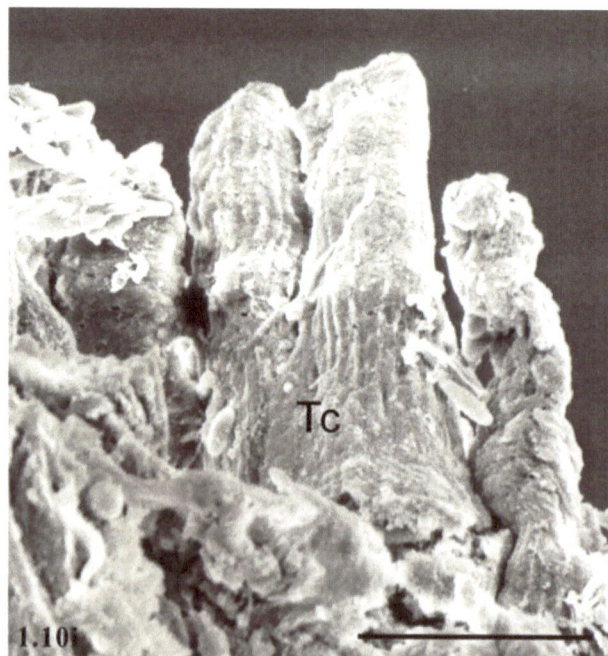

Figure 1.10i.

A twin cone (Tc) with massive inner segments is noted. The inner segments are of similar height and sizes. Bar = 5 μm.

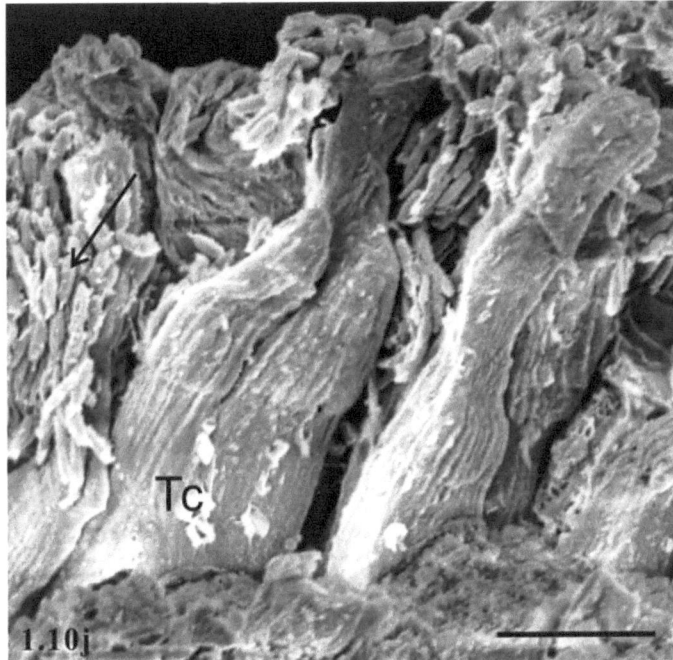

Figure 1.10j.

Another twin cone (Tc) is identified in a different region. The visual cells shown are still covered by the pigment epithelium, and its processes are indicated by an arrow.

Bar = 5 μm.

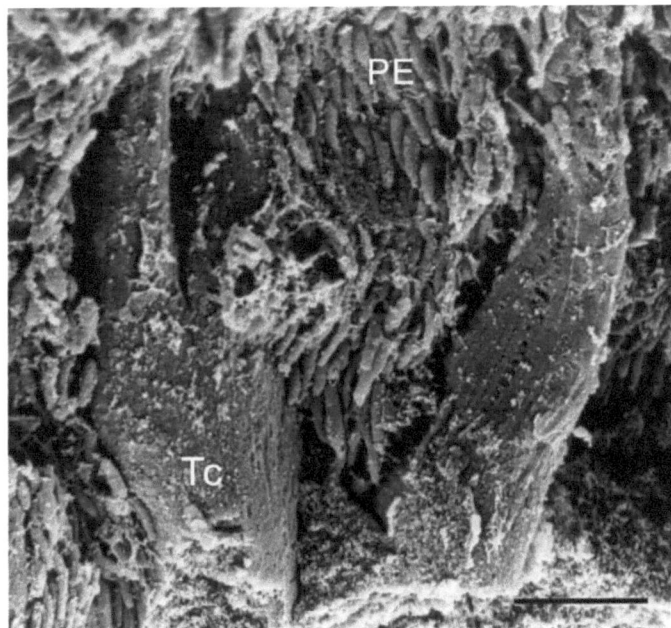

Figure 1.10k.

This figure shows another twin cone (Tc). The distal outer segments are covered by the pigment granules of the epithelium (PE). Bar = 3 μm.

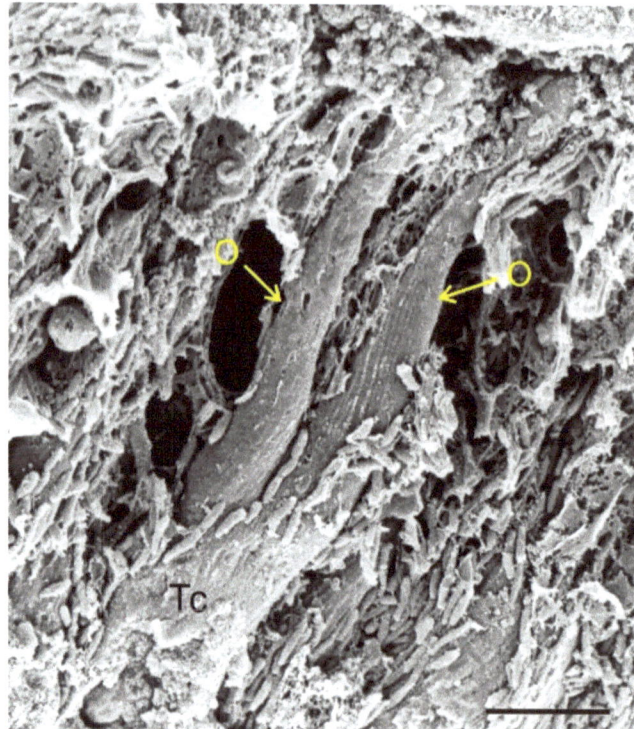

Figure 1.10l.

This figure also shows a twin cone (Tc) but with longer outer segments (O). The outer segments are uncovered and are tapered. Bar = 5 μm.

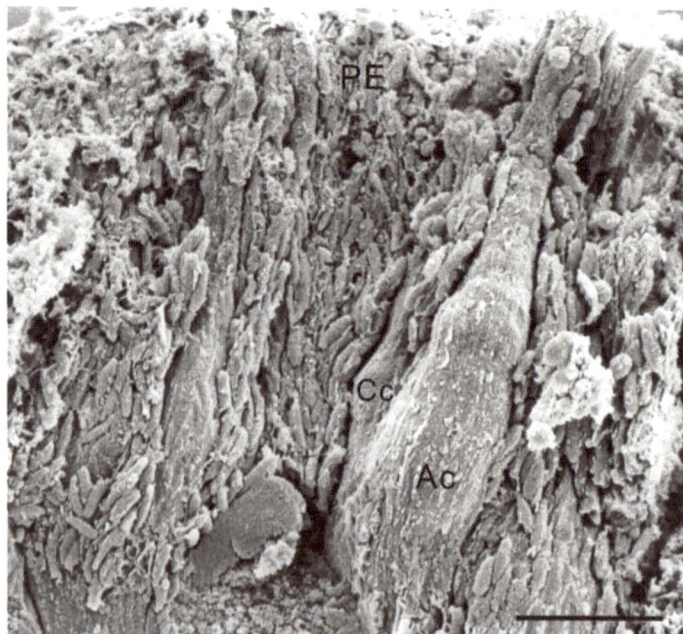

Figure 1.10m.

A double cone with a large accessory cone (Ac) and a comparatively small chief cone (Cc) is shown. Bar = 5 mm.

(PE - Pigment epithelium).

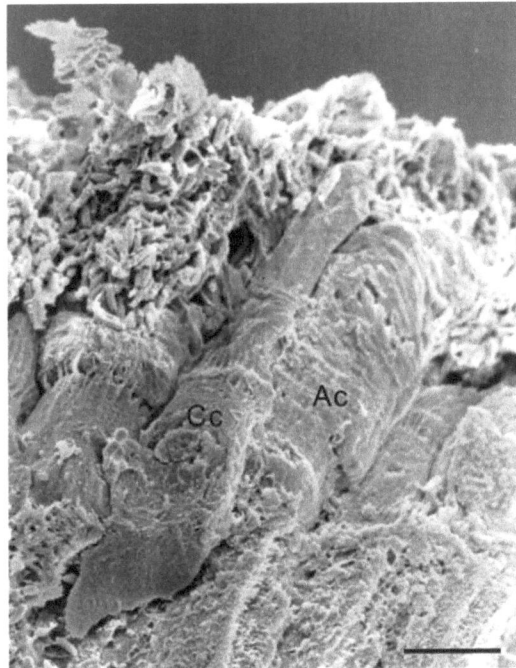

Figure 1.10n.

Another pair of double cones is shown. Bar = 5 μm.

(Ac - Accessory cone; Cc - Chief cone).

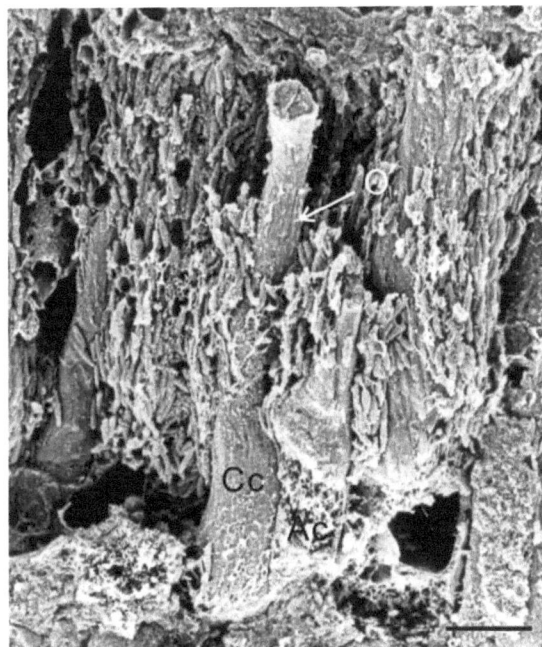

Figure 1.10o.

A double cone of the salamander's retina is shown with a shorter accessory cone (Ac) and a taller chief cone (Cc) with a long outer segment (O). In the salamander, the accessory component of the double cone may not be very broad. Bar = 10 μm.

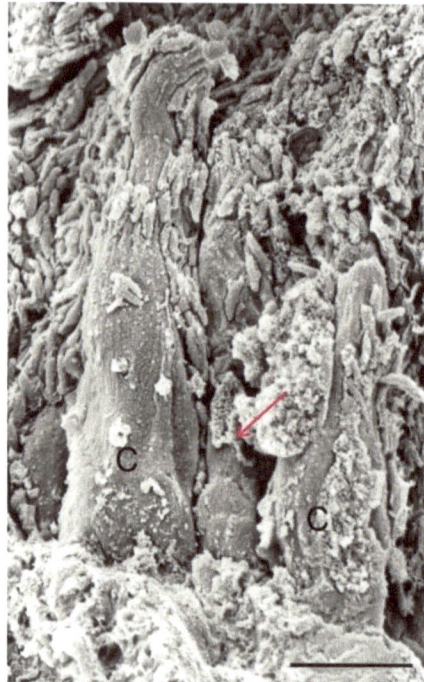

Figure 1.10p.

A small budding cone (red arrow) is seen between two cones (C) in this salamander's retina, perhaps indicating constant renewal. Bar = 5 mm.

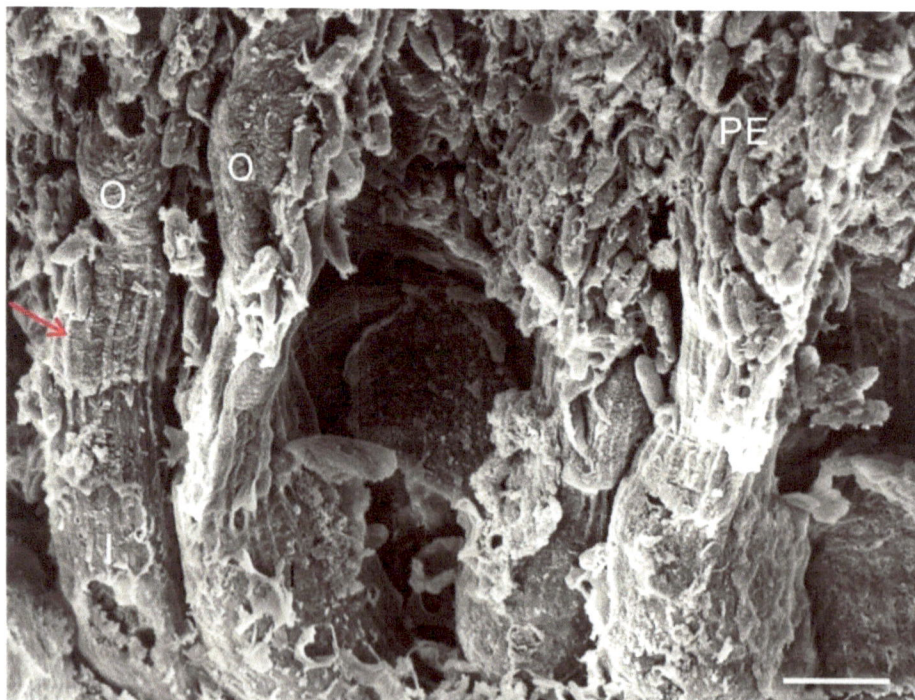

Figure 1.10q.

The outer (O) and inner (I) segments of the visual cells are identified. The distal outer segments of some visual cells are still covered by the pigment epithelium (PE). The typical microvilli at the proximal end of the outer segment are also clearly seen (red arrow). Bar = 2 μm.

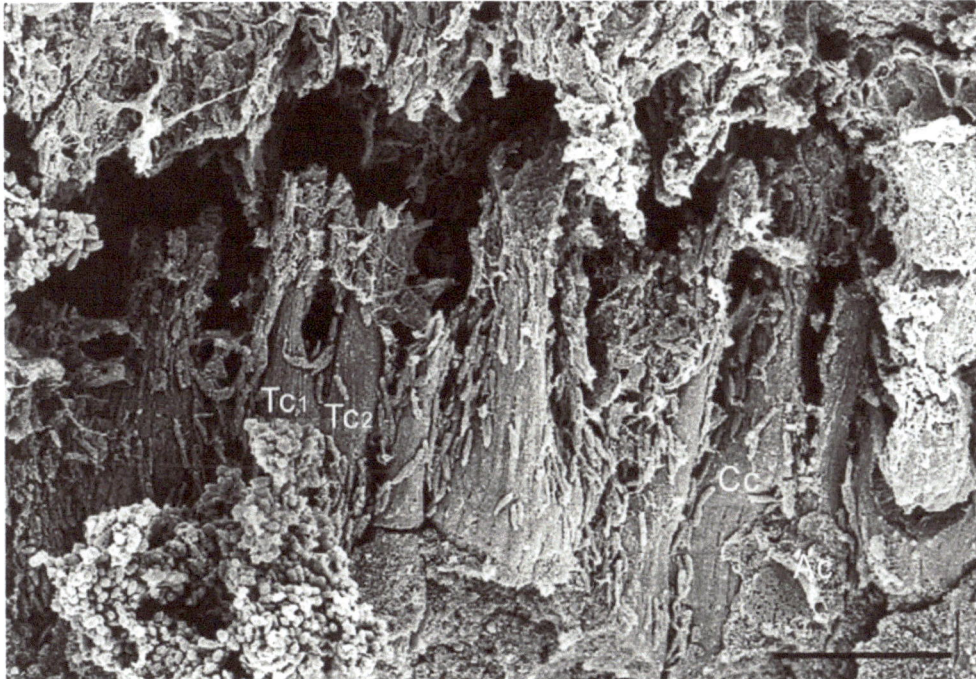

Figure 1.10r.

A pair of double cones with an accessory cone (Ac) and a chief cone (Cc). A pair of identified twin cones (Tc1 and Tc2) is also shown. Bar = 10 μm.

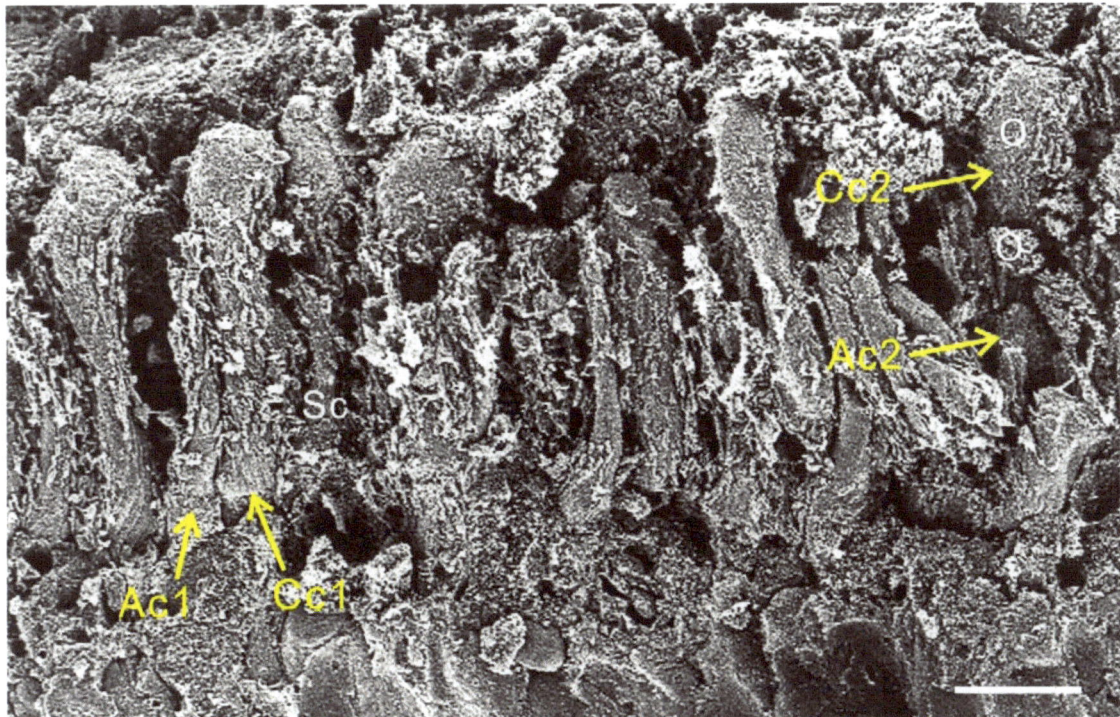

Figure 1.10s.

This figure shows a single cone (Sc) beside a double cone comprised of an accessory cone (Ac1) and a chief cone (Cc1). Another pair of double cones with the inner segments and outer segments (O) of an accessory cone (Ac2) and a chief cone (Cc2) are shown. This latter pair of double cones is at a right angle to the cut surface. Bar = 10 μm.

11. CHINESE EDIBLE FROG

The Chinese edible frog has visual cells containing oil droplets. This animal has a thin outer nuclear layer and a folded thicker inner nuclear layer. Ganglion cells are moderate in number and occupy only one layer. Many visual cells are rods with short inner segments. Double cones are also one of the cone types seen.

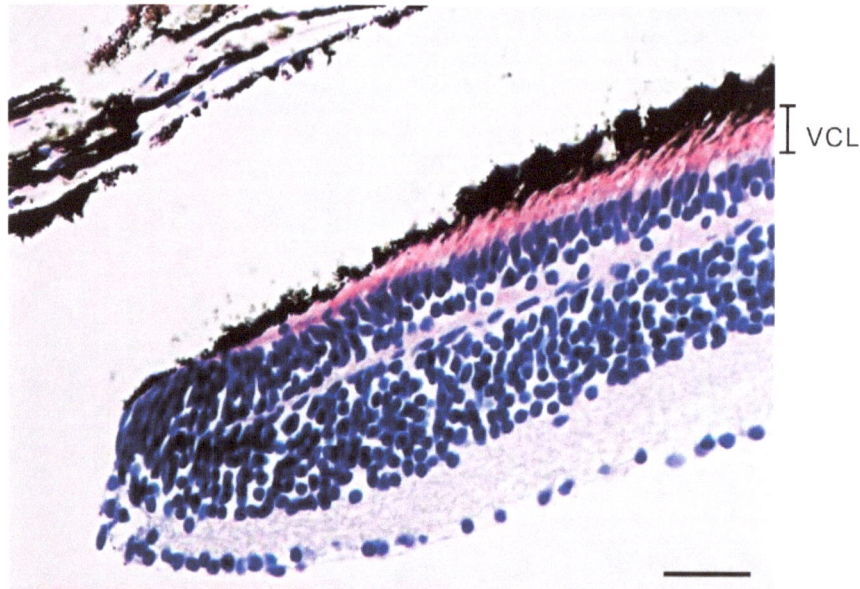

Figure 1.11a. *Anterior retina.*

This figure shows the anterior retina of a Chinese edible frog with a decreasing thickness of visual cell layer (VCL). Bar = 50 μm.

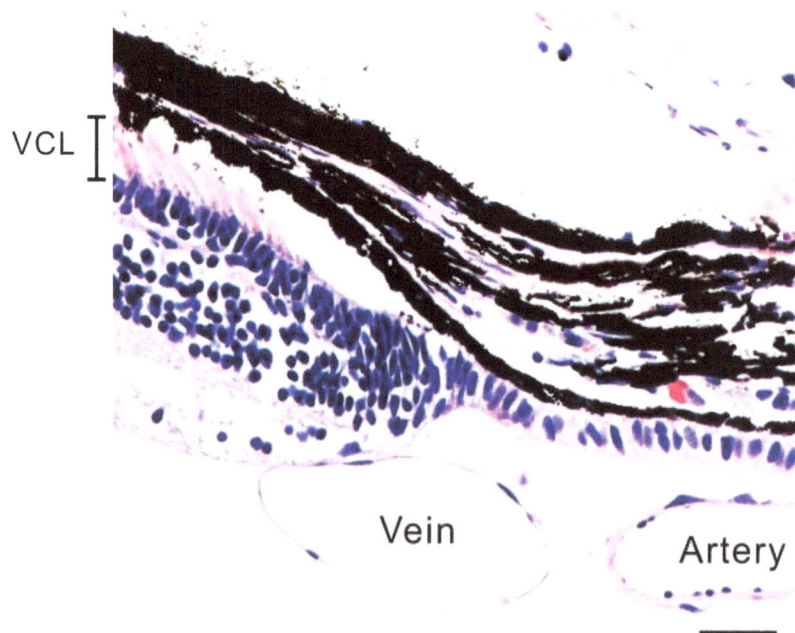

Figure 1.11b. *Ora serrata.*

Note the gradual transition into the ora serrata. The visual cell layer (VCL) is absent and the retinal layers become a single layer of cells. Note the large artery and vein inner to the retina. Bar = 50 μm.

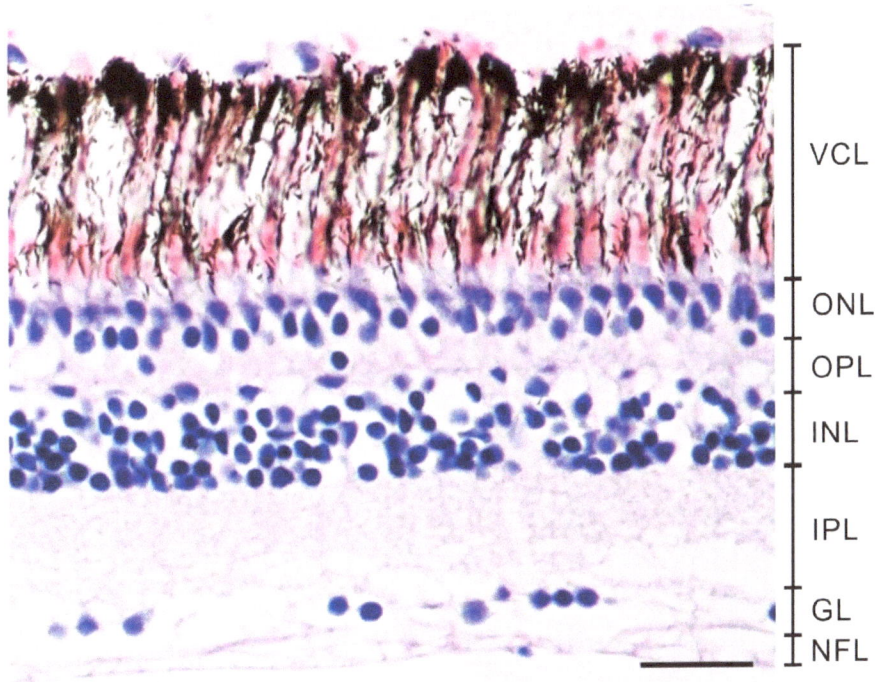

Figure 1.11c. *Peripheral retina.*

Layers of the Chinese edible frog's retina are identified. Bar = 50 µm.

(GL - Ganglion layer; INL - Inner nuclear layer; IPL - Inner plexiform layer; NFL - Nerve fiber layer; ONL - Outer nuclear layer; OPL - Outer plexiform layer; VCL - Visual cell layer).

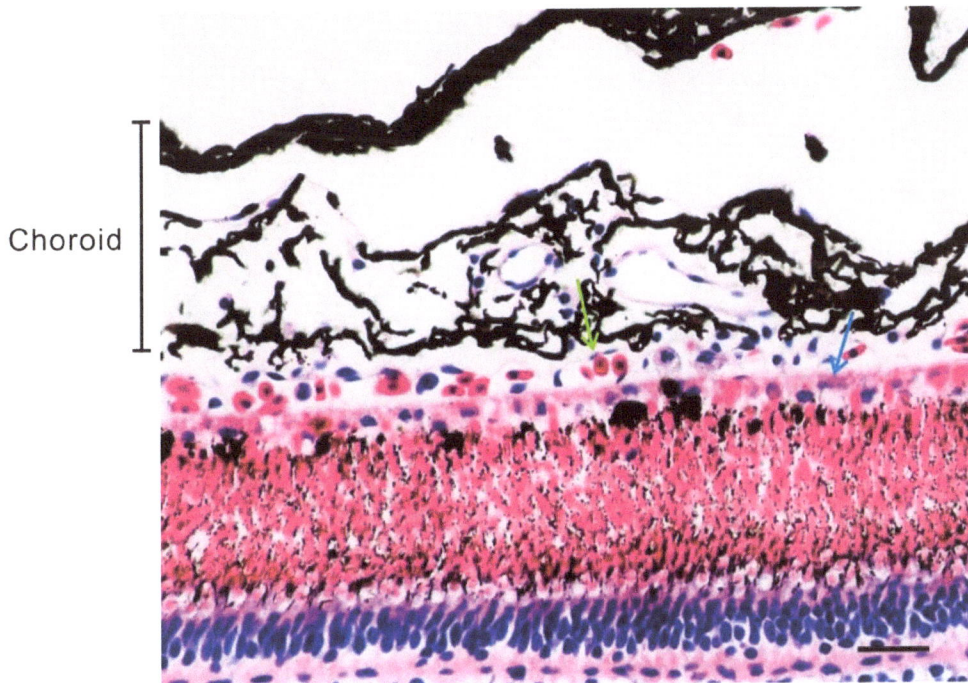

Figure 1.11d. *Peripheral retina.*

External to the retina is a layer of epithelial cells (blue arrow). Blood vessels with plasma cells inside (yellow arrow) and pigmented choroid are also noted. Bar = 50 mm.

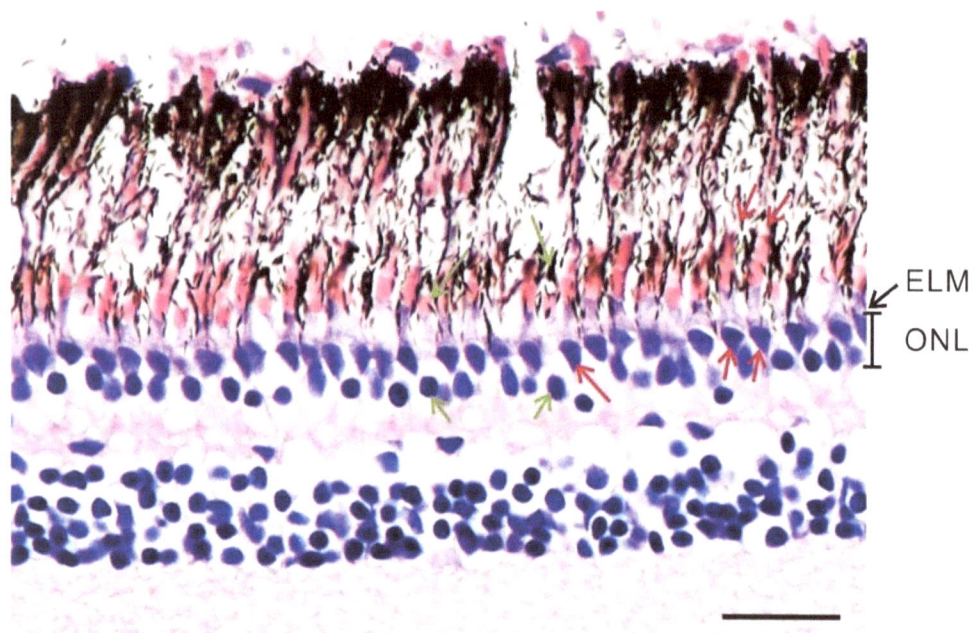

Figure 1.11e. *Peripheral retina.*

Two types of cone cells are identified by the different height and positional level of their nuclei in the outer nuclear layer (ONL). The taller cones with nuclei close to the external limiting membrane (ELM) are indicated with red arrows. The shorter cones with their nuclei at a lower level are indicated with green arrows. Bar = 50 μm.

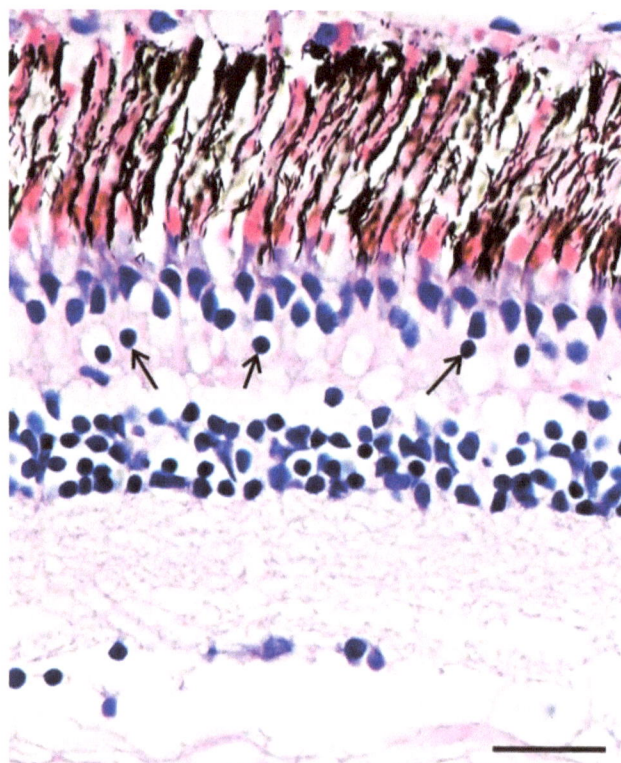

Figure 1.11f. *Peripheral retina.*

Rods do not predominate the retina. Note the positions of their nuclei (arrows) and compare them with the nuclei of different cones lying above. Bar = 50 μm.

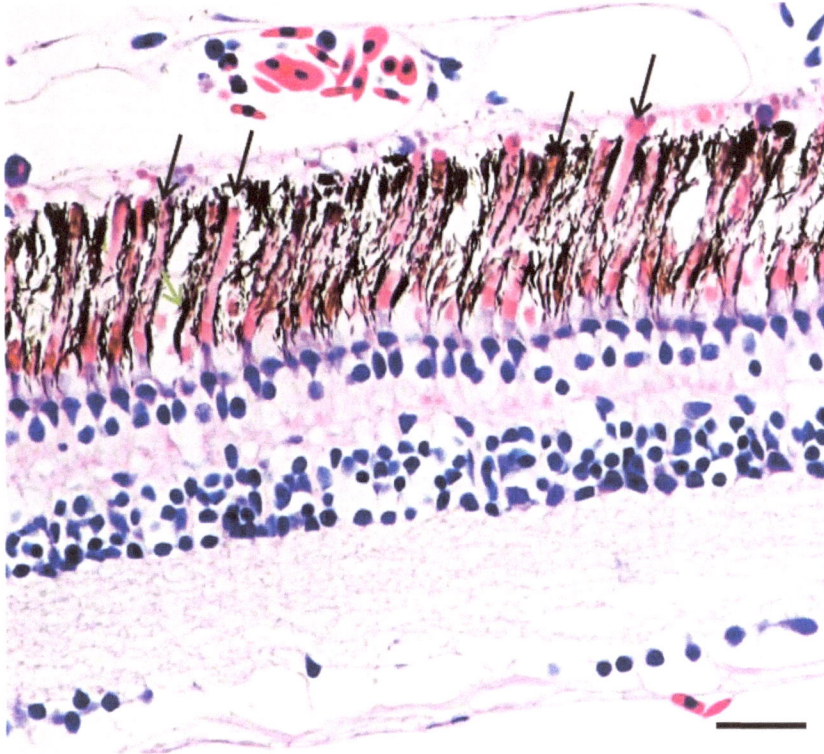

Figure 1.11g. *Peripheral retina.*

The long outer segments of the tall cone cells are clearly shown (arrows). A small cone cell with a short tapered outer segment is also noted (green arrow). Bar = 50 µm.

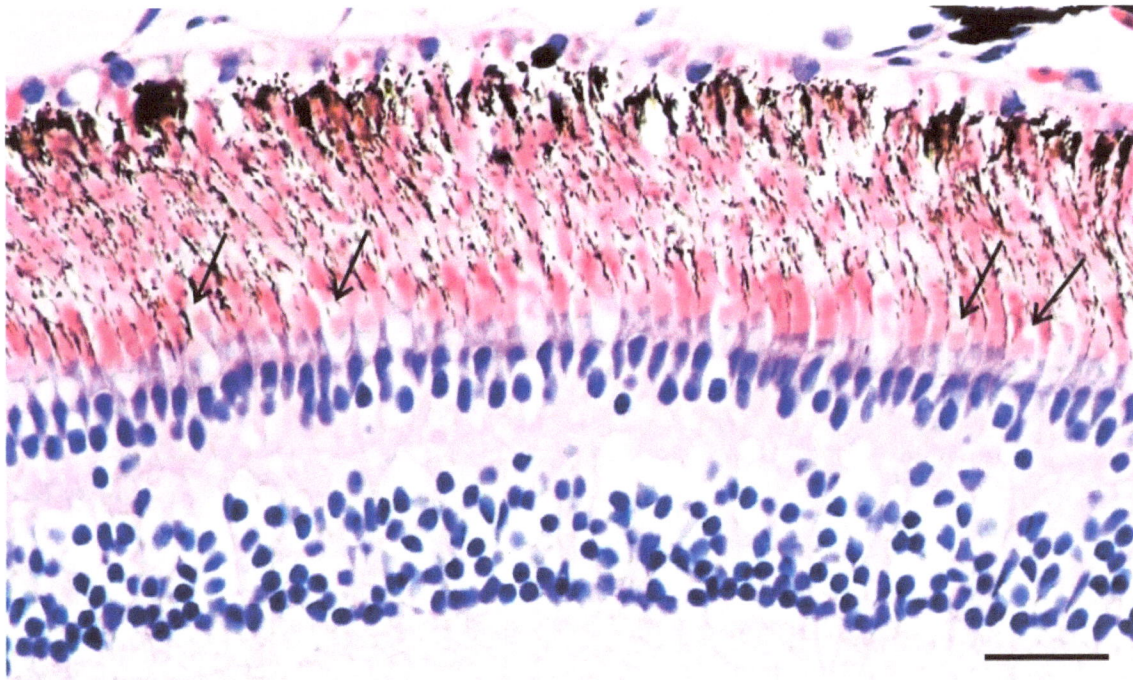

Figure 1.11h. *Central retina.*

In this figure, oil droplets (arrows) are seen in some cone cells. Bar = 50 µm.

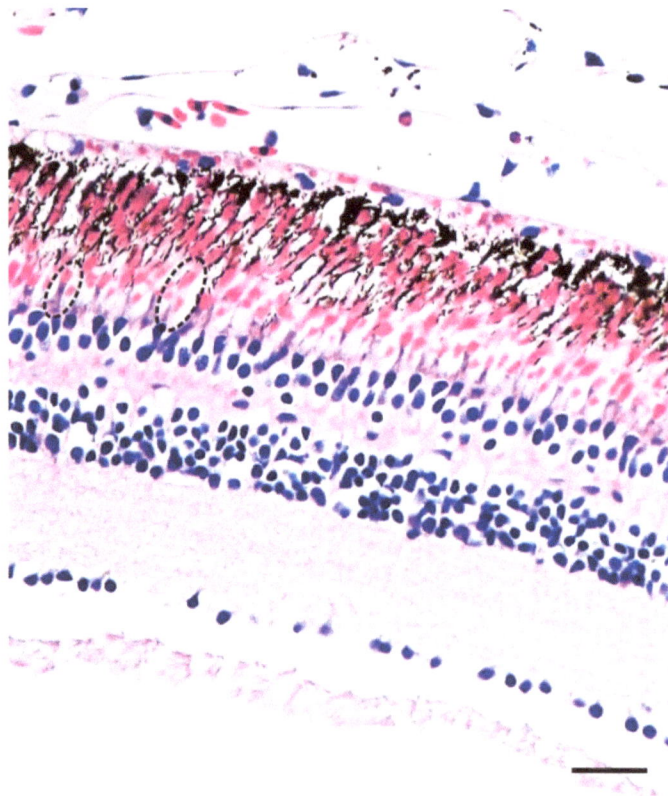

Figure 1.11i. *Central retina.*

Double cones (circles) are seen in the central retina. The tall ones represent the chief cones whereas the short ones are the accessory cones. Bar = 50 μm.

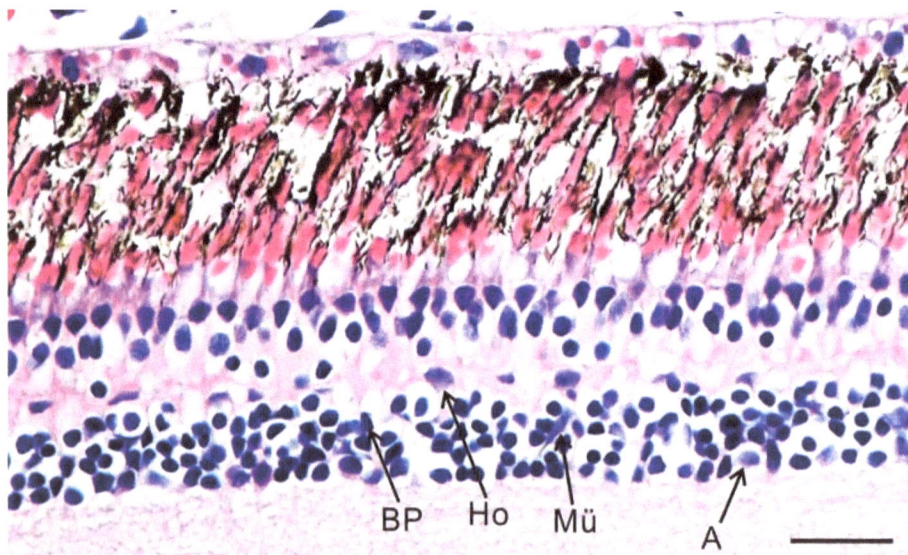

Figure 1.11j. *Central retina.*

Some retinal cells in the inner nuclear layer are identified. Bar = 50 μm.

(A - Amacrine cell; BP - Bipolar cell; Ho - Horizontal cell; Mü - Müller cell).

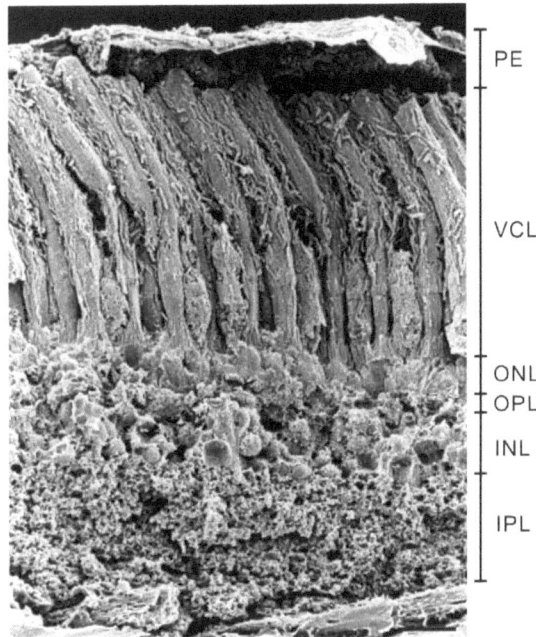

Figure 1.11k.

Scanning electron microscopy showing the retinal layers of the Chinese edible frog. Two distinct types of visual cells are noted. Bar = 10 μm.

(INL - Inner nuclear layer; IPL - Inner plexiform layer; ONL - Outer nuclear layer; OPL - Outer plexiform layer; PE - Pigment epithelium; VCL - Visual cell layer).

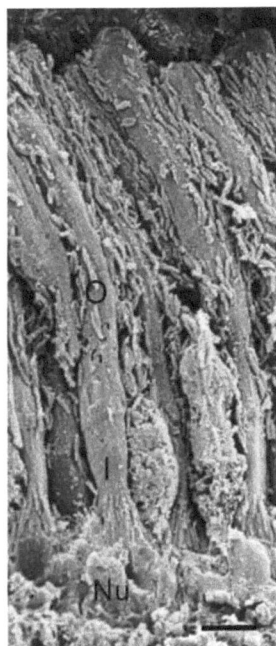

Figure 1.11l.

A cone cell is illustrated. Both the inner (I) and outer (O) segments are elongated; however, its inner segment is extremely short as compared with the outer segment. The cone cell nucleus (Nu) is also noted. Bar = 10 μm.

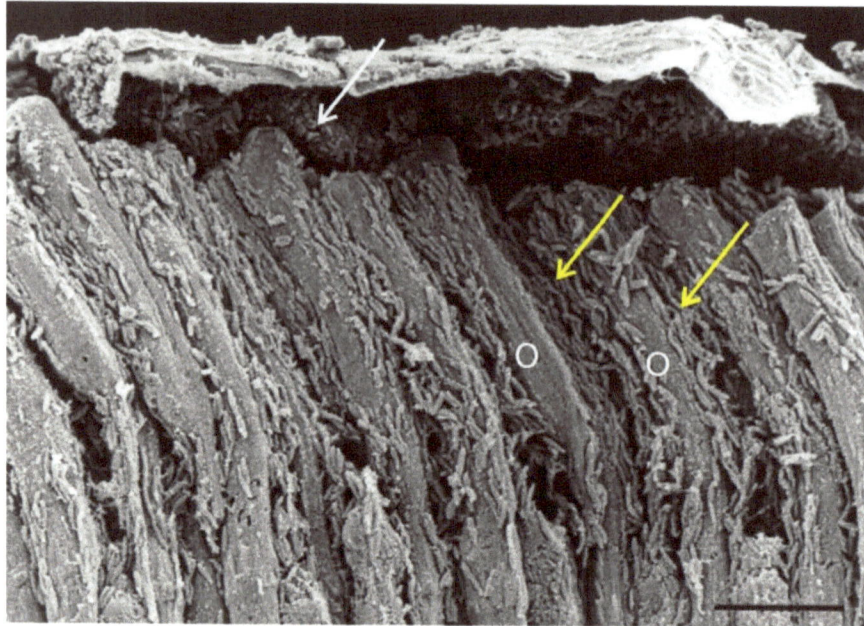

Figure 1.11m.

The layer of pigment epithelium covering the visual cells is clearly illustrated (white arrow). Spaces between the outer segments (O) are fully occupied by the pigment granules of this epithelial layer (yellow arrows). Bar = 10 μm.

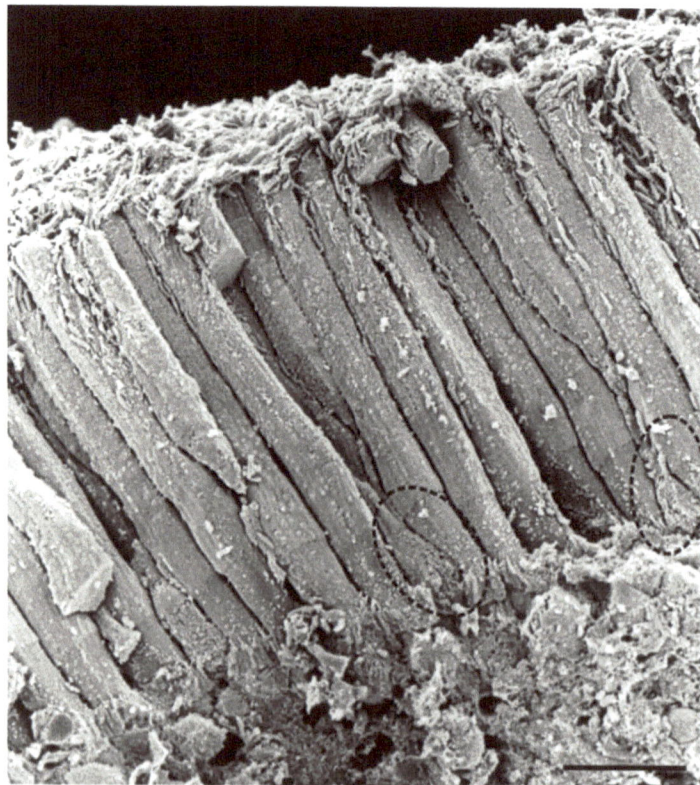

Figure 1.11n.

Another region of the retina again showing many long and straight visual cells, but with fewer pigment granules around the outer segments. A few double cones are noted. Circles indicate the basal part of the double cones. Bar = 10 μm.

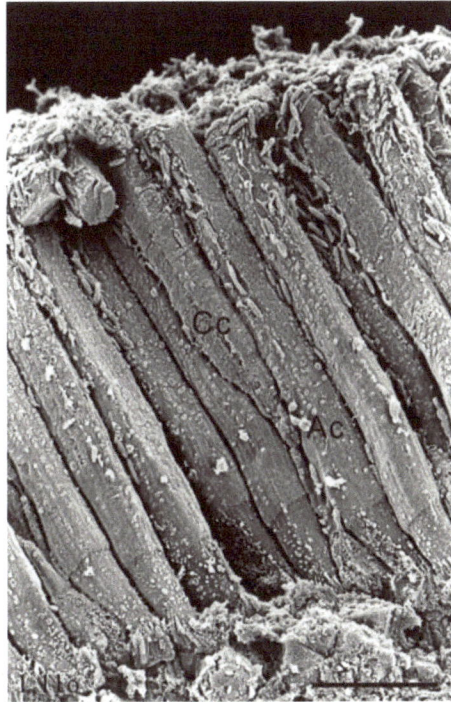

Figure 1.11o.

A higher magnification of the double cone. The chief cone (Cc) has a long outer segment as does the accessory cone (Ac); however, its outer segment is thin and slender at the proximal part then becomes thick and rod-like distally. Bar = 10 μm.

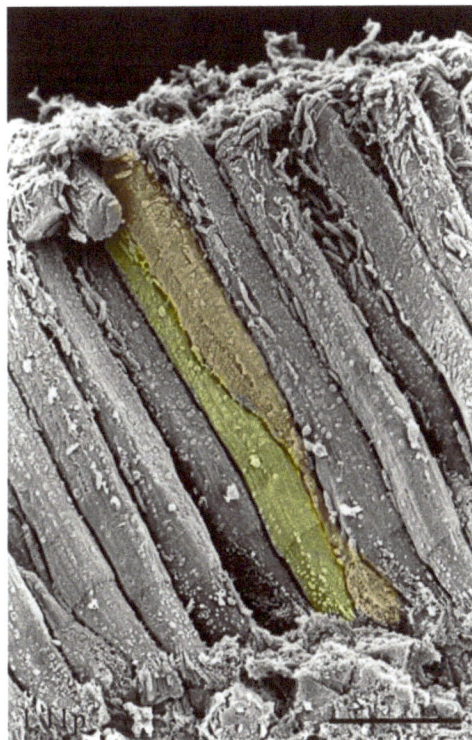

Figure 1.11p.

Same as figure 1.11o. The chief cone is colored in orange; the accessory cone is colored in yellow. Bar = 10 μm.

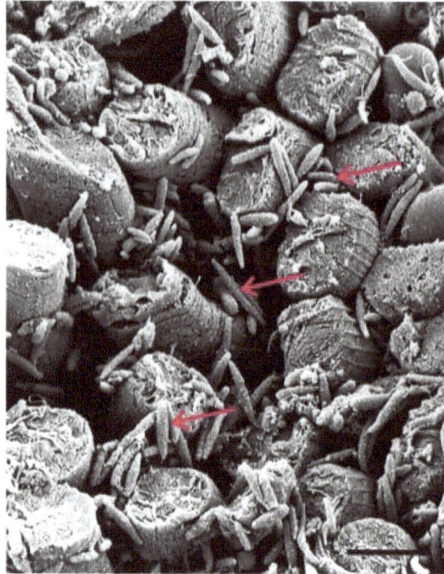

Figure 1.11q.

This figure shows the cross section of the visual cell outer segments. Surrounding the outer segments are many tiny pigment granules (red arrows) from the pigment epithelial layer. Bar = 1 μm.

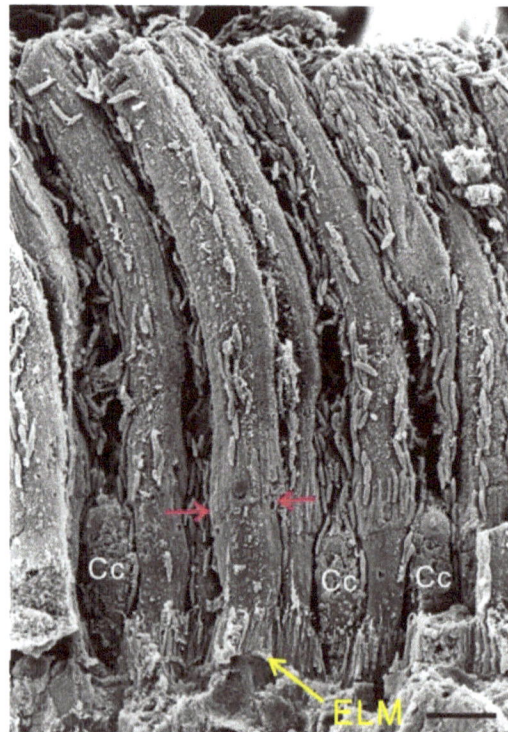

Figure 1.11r.

Three chief cone (Cc) inner segments are noted. The external limiting membrane (ELM) contains many Müller cell processes covering parts of the lower inner segments. The two red arrows indicate the boundary between the inner and outer segments of the visual cell. Again, there are microvilli surrounding the proximal outer segments. Bar = 5 mm.

12. AFRICAN CLAWED FROG

The African clawed frog is a freshwater frog species that spend most their time in water. This animal has a thin retina with only a single row of outer nuclear cells. The inner nuclear layer is about 2 to 3 layers thick. The visual cells, usually rods, are few in number but are rather thick individually. As in the bullfrog, the inner segment is distinctly short while the outer segment is long.

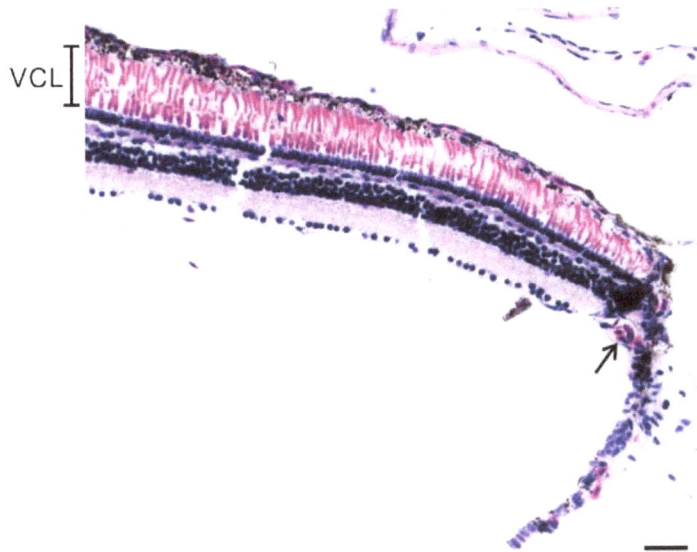

Figure 1.12a. *Anterior retina, near ora serrata.*

There is no gradual decrease of visual cells in the anterior retina of this animal. However, the height of the visual cells near the ora serrata appear slightly shorter than the ones away from the ora serrata. A blood capillary (arrow) is noted at the transitional zone between the anterior retina and ora serrata. Bar = 30 μm.

(VCL - Visual cell layer).

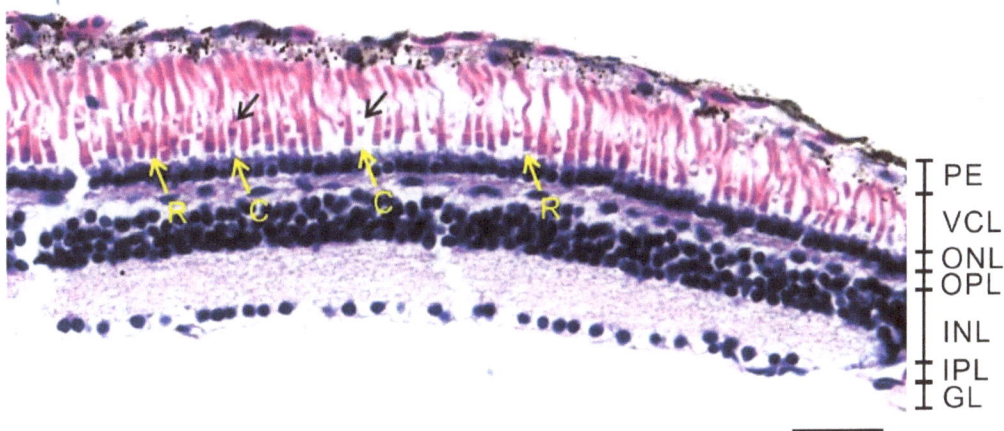

Figure 1.12b. *Anterior retina.*

Both cones (C) and rods (R) are noted in the anterior retina. Cones can be identified by oil droplets present in the distal inner segment (black arrows). Bar = 30 μm.

(GL - Ganglion cell layer; INL - Inner nuclear layer; IPL - Inner plexiform layer; ONL - Outer nuclear layer; OPL - Outer plexiform layer; PE - Pigment epithelium; VCL - Visual cell layer).

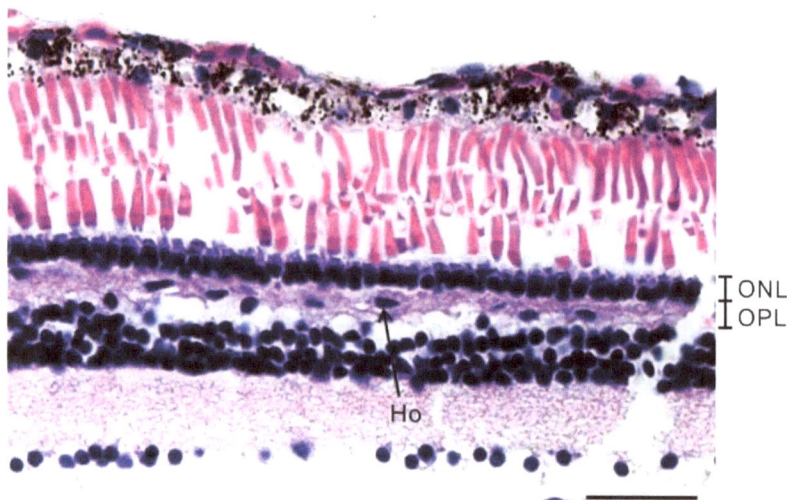

Figure 1.12c. *Peripheral retina.*

There are not much morphological differences between the anterior and peripheral retina. The regularity of the visual cell distribution is indicated by the homogenous arrangement of the cell nuclei in the outer nuclear layer (ONL). A few horizontal cells (Ho) are seen in the outer plexiform layer (OPL). Bar = 30 μm.

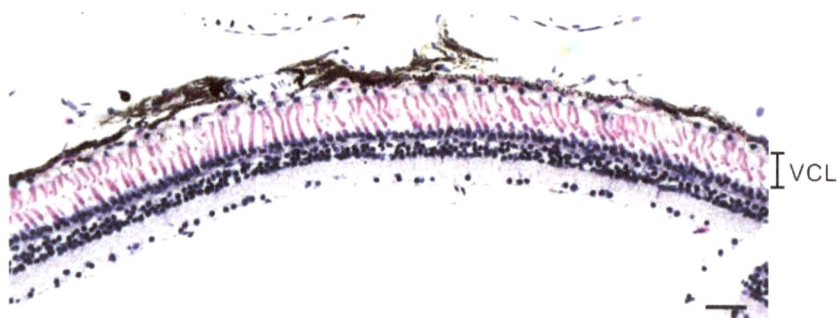

Figure 1.12d. *Central retina.*

The visual cells in even the central retina of this animal are not highly packed. Bar = 30 μm.

(VCL - Visual cell layer).

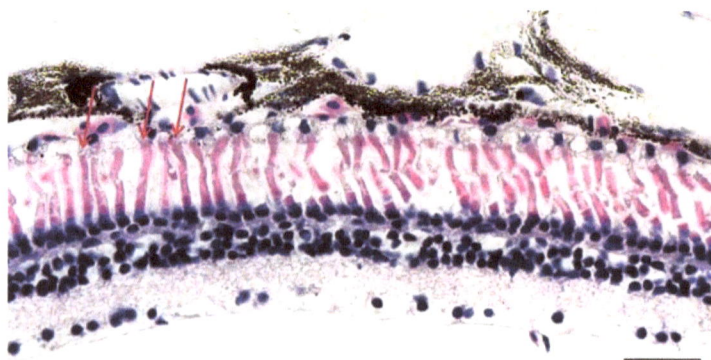

Figure 1.12e. *Central retina.*

There are many rod cells (red arrows) in the central retina. Both the inner and outer segments of these cells appear to be cylindrical. Bar = 30 μm.

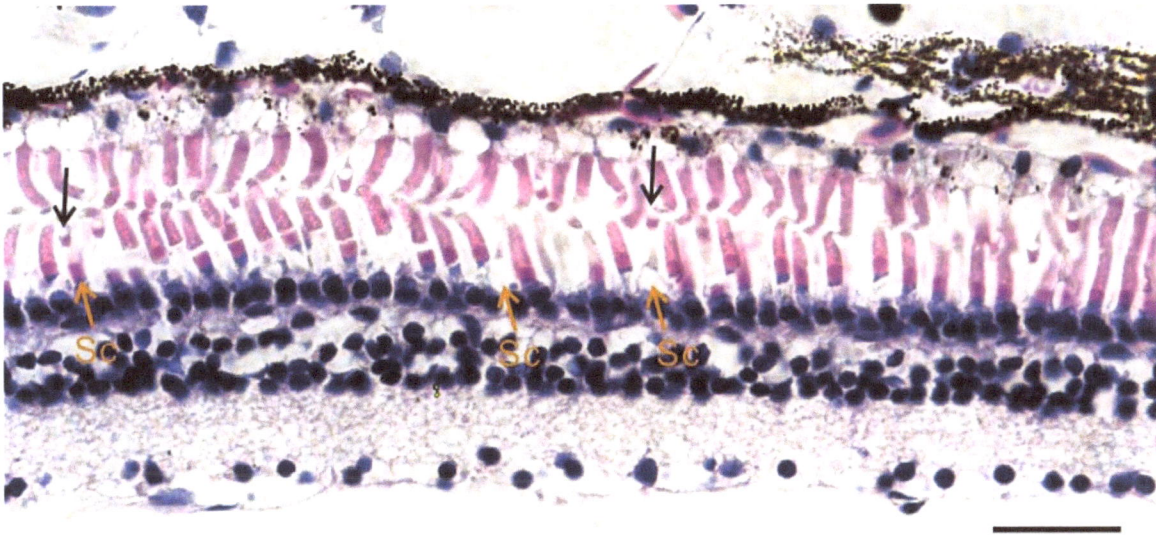

Figure 1.12f. *Central retina.*

There are a few single cones (Sc) noted among the rods. These cone cells have spherical proximal inner segments bearing a long and slender distal part. At the distal end, oil droplets are seen (black arrows). Bar = 30 μm.

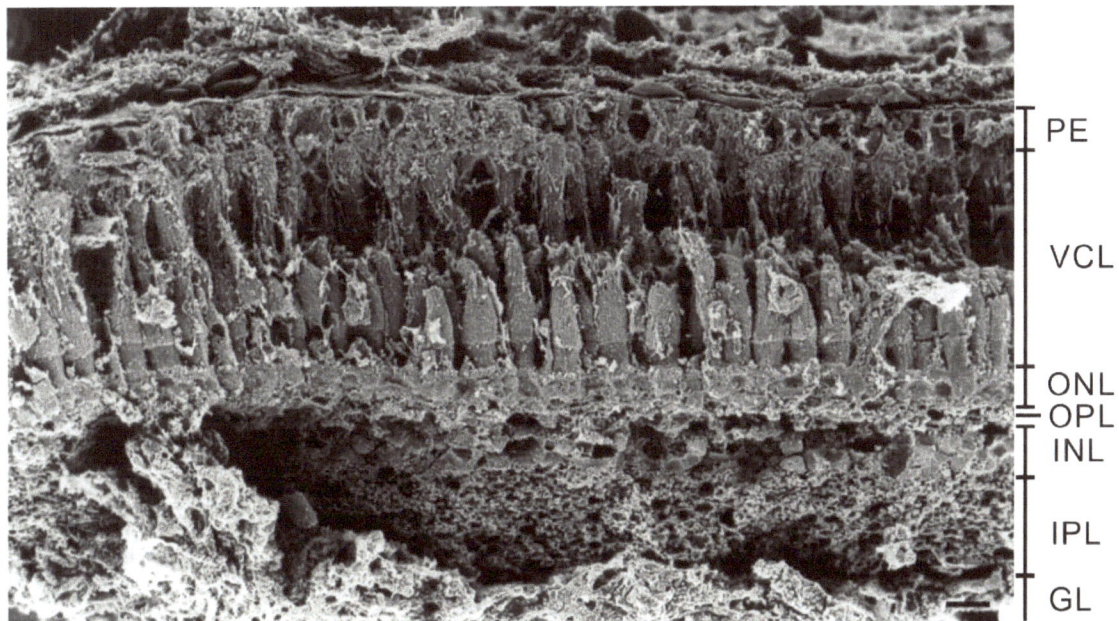

Figure 1.12g.

A scanning electron micrograph showing the various layers of the neural retina and the pigment epithelium of an African clawed frog. The outer and inner nuclear layers of this animal are thin with fewer number of cell nuclei. The visual cells in the front layer of this figure have lost the distal parts of their outer segments. Bar = 10 μm.

(GL - Ganglion cell layer; INL - Inner nuclear layer; IPL - Inner plexiform layer; ONL - Outer nuclear layer; OPL - Outer plexiform layer; PE - Pigment epithelium; VCL - Visual cell layer).

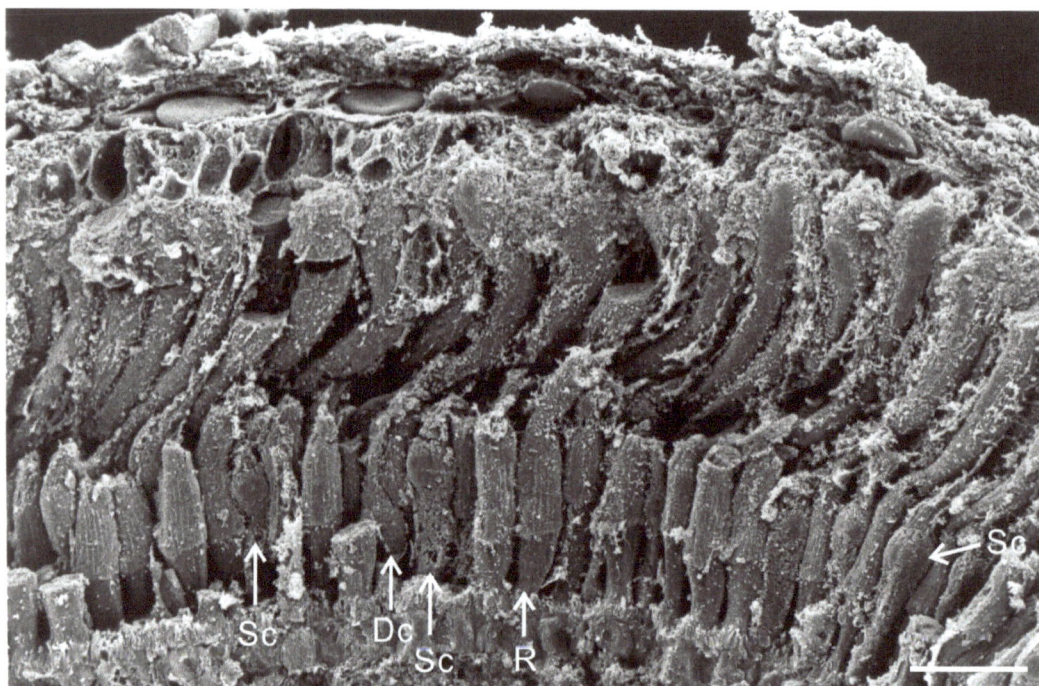

Figure 1.12h.

In this figure, different types of visual cells such as double cone (Dc), single cone (Sc) and rod (R) can be identified. Some visual cells have shown a complete set of outer segments, which are about six times longer than the inner segments. Bar = 10 μm.

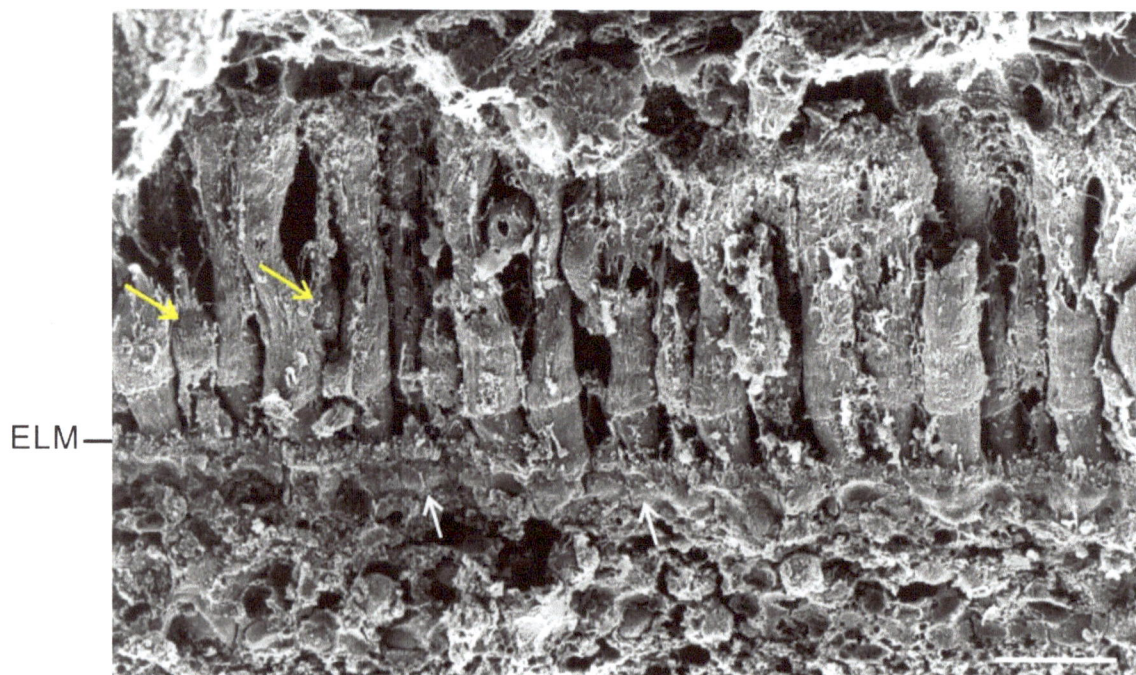

Figure 1.12i.

In this figure, oil droplets of the cone cells can be seen (yellow arrows). There is no oil droplet in the rod cells. Along the external limiting membrane (ELM), only short microvilli are seen. Below the ELM are nuclei of the visual cells (white arrows). Bar = 10 μm.

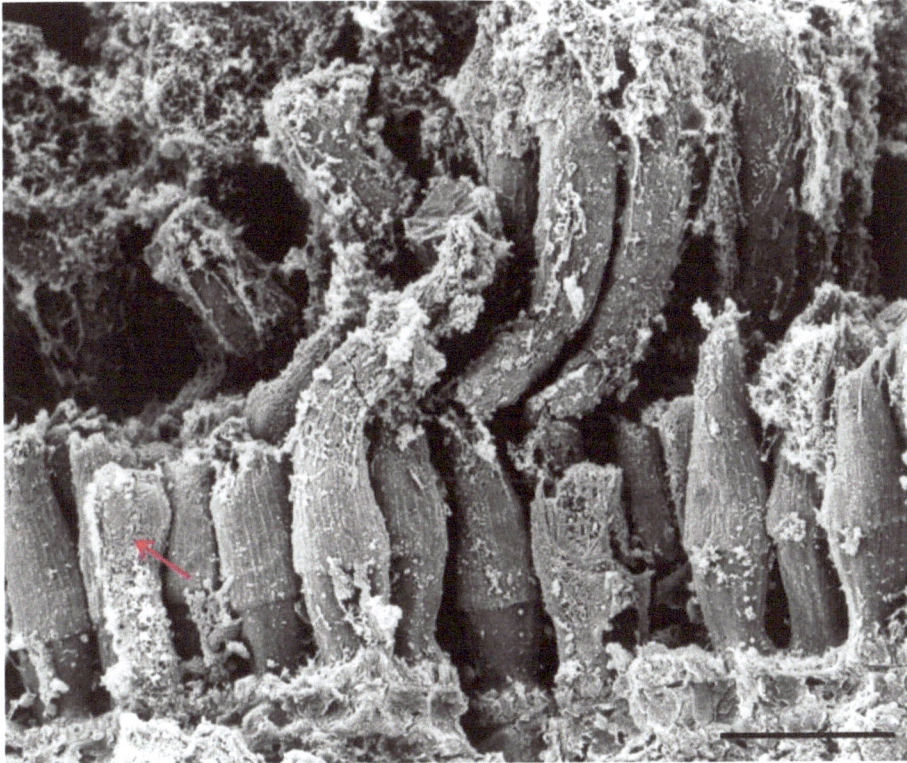

Figure 1.12j.

Again, a few rods with their long outer segments are shown. The visual cell with a broken outer segment (red arrow) is a single cone whose inner segment has a dilated distal end and houses an oil droplet. Bar = 10 μm.

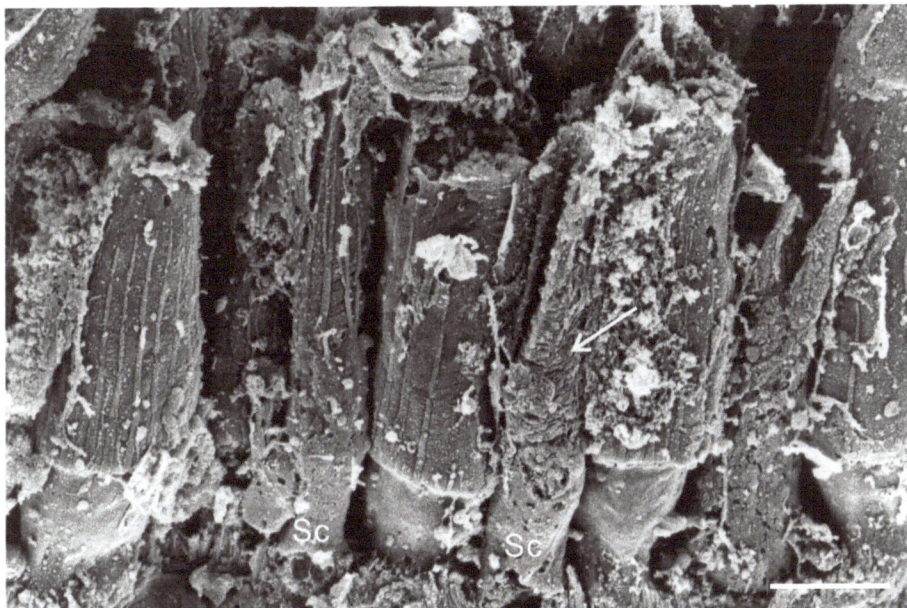

Figure 1.12k.

In between some rod cells are another type of single cones (Sc). Their inner segments appear shorter and smaller in diameter than the rods. Moreover, their outer segments are conical in shape. In one of the outer segment of these single cones (white arrow), stacks of membrane are clearly displayed. Bar = 3 μm.

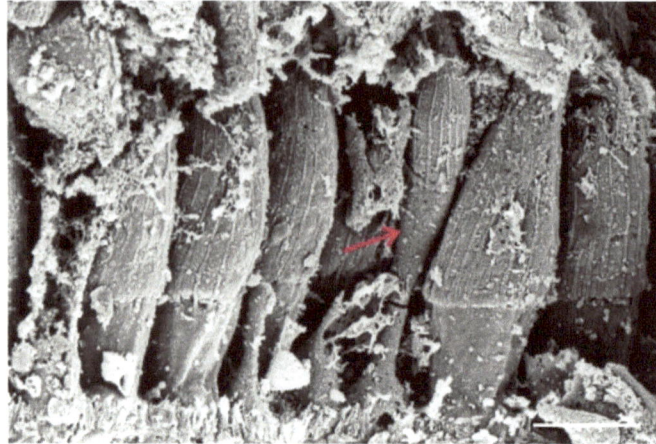

Figure 1.12l.

Another less dominant type of visual cell is noted in this figure (red arrow). It has a long but thin inner segment as compared to the ones seen in the previous figure. This might be a different type of rod cell as no oil droplet is noted in its inner segment.

Bar = 10 μm.

13. CHINESE POND TURTLE

The retina of the Chinese pond turtle has a single external layer of cone cells with the occasional rod cell bodies internally placed. Among the cones, there are some double cones. The chief and accessory members of the double cones appear to share the proximal part of the inner segments. Inside some visual cells, oil droplets are observed. Despite being classified into the same class - reptile, the turtle has an inner nuclear layer much thinner than that of the crocodile. The ganglion cells in this animal are moderate in number and are distributed in a scattered pattern in the layer they belong to.

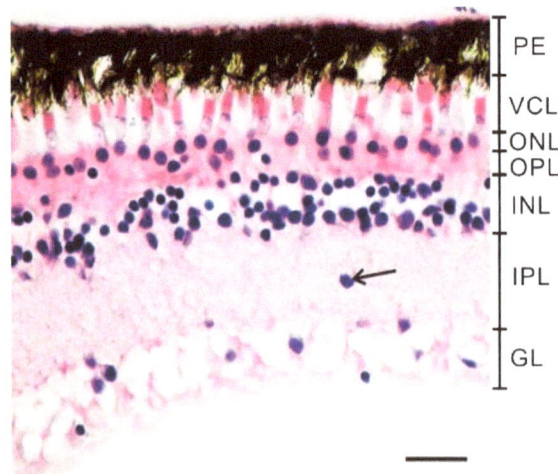

Figure 1.13a. *Anterior retina.*

Layers of the retina in the Chinese pond turtle are shown. The pigment epithelial layer (PE) is still contacting with the visual cell layer (VCL). The visual cells as shown are sparsely separated. There is a displaced ganglion cell in the inner plexiform layer (arrow). Bar = 50 μm.

(GL - Ganglion cell layer; INL - Inner nuclear layer; IPL - Inner plexiform layer; ONL - Outer nuclear layer; OPL - Outer plexiform layer; PE - Pigment epithelium; VCL - Visual cell layer).

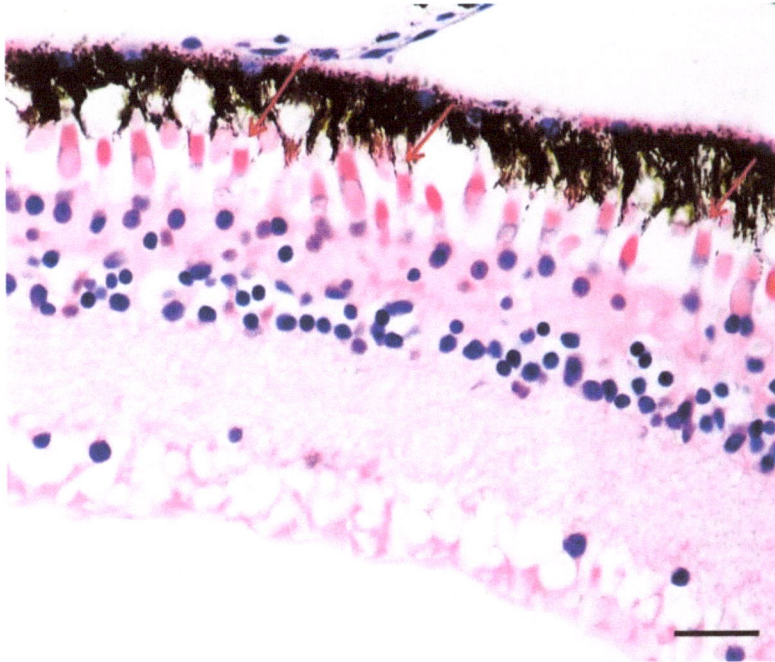

Figure 1.13b. *Anterior retina.*

Anterior retina of the Chinese pond turtle showing many cones. In some cone cells, oil droplets are present (red arrows). Bar = 50 μm.

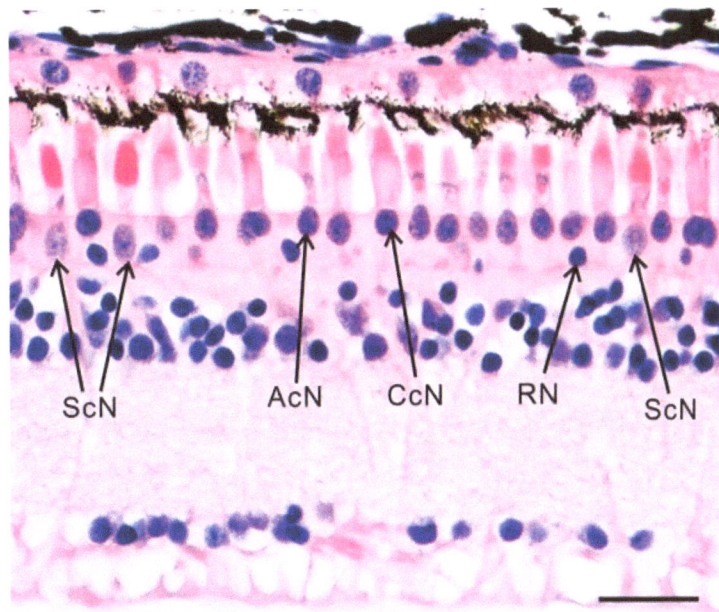

Figure 1.13c. *Peripheral retina.*

In the peripheral retina, cones are still more plentiful than rods. This figure illustrates the different nuclei of the different types of visual cells and their relative positions in the outer nuclear layer. Bar = 50 μm.

(ScN - Single cone nucleus; RN - Rod nucleus; CcN - Chief cone nucleus; AcN - Accessory cone nucleus).

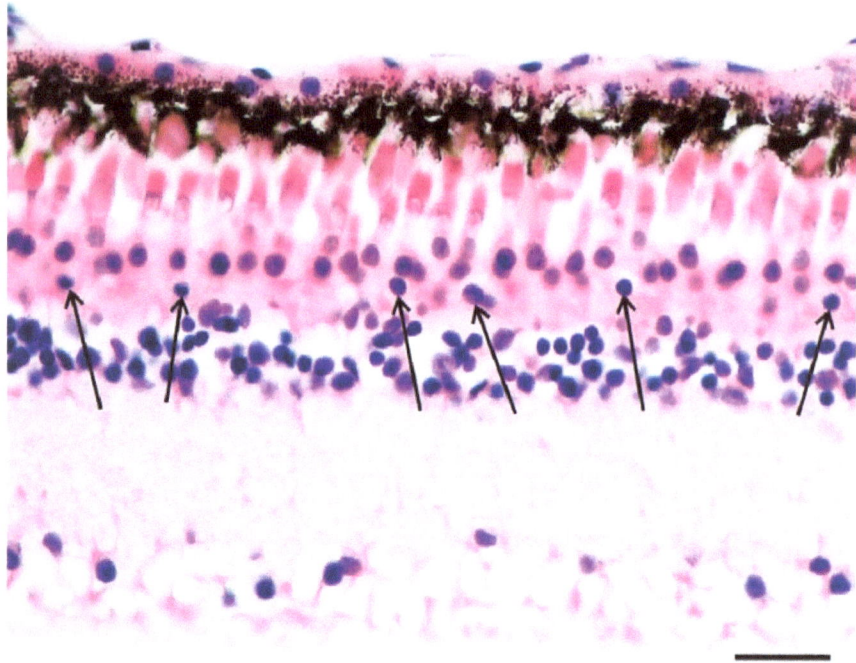

Figure 1.13d. *Peripheral retina.*

Rod cell nuclei (arrows) are limited in the peripheral retina of the Chinese pond turtle. Bar = 50 μm.

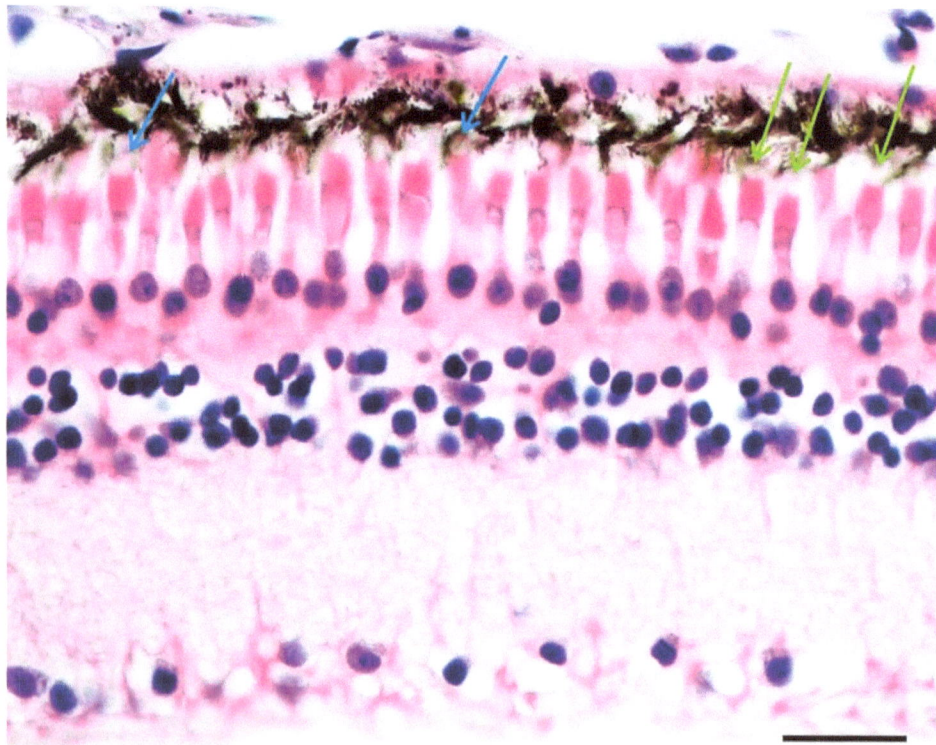

Figure 1.13e. *Peripheral retina.*

Oil droplets are present in the inner segment of chief cones (blue arrows) and single cones (green arrows). Bar = 50 μm.

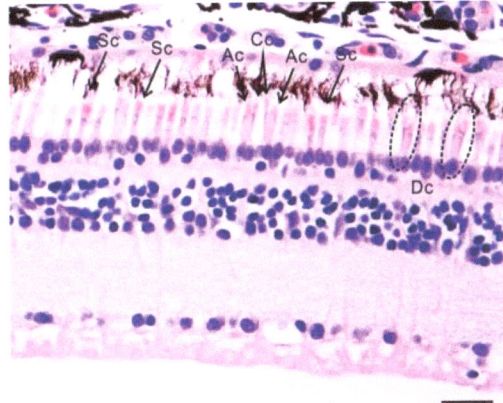

Figure 1.13f. *Central retina.*

The central retina of the turtle illustrates many cones - double cones (Dc; some are in circles), consisting of chief cones (Cc) and accessory cones (Ac). Single cones (Sc) are also present. These visual cells are scattered and are relatively fewer in number than in other animals. Bar = 50 µm.

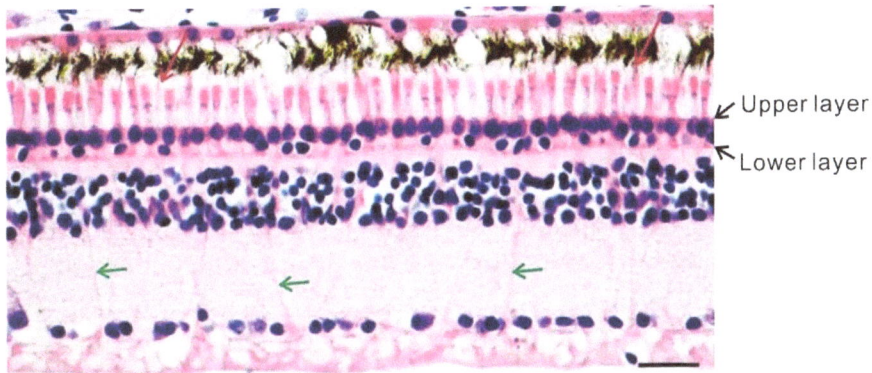

Figure 1.13g. *Central retina.*

Note the ratio of rod nuclei to cone nuclei in the turtle retina. Cone nuclei occupy the upper layer and the rod nuclei dominate the lower layer. The red arrows indicate the rods. The green arrows point to the Müller fibers going down to form internal limiting membrane. Bar = 50 µm.

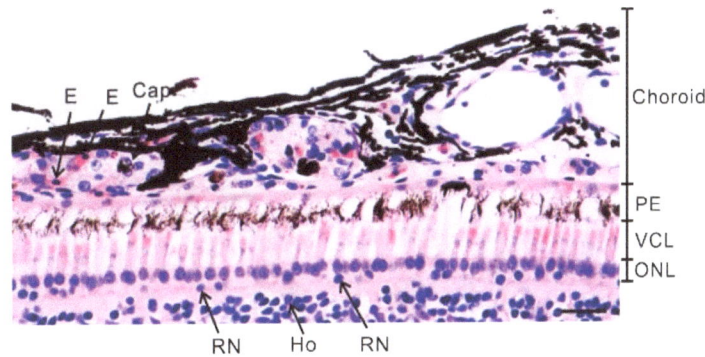

Figure 1.13h. *Central retina.*

Choroid and retina of the Chinese pond turtle. Note the presence of the nuclei of rod cells (RN) and horizontal cells (Ho). Also observe the nucleated red blood cells (E) in the choriocapillaries (Cap). Bar = 50 µm.

(ONL - Outer nuclear layer; PE - Pigment epithelium; VCL - Visual cell layer).

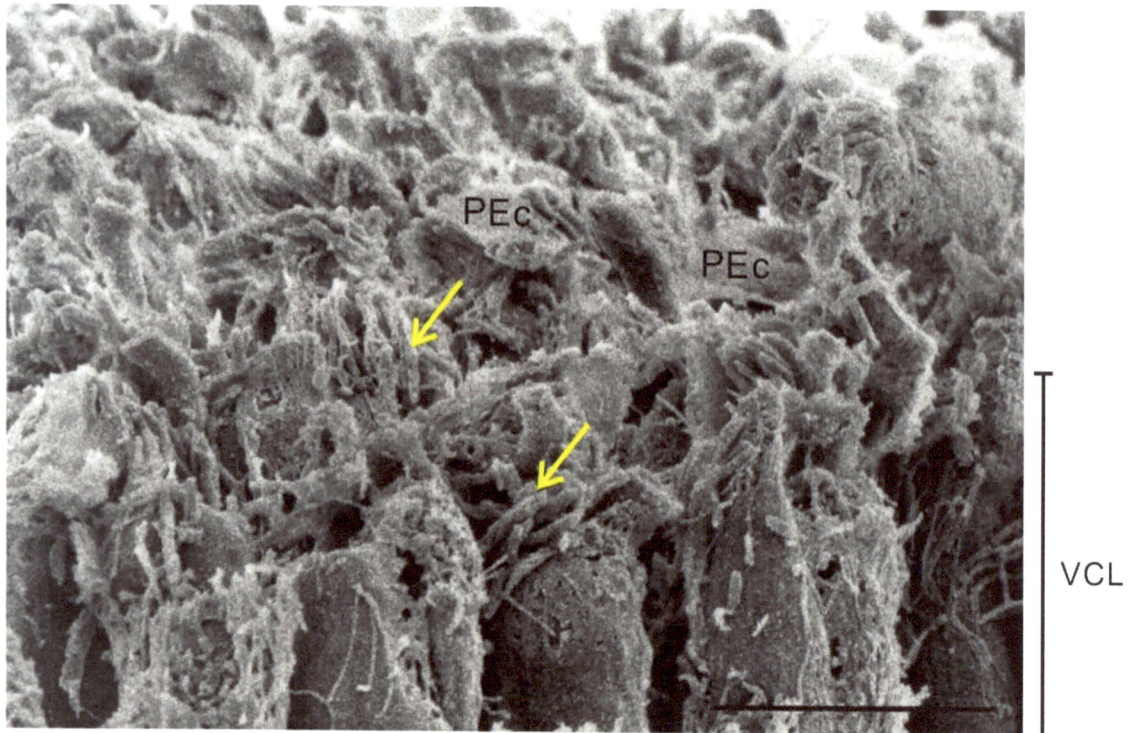

Figure 1.13i.

A layer of pigment epithelium lying above the visual cell layer (VCL). The yellow arrows indicate the processes of the epithelial cells (PEc). Bar = 10 μm.

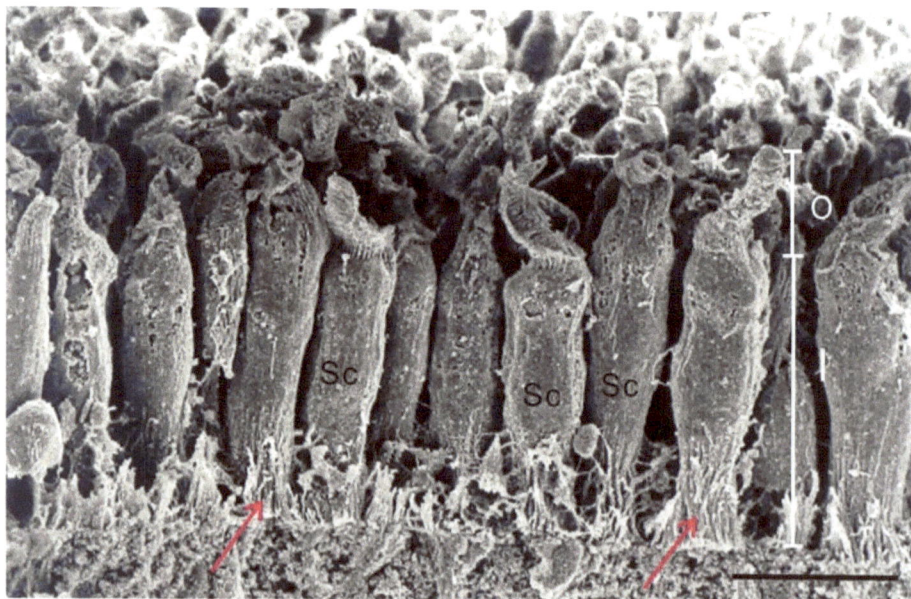

Figure 1.13j.

Single cones (Sc) in Chinese pond turtle retina are shown in this scanning electron micrograph. The red arrows show the processes of the Müller cells. Bar = 10 μm.

(I - Inner segment; O - Outer segment).

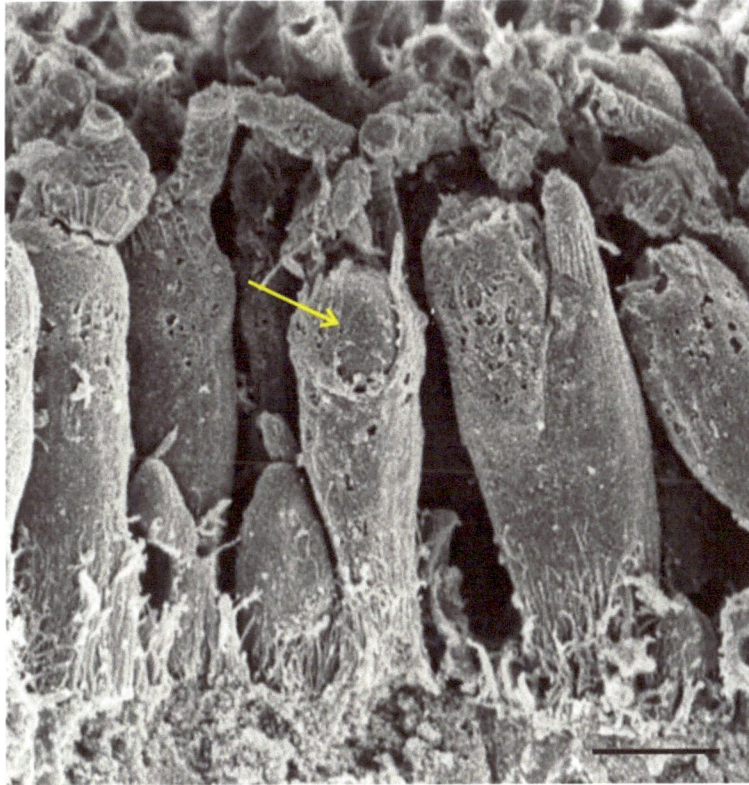

Figure 1.13k.

An oil droplet in the ellipsoid region of a single cell is exposed (yellow arrow). Bar = 5 μm.

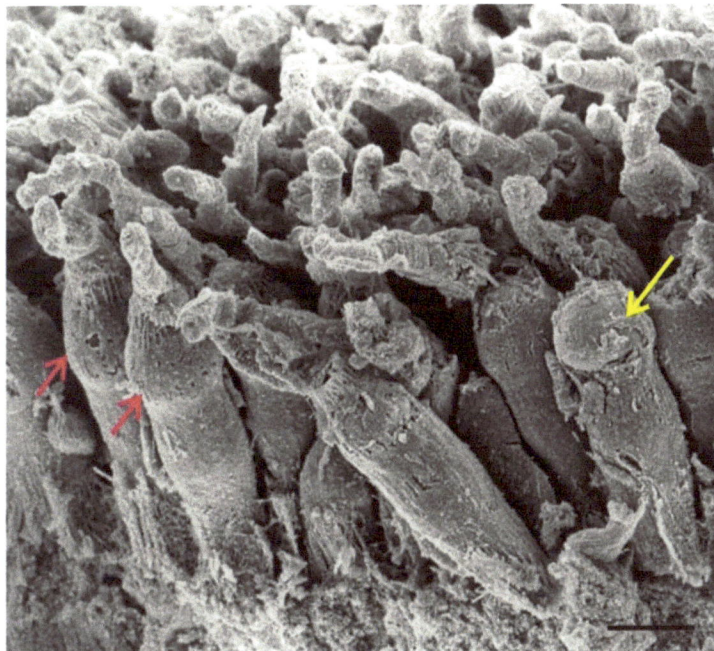

Figure 1.13l.

Another exposed oil droplet is seen (yellow arrow). The enlarged regions of two single cones on the left of this micrograph also indicate the presence of oil droplets (red arrows). Bar = 5 μm.

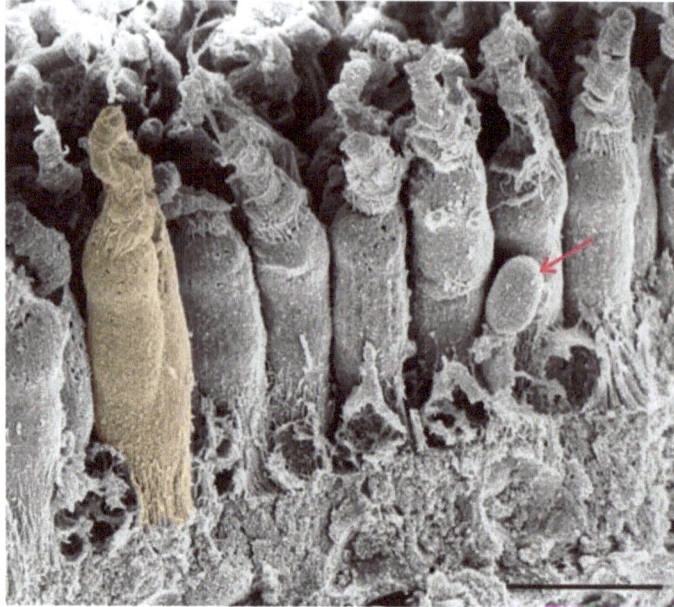

Figure 1.13m.

A double cone (colored) is shown among the single cones. Note also a small budding visual cell (red arrow). Bar = 10 μm.

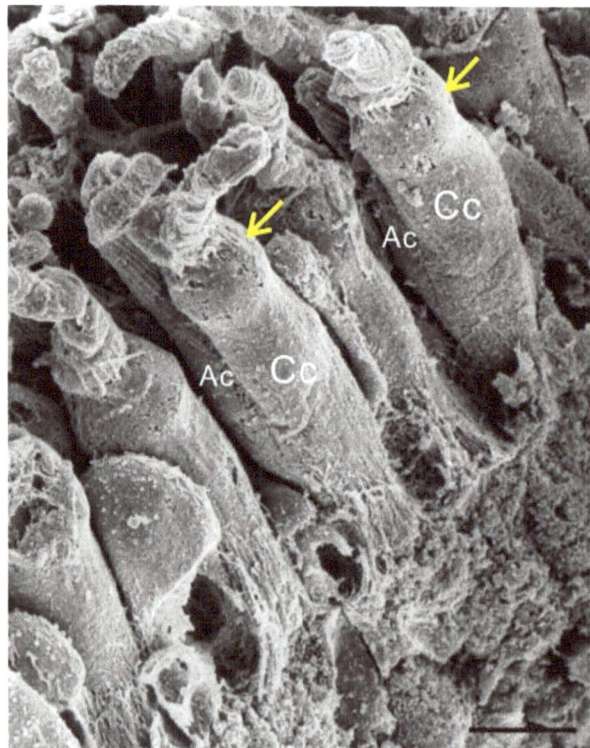

Figure 1.13n.

The chief cones (Cc) and accessory cones (Ac) of the double cones are identified. Inside the ellipsoid region of the chief cones is a round oil droplet (yellow arrows). Bar = 5 μm.

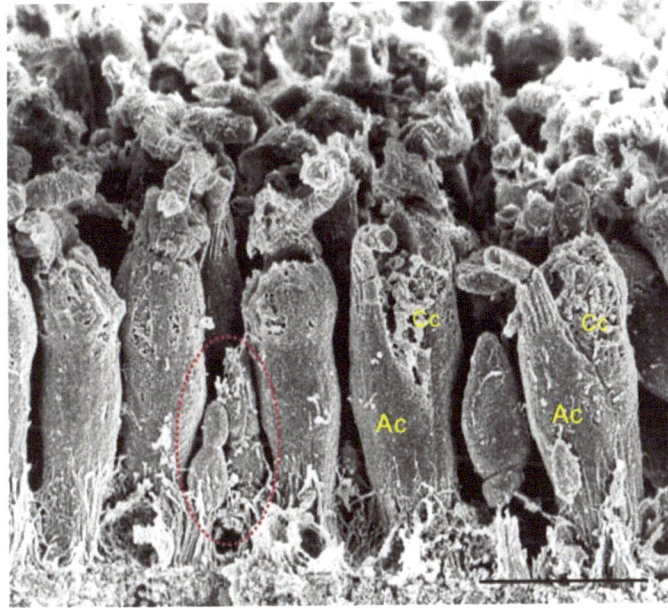

Figure 1.13o.

Two smaller visual cells with inner and outer segments (circle) are observed in between two single cones. On the right of this micrograph are two double cones. Bar = 5 µm.

(Ac - Accessory cone; Cc - Chief cone).

14. CROCODILE

The crocodile displays the retina with the thinnest outer nuclear (one layer thick approximately), contrasting with its thick inner nuclear layer with a moderate number of cells. The Müller fibers are clearly observed, even under light microscopy. A relatively high number of ganglion cells is seen, sometimes is more than one layer.

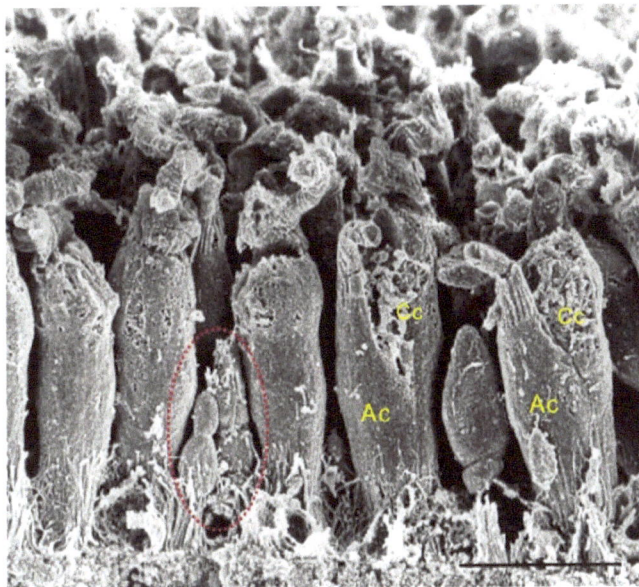

Figure 1.14a. *Anterior retina near ora serrata.*

This figure shows the anterior retina of the crocodile with a reduction in number of visual cells. Bar = 100 µm.

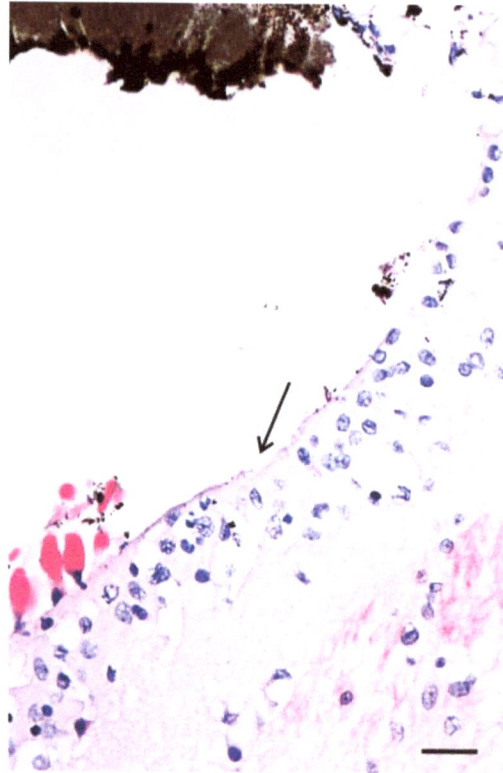

Figure 1.14b. *Anterior retina.*

A higher magnification of the anterior retina. An arrow indicates the region depleted of visual cells while on the left of this figure, indicating the presence of visual cells. Bar = 50 μm.

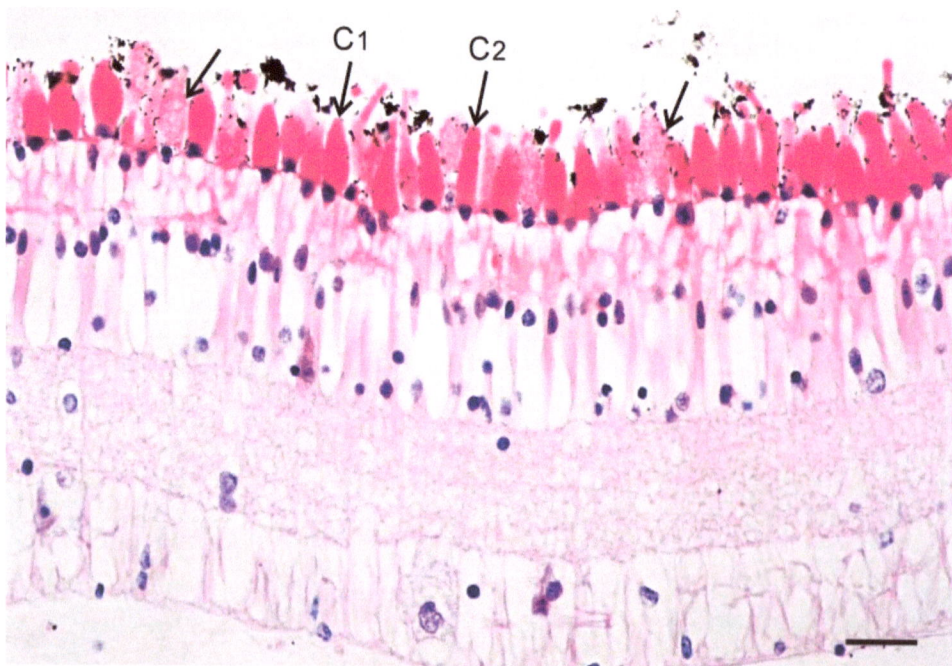

Figure 1.14c. *Anterior retina.*

The anterior retina of the crocodile shows two different types of cone cells, one with a pear shaped inner segment (C1) and the other with a rod shaped inner segment (C2). Some areas shows autolytic cone cells (arrows). Bar = 50 μm.

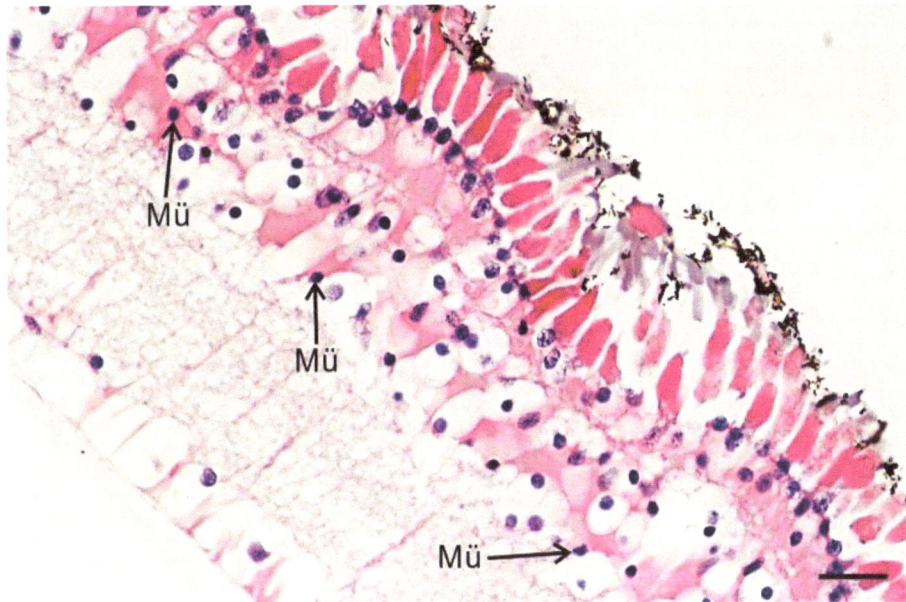

Figure 1.14d. *Anterior retina.*

"Mü" denotes Müller cells in the inner nuclear layer of the retina. They can be identified by the dark nuclei and eosinophilic cytoplasm. Bar = 50 μm.

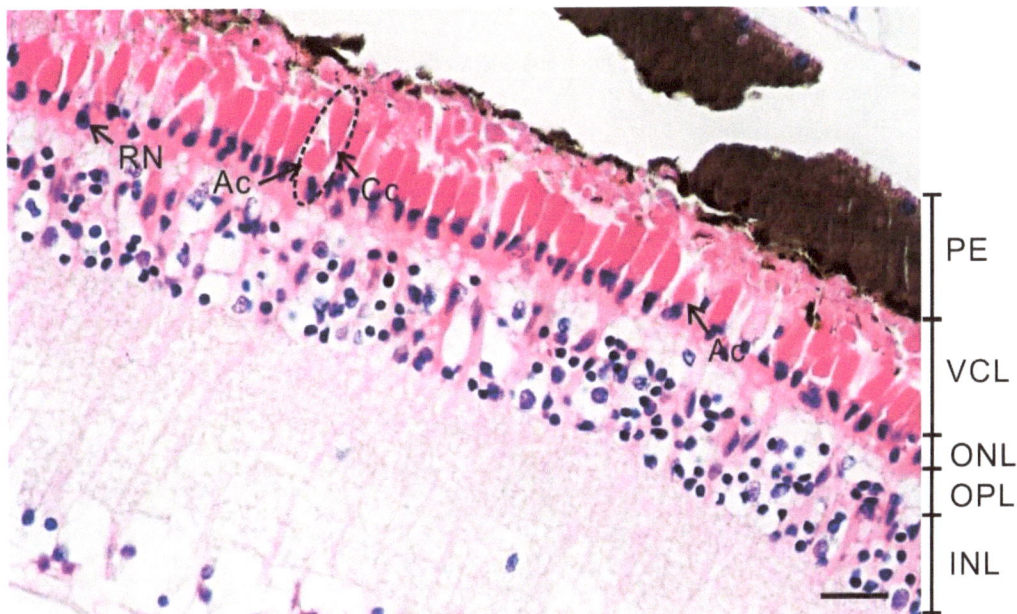

Figure 1.14e. *Peripheral retina.*

In this peripheral region, a double cone (circle) is observed. The shorter, pear shaped one is an accessory cone (Ac) whereas the taller one is a chief cone (Cc). On the right, there is one more accessory cone (Ac). Even in the peripheral retina, rods are few in number. A rod with its nucleus (RN) located at a lower level of the outer nuclear layer (ONL) is also observed on the left. The outer nuclear layer is always much thinner than that of the inner nuclear layer (INL). Bar = 50 μm.

(INL - Inner nuclear layer; ONL - Outer nuclear layer; OPL - Outer plexiform layer; PE - Pigment epithelium; VCL - Visual cell layer).

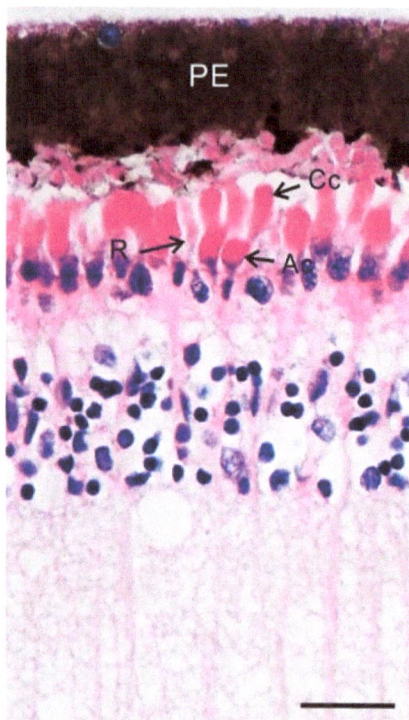

Figure 1.14f. *Peripheral retina.*

The pigment epithelial layer (PE) of this reptile is thick and does not show many processes going into the visual cell layer. In this figure, a rod (R) and a double cone are seen. "Ac" denotes the accessory cone; "Cc" denotes the chief cone. Bar = 50 μm.

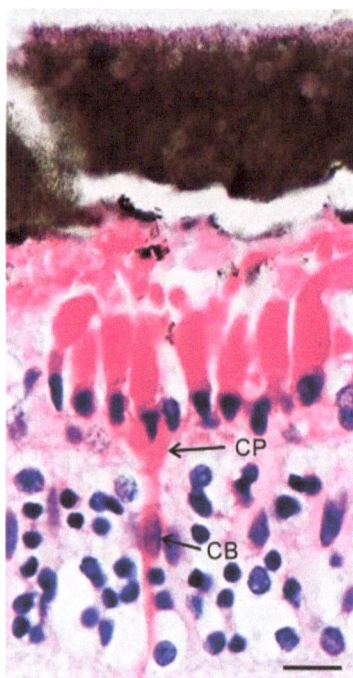

Figure 1.14g. *Peripheral retina.*

A cone pedicle (CP) and a cone bipolar (CB) can be clearly recognized. Bar = 25 μm.

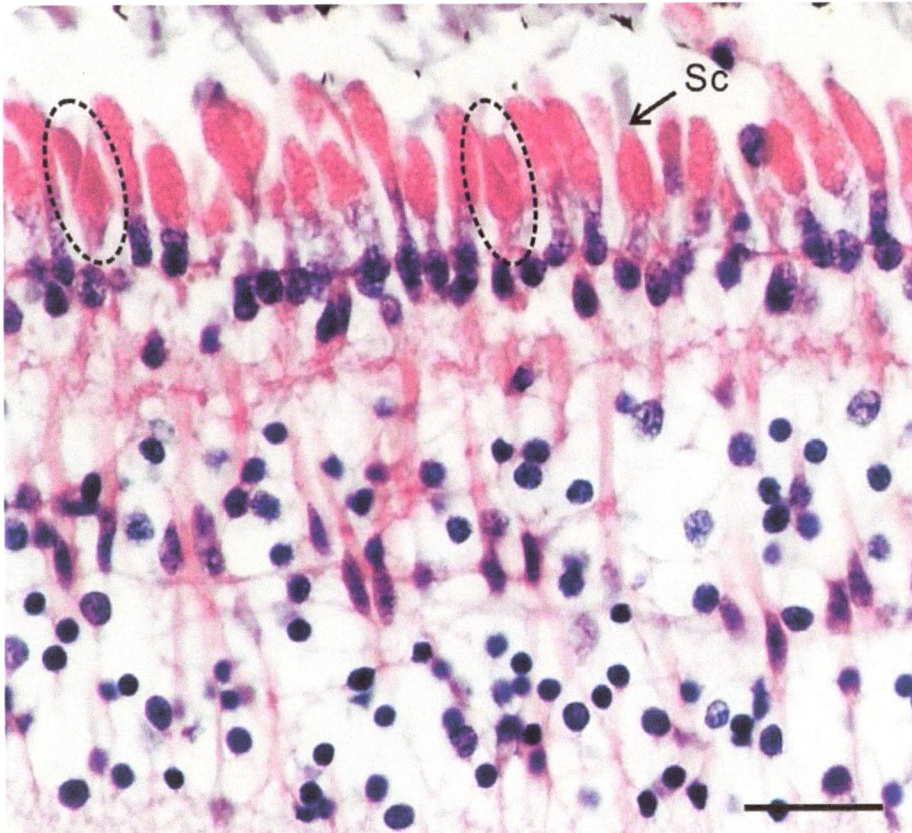

Figure 1.14h. *Peripheral retina.*

Note that the peripheral retina contains more double cones (circles) as well as single cone (Sc). Bar = 50 μm.

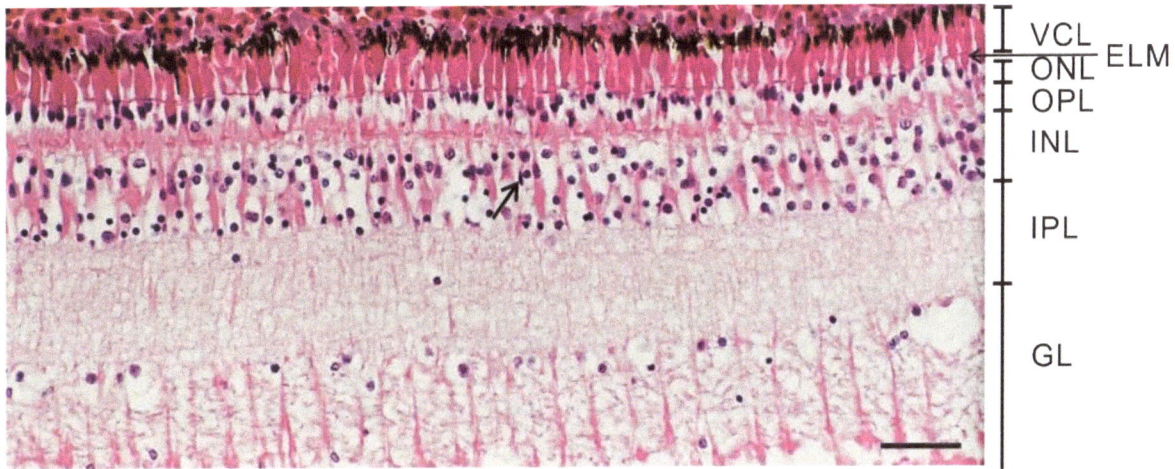

Figure 1.14i. *Central retina.*

Visual cells are distributed fairly regularly in the central retina and the density is not high. The external limiting membrane (ELM) is distinct, appearing as a horizontal line in this figure. Some bipolar cells (arrow) are seen in the inner nuclear layer (INL). Bar = 100 μm.

(ELM - External limiting membrane; GL - Ganglion cell layer; INL - Inner nuclear layer; IPL - Inner plexiform layer; ONL - Outer nuclear layer; OPL - Outer plexiform layer; VCL - Visual cell layer).

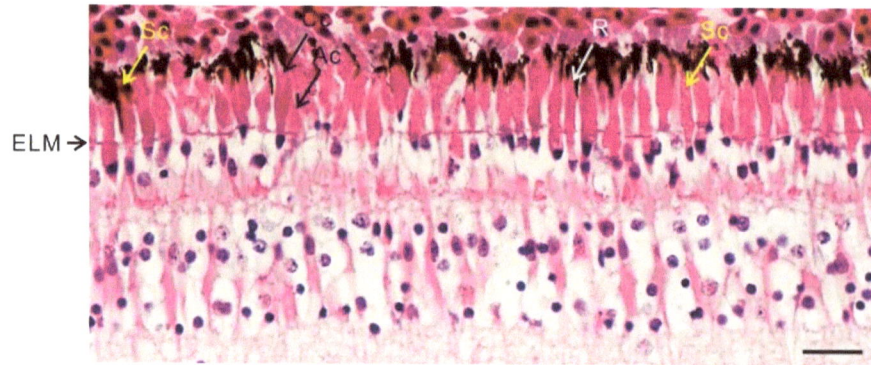

Figure 1.14j. *Central retina.*

Chief cones (Cc), accessory cones (Ac), and single cones (Sc) in the central region of the retina of crocodile. Note the different visual cell nuclei positions. The nuclei of the double cones are closer to the external limiting membrane (ELM). The nuclei of the single cones are in the middle, whereas the nuclei of the rods are in the lowest. Some degree of autolysis is present in this tissue. Bar = 50 μm.

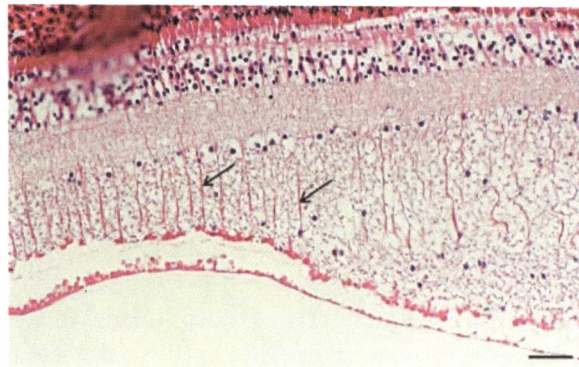

Figure 1.14k. *Near fovea.*

Even at this lower magnification, many vertically oriented Müller fibers are seen (arrows), forming the internal limiting membrane. Bar = 50 μm.

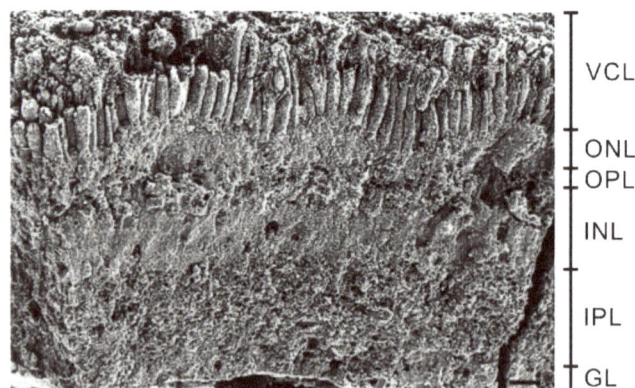

Figure 1.14l.

The retina of crocodile is shown by scanning electron microscopy. Various retinal layers in different thickness are identified. Bar = 10 μm.

(GL - Ganglion cell layer; INL - Inner nuclear layer; IPL - Inner plexiform layer; ONL - Outer nuclear layer; OPL - Outer plexiform layer; VCL - Visual cell layer).

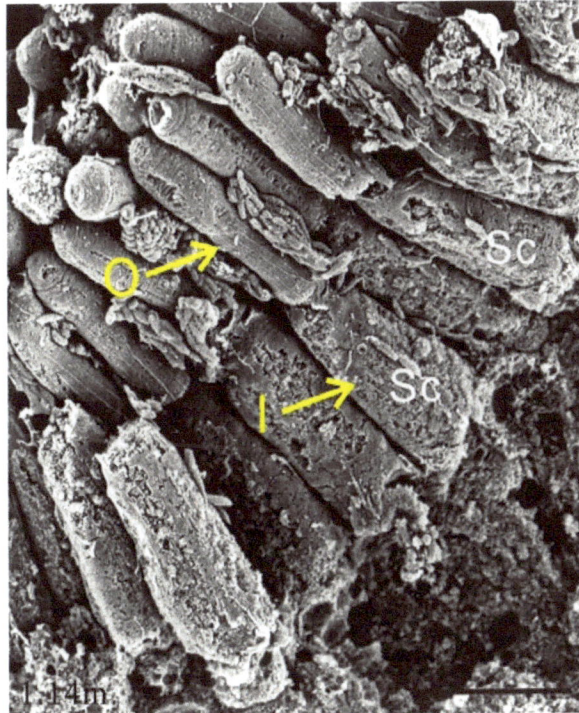

Figure 1.14m.

Single cones of the crocodile's retina are shown. The height of the outer (O) and.

inner (I) segments appears to be similar. Bar = 10 μm.

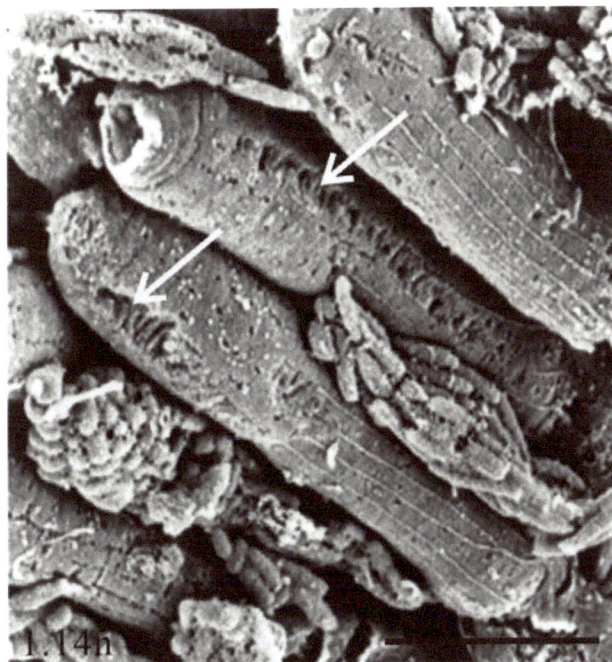

Figure 1.14n.

A higher magnification of figure 1.14m shows the outer segments of the single cones. Parts of the membrane in both single cones are lost (white arrows), displaying the internal multiple stacks of membrane. Bar = 5 μm.

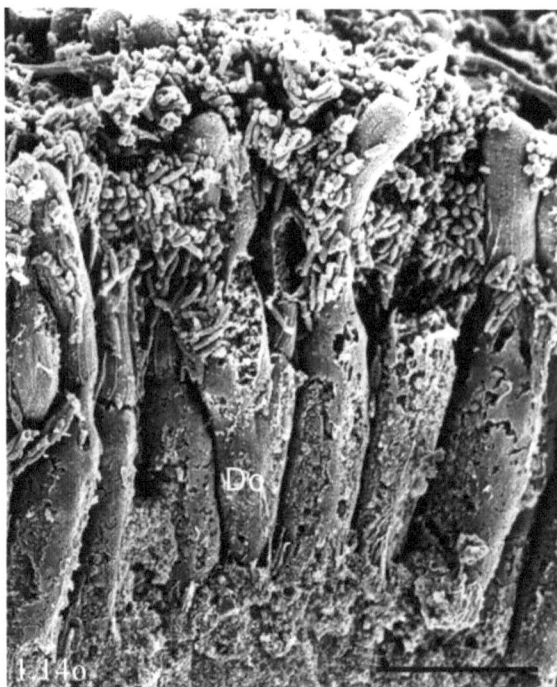

Figure 1.14o.

A double cone (Dc) is shown. Bar = 10 μm.

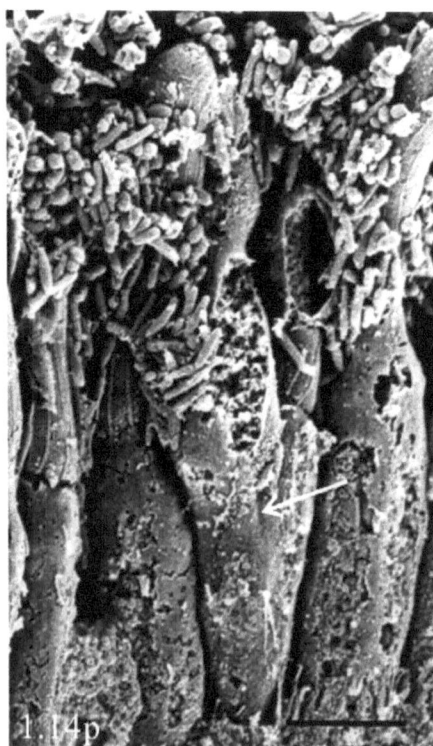

Figure 1.14p.

A higher magnification of the double cone indicated in figure 1.14o. The arrow shows a partition between the two components. Bar = 5 μm.

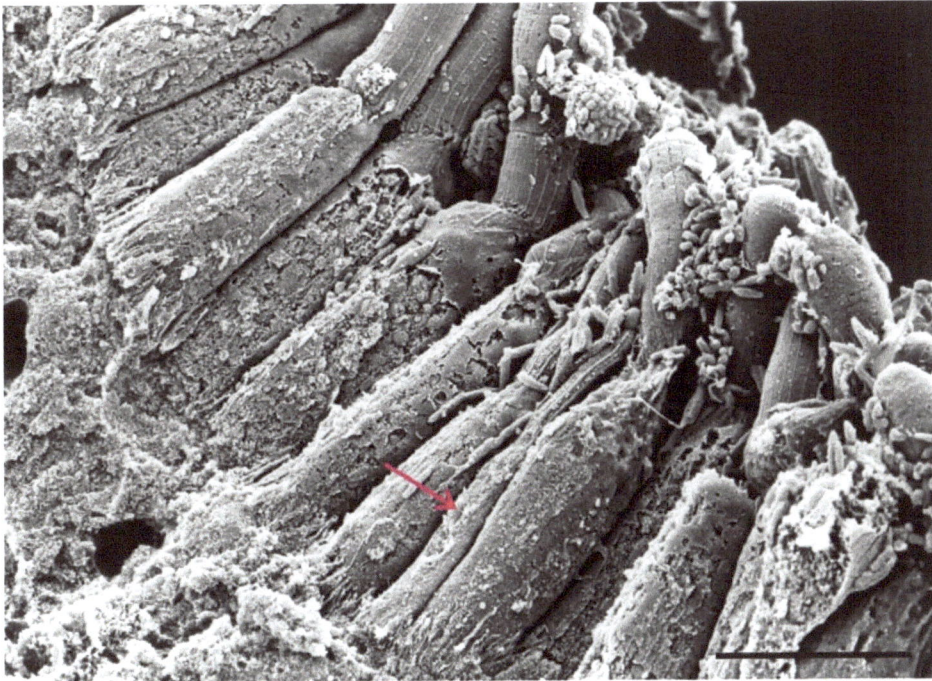

Figure 1.14q.

Smaller cone (red arrow) with a thin inner segment and a tapering outer segment is sometimes noted among the dominant broader cones. Bar = 10 μm.

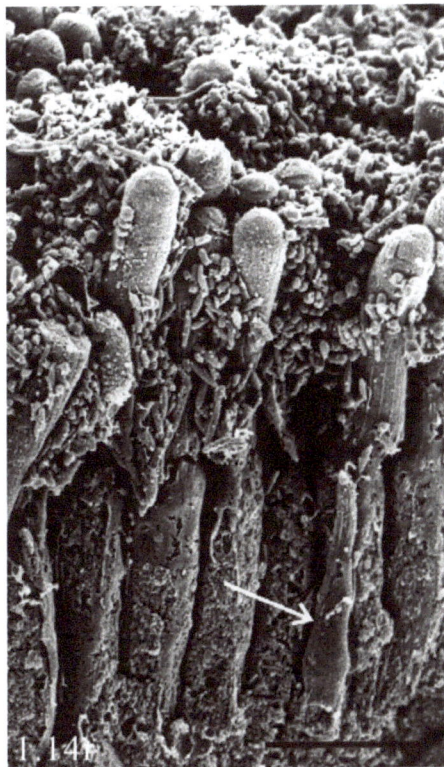

Figure 1.14r and 1.14s.

Another smaller cones are shown (white arrows); note their tapering shape outer segments. Bar = 10 μm.

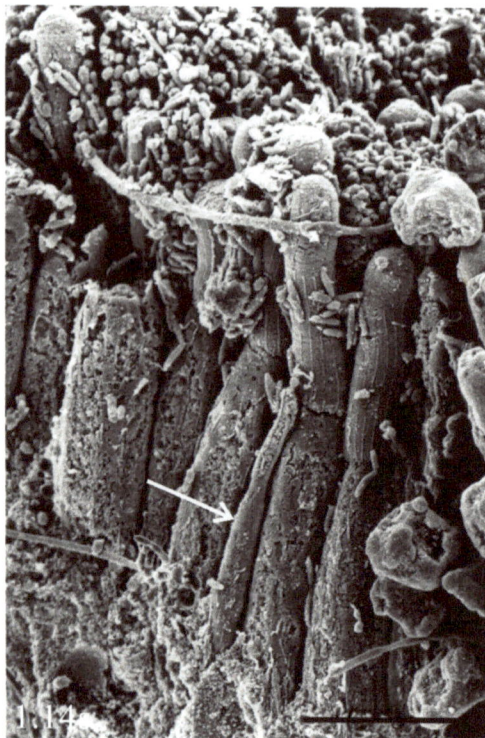

Figure 1.14t.

The inner segments of a possible double cone are shown. "Ac" denotes the accessory cone and "Cc" denotes the chief cone. Another possible accessory cone (arrow) is also observed on the right of this figure. Bar = 10 μm.

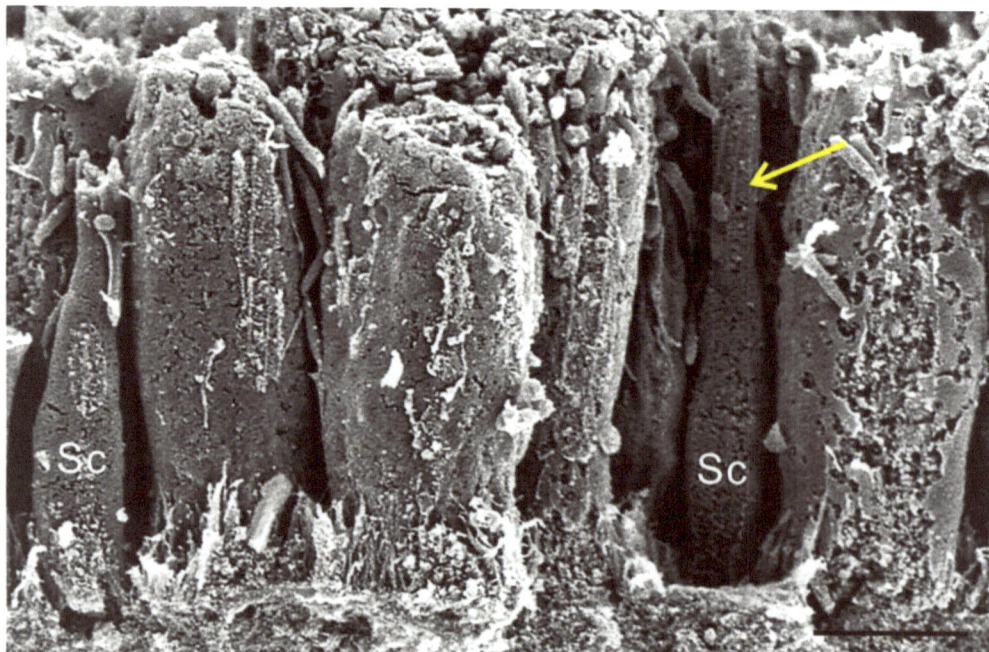

Figure 1.14u.

Two small single cones (Sc) are noted. The yellow arrow indicates the microvilli surrounding the outer segment. Bar = 5 μm.

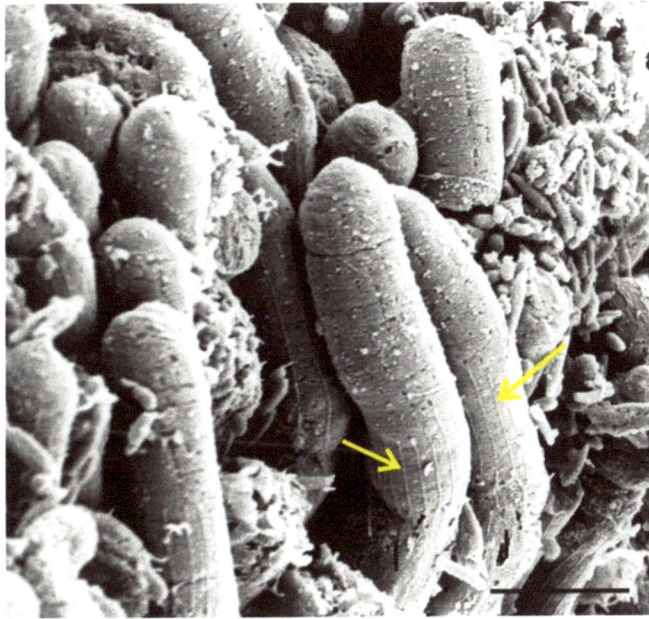

Figure 1.14v.

The outer segments of the visual cells are shown. As in other animals, the outer segments of the crocodile visual cells are encircled by microvilli (yellow arrows) at the base. "I" denotes the inner segments. Bar = 5 μm.

15. SNAKE

The pattern of the retinal layers of the snake is quite similar to that of the Chinese pond turtle except they have a more organized outer nuclear layer. The outer nuclear layer in this animal is a single distinct layer. The inner nuclear layer is comparatively thicker but the ganglion cells are only in few number. The visual cells of this animal are formed by short and fat inner segments along with tiny outer segments.

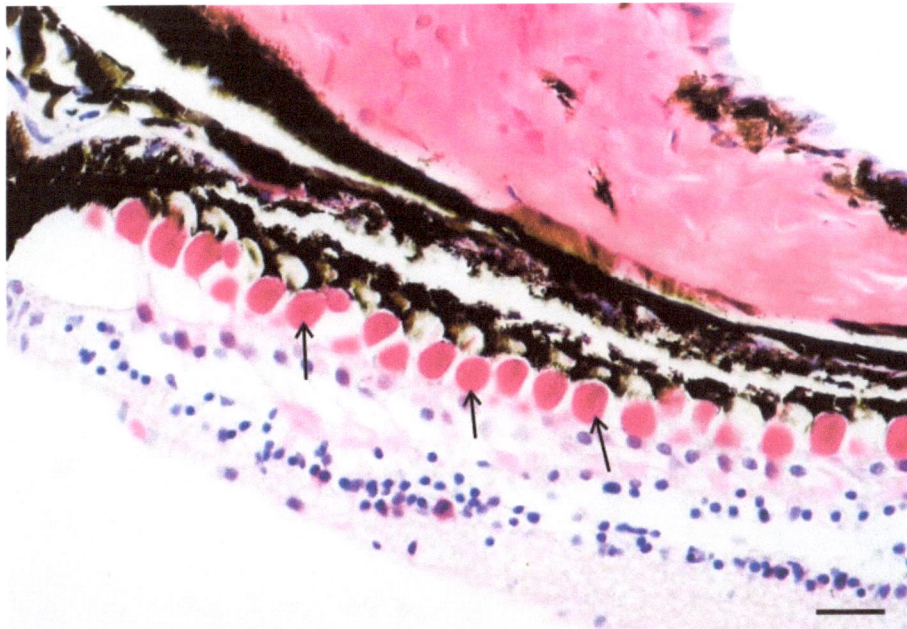

Figure 1.15a. *Anterior retina near ora serrata.*

The anterior retina of the snake with large conical inner segments (arrows) is shown. Bar = 50 μm.

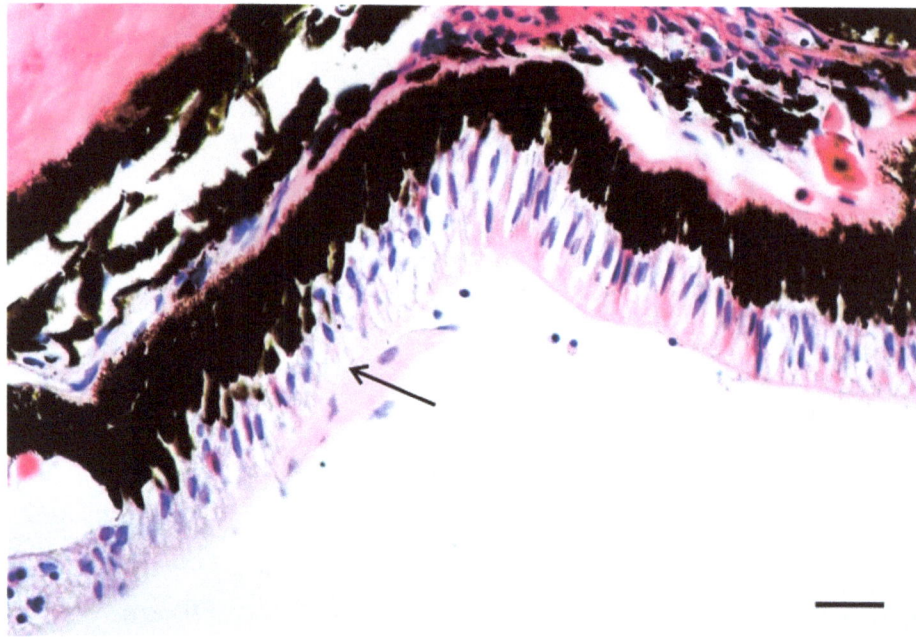

Figure 1.15b. *Ora serrata.*

The ora serrata of the snake shows a gradual transition from the anterior retina (arrow) to the ora serrata. Bar = 50 μm.

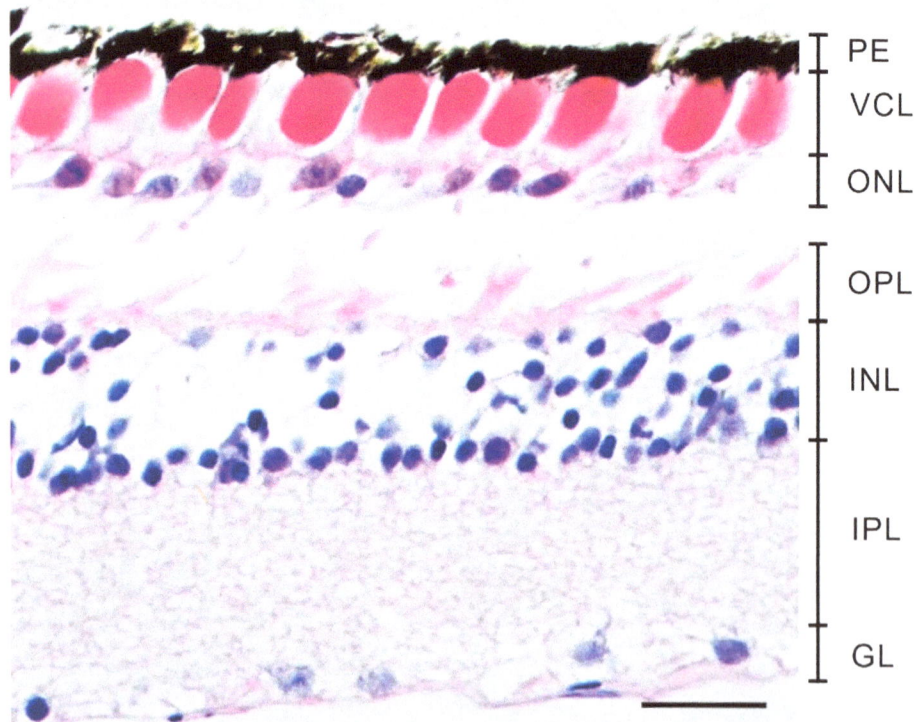

Figure 1.15c. *Peripheral retina.*

Different retinal layers are shown. A very thin outer nuclear layer (ONL) with a small number of visual cells is noted in this animal. Bar = 50 μm.

(GL - Ganglion cell layer; ONL - Outer nuclear layer; OPL - Outer plexiform layer; PE - Pigment epithelium; INL - Inner nuclear layer; IPL - Inner plexiform layer).

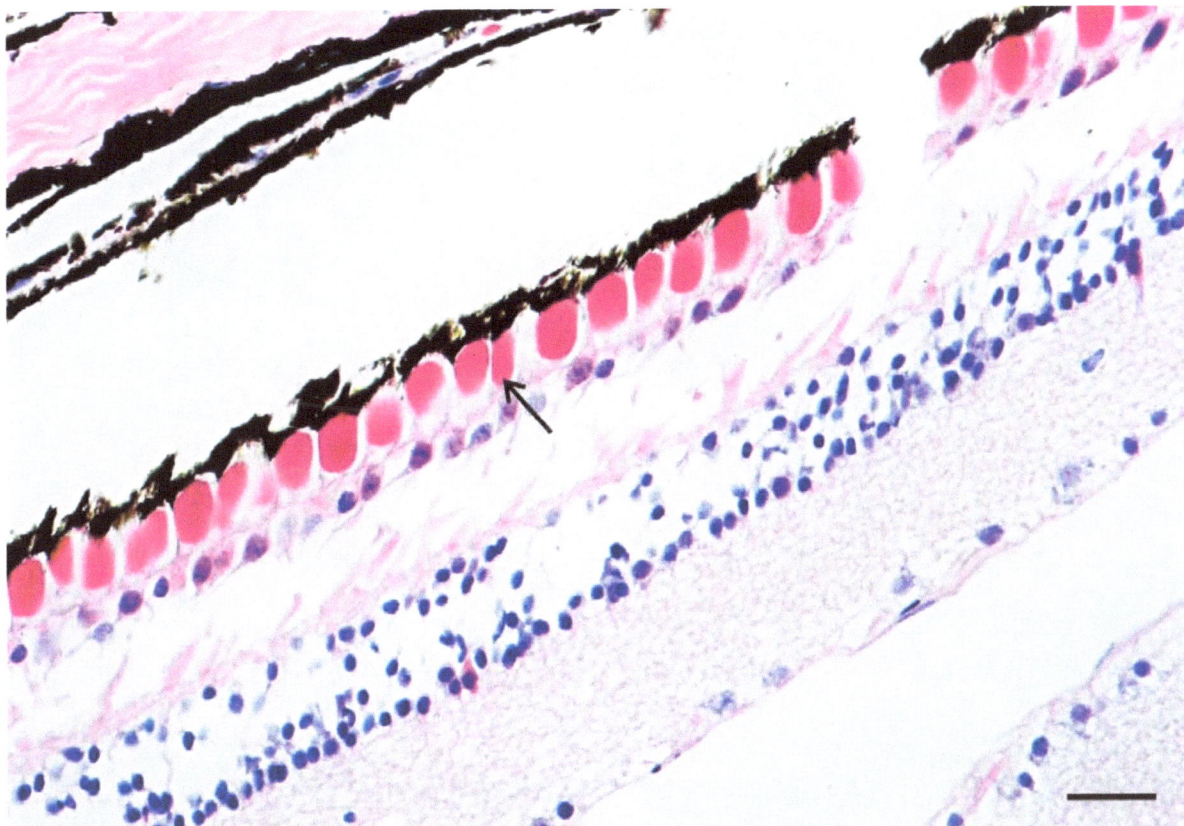

Figure 1.15d. *Peripheral retina.*

In the peripheral retina, rod-like inner segments of visual cells (arrow) begin to appear. Bar = 50 µm.

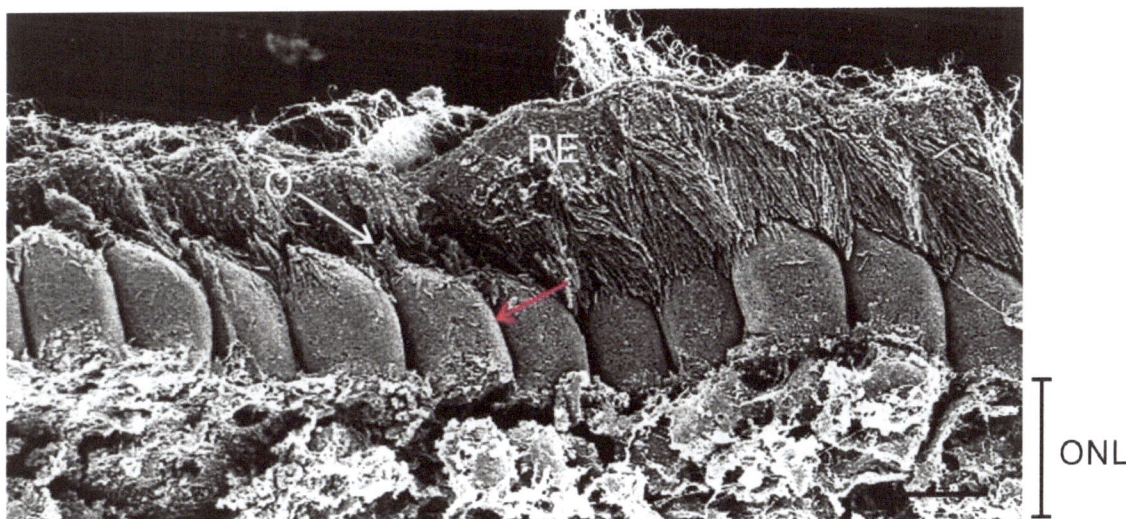

Figure 1.15e.

A layer of "fat" and "short" cone cells (red arrow) with short outer segments (O) is featured in the central retina of the snake. Covering the cone cells is a layer of pigmental cells of the pigment epithelium (PE). "ONL" denotes the outer nuclear layer. Bar = 10 µm.

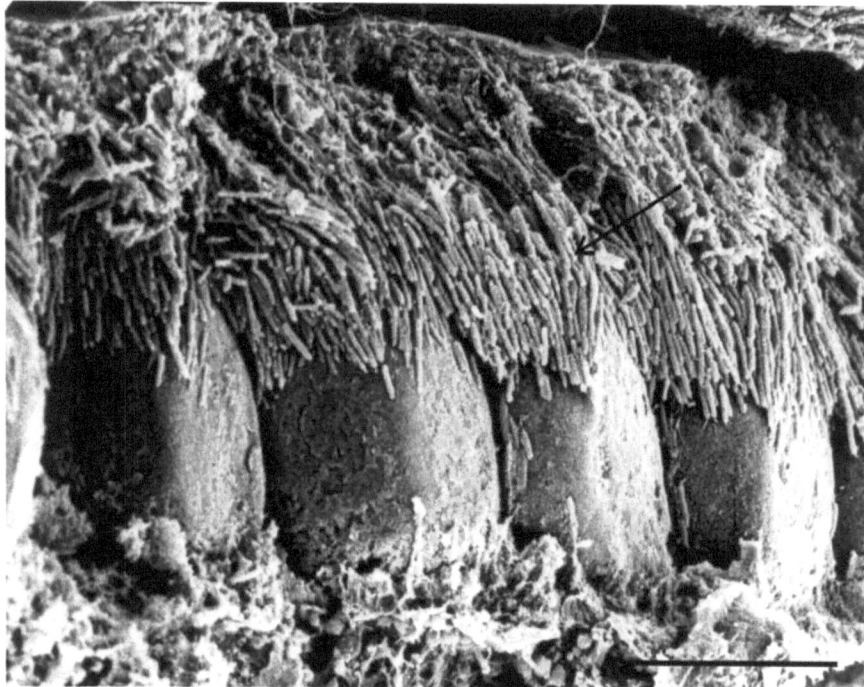

Figure 1.15f.

Note the very long pigment granules in the microvilli interdigitating between the visual cells (arrow), covering the outer portion of the cells. Bar = 10 μm.

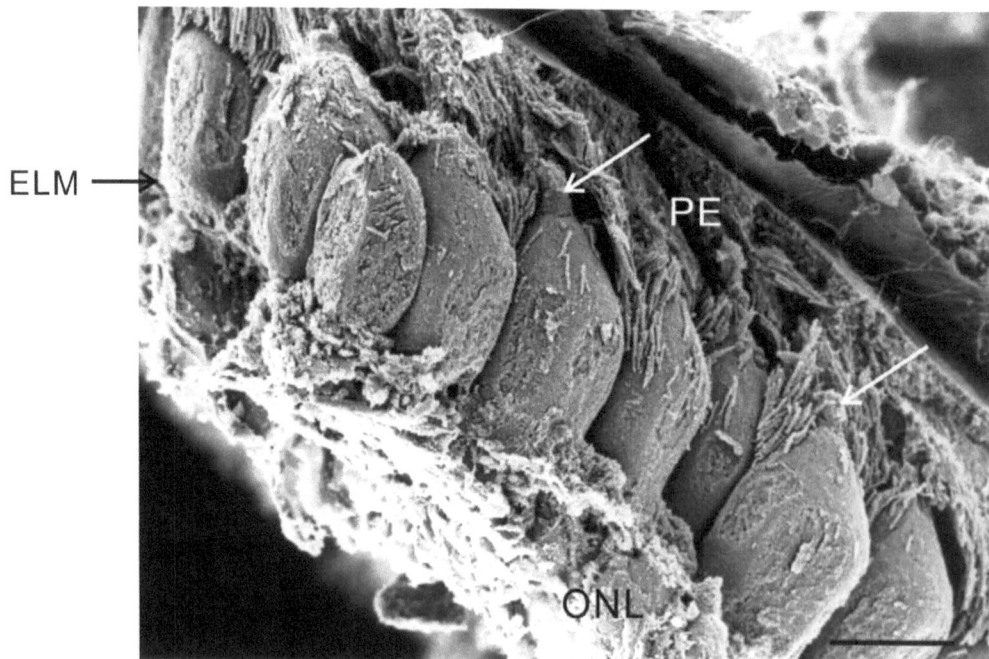

Figure 1.15g.

Two cone cells with tiny outer segments (white arrows) are shown. Note the minute amount of microvilli extending from the external limiting membrane (ELM) in the snake. Bar = 10 μm.

(ELM - External limiting membrane; ONL - Outer nuclear layer).

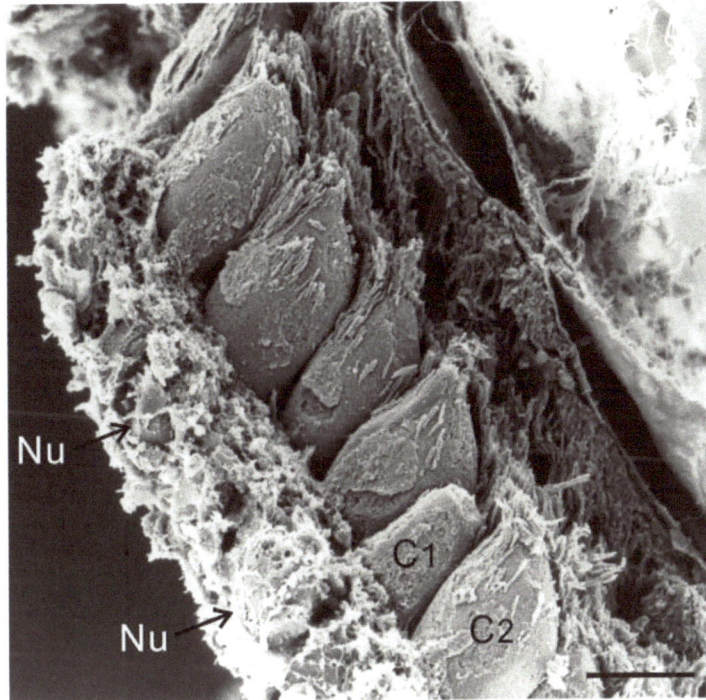

Figure 1.15h.

At least two types of cone cells (C1 and C2) are seen in this figure. "C1" has a rectangular inner segment whereas "C2" has an oval inner segment. Spherical cone cell nuclei (Nu) inside the inner nuclear layer (INL) are also noted. Bar = 10 μm.

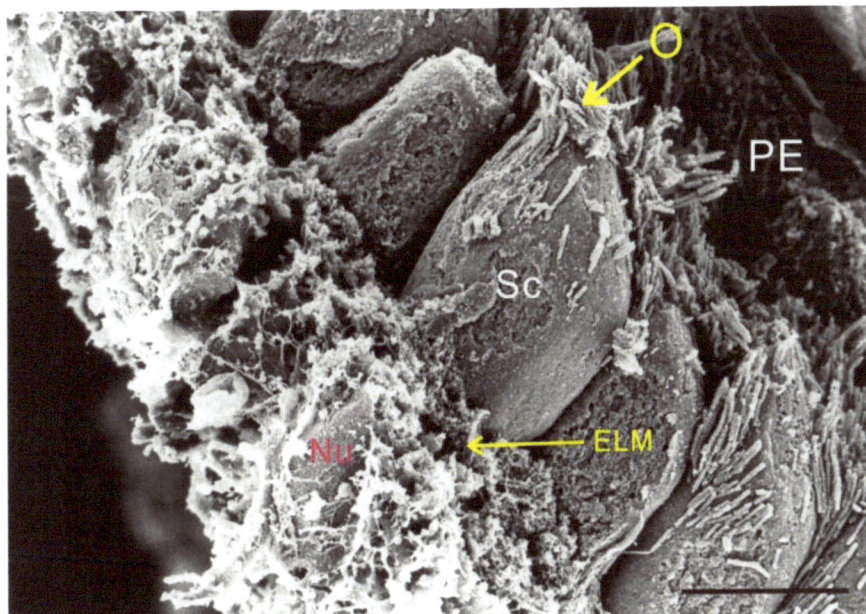

Figure 1.15i.

A single cone (Sc) with its nucleus (Nu) is shown. Its outer segment (O) is still covered by the pigment granules of the pigment epithelium (PE). Bar = 10 μm.

(ELM - External limiting membrane).

16. GOLDEN GECKO

The golden gecko's retina has an outer nuclear layer with alternating darker and lighter cell bodies. The inner nuclear layer is thicker and consisting of about 4 to 5 layers of cells. As compared with other reptiles such as the snake, more ganglion cells are noted. The inner segments of the visual cells are small and conical, but the outer segments appear to be of medium height with much thicker diameter than that of other reptiles. Many double cones are visible in this animal. Interestingly, the distribution of the single and double cones forms an alternate pattern.

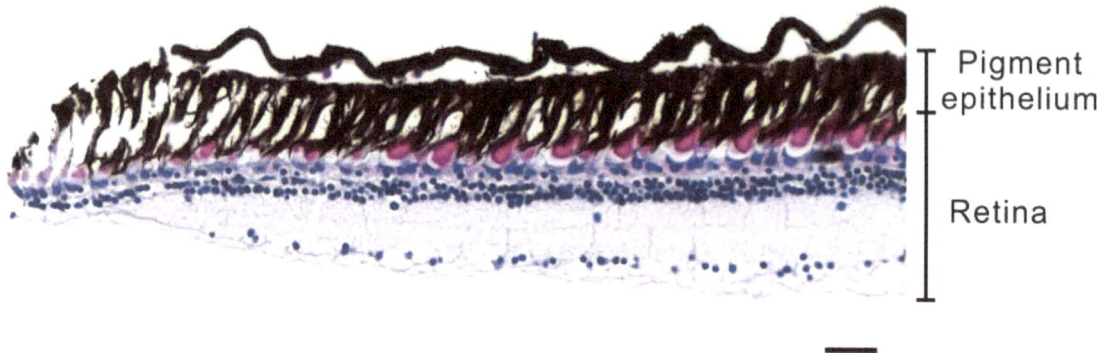

Figure 1.16a. *Anterior retina.*

This figure shows the anterior retina of the lizard. Both the thickness and size of visual cells are noted to decrease gradually towards the anterior region of the eye. Bar = 30 µm.

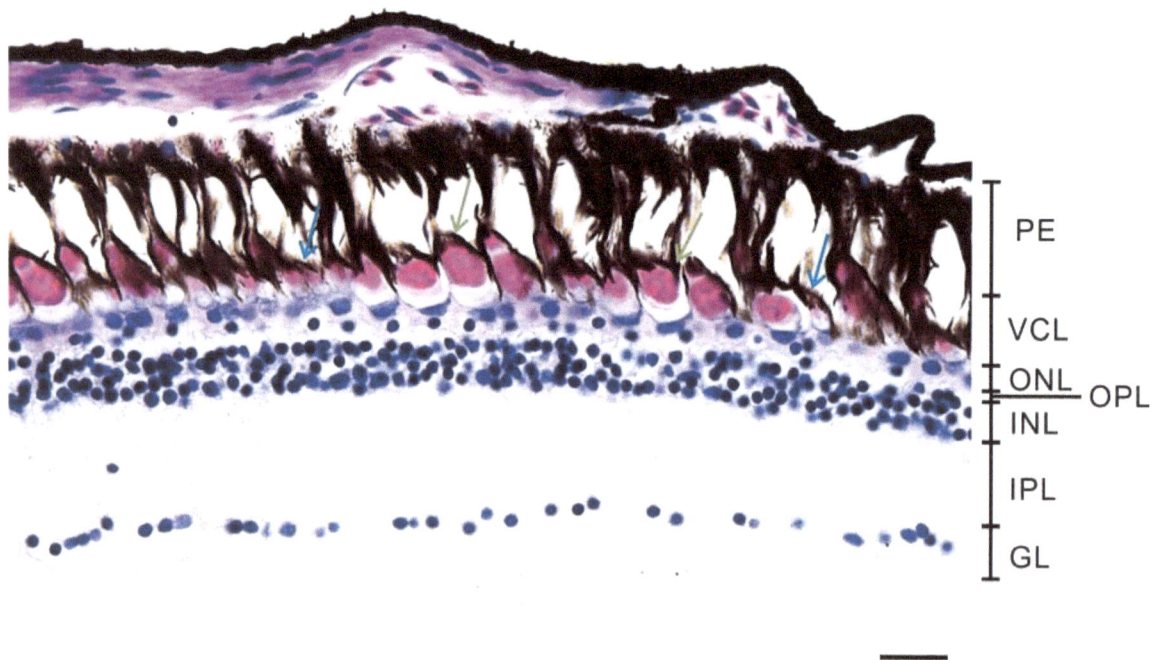

Figure 1.16b. *Anterior retina.*

A row of round visual cells with different sizes is noted (large - green arrows; small - blue arrows). Some visual cells are still covered by the black pigment epithelial processes. The outer nuclear layer (ONL) in this animal is thin, having fewer number of cell nuclei as compared with the inner nuclear layer (INL). Bar =20 µm.

(GL - Ganglion cell layer; INL - Inner nuclear layer; IPL - Inner plexiform layer; ONL - Outer nuclear layer; OPL - Outer plexiform layer; PE - Pigment epithelium; VCL - Visual cell layer).

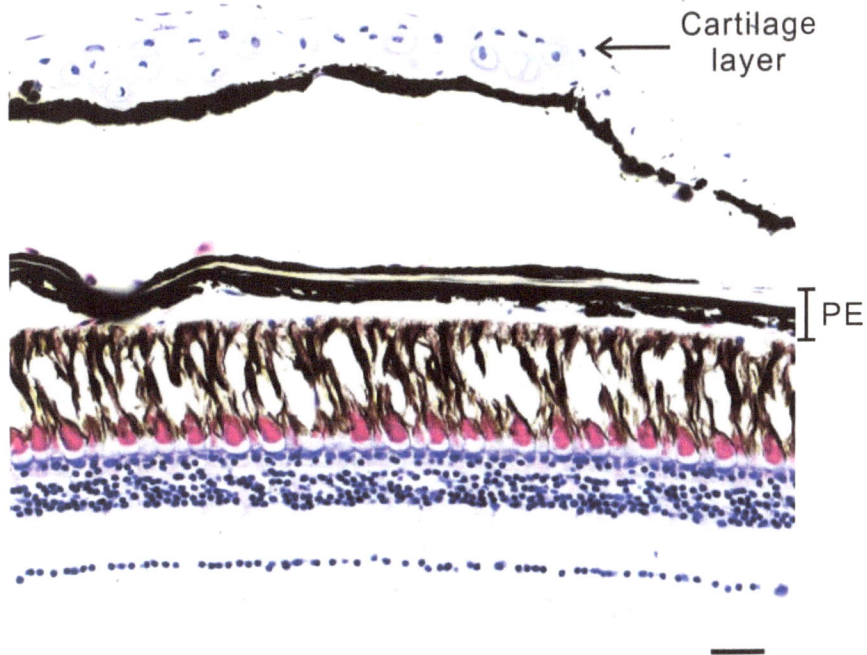

Figure 1.16c. *Peripheral retina.*

At a low magnification, a layer of cartilage is seen exterior to the pigment epithelium (PE). Bar = 30 μm.

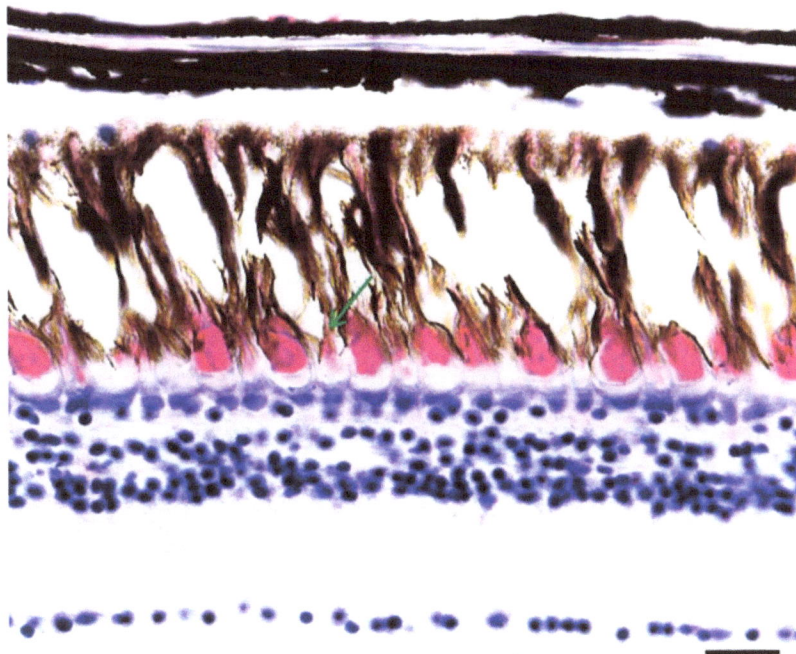

Figure 1.16d. *Peripheral retina.*

Both large and small (green arrow) cone cells are seen in the peripheral retina.

Bar = 20 μm.

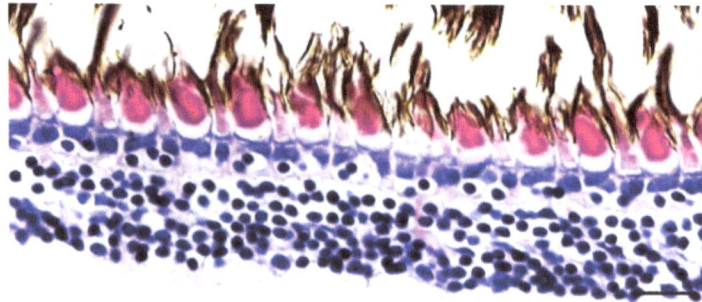

Figures 1.16e. *Central retina.*

At the central region of the retina, an alternative pattern of large and small cone cells is seen. Rod cells are rarely observed. Bar = 20 μm.

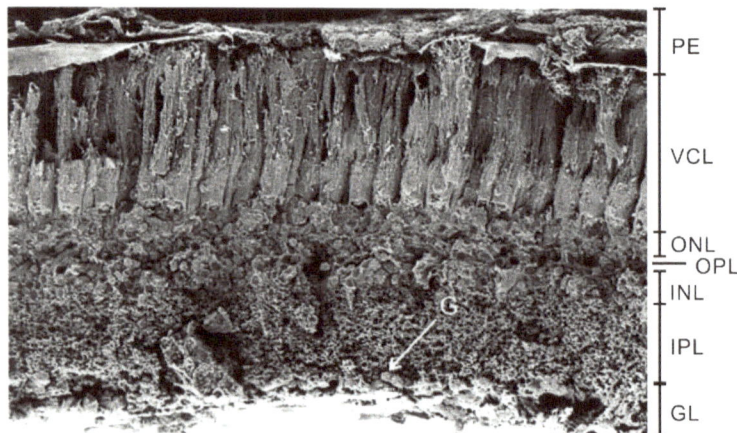

Figure 1.16f.

Retinal layers of the golden gecko at different thickness are shown by scanning electron microscopy. The extremely thin outer plexiform layer (OPL) noted in the tissue sections can also be seen in this micrograph. "G" denotes a potential ganglion cell in the inner most layer. Bar = 10 μm.

(GL - Ganglion cell layer; INL - Inner nuclear layer; IPL - Inner plexiform layer; ONL - Outer nuclear layer; OPL - Outer plexiform layer; PE - Pigment epithelium; VCL - Visual cell layer).

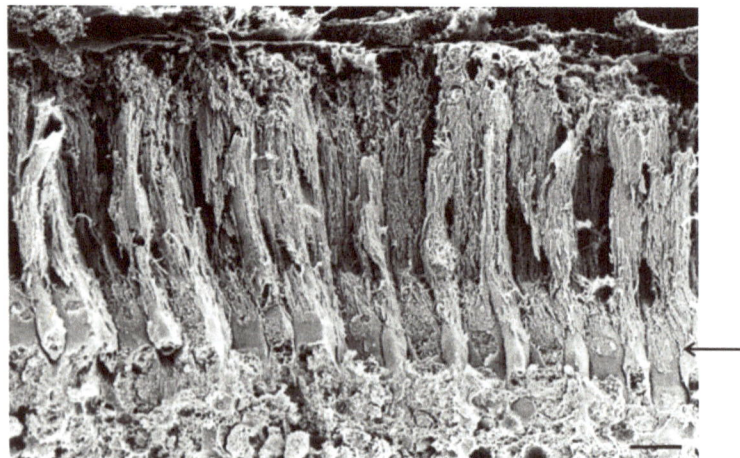

Figure 1.16g.

A row formed predominantly by cone cells (arrow) is noted in the central retina of the golden gecko. Bar = 10 μm.

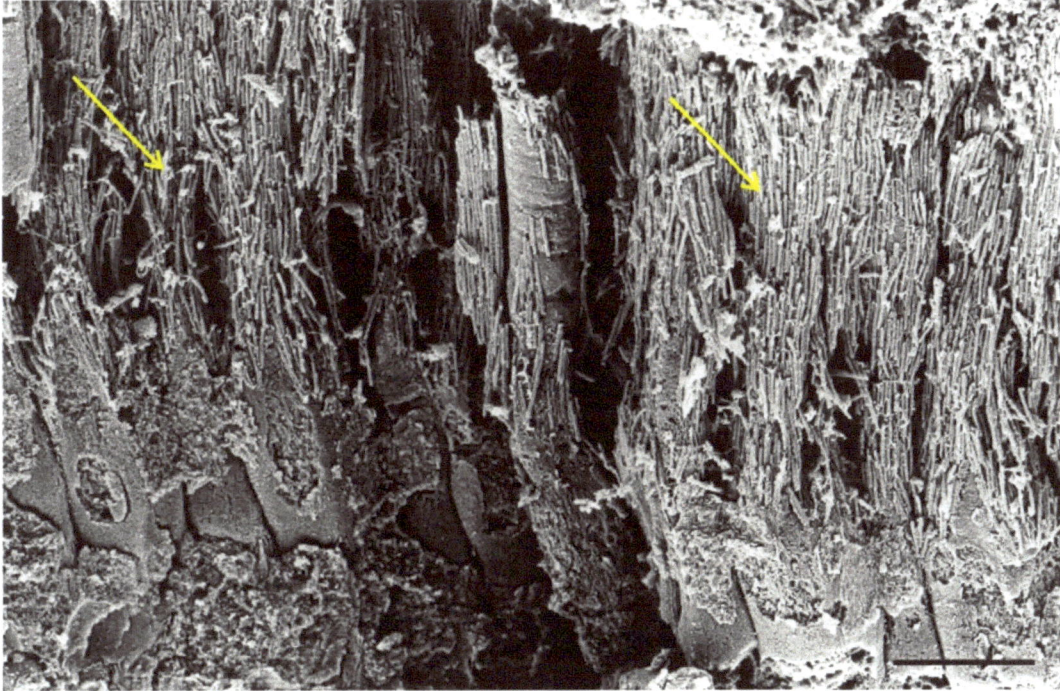

Figure 1.16h.

Note the elongated pigment granules in the processes of the pigment cells (yellow arrows). These granules cover the entire bodies of the visual cell outer segments. Bar = 10 μm.

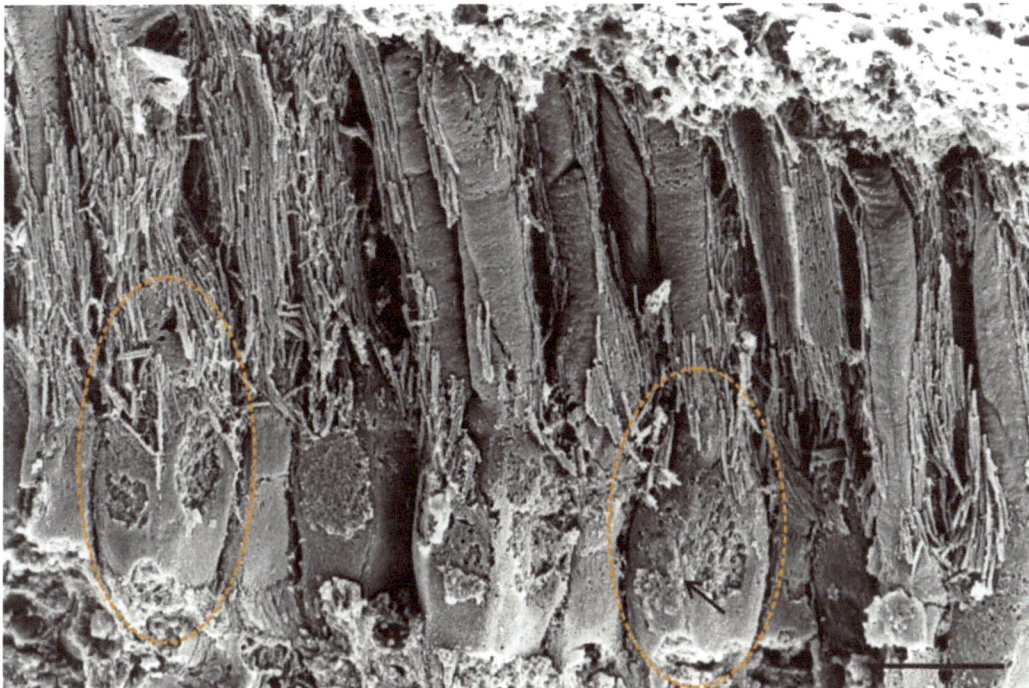

Figure 1.16i.

Circles indicate two double cone cells in the golden gecko. Note the junction (arrow) between the two cells. Bar = 10 μm.

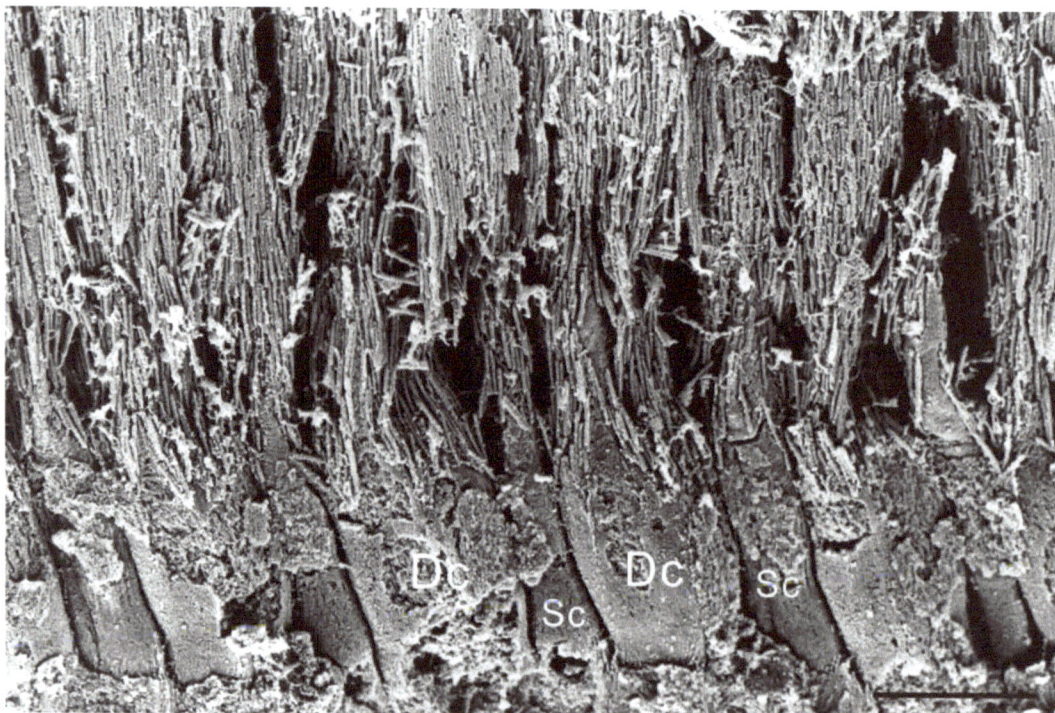

Figure 1.16j.

Single cones (Sc) are noted in between the double cones (Dc). Bar = 10 mm.

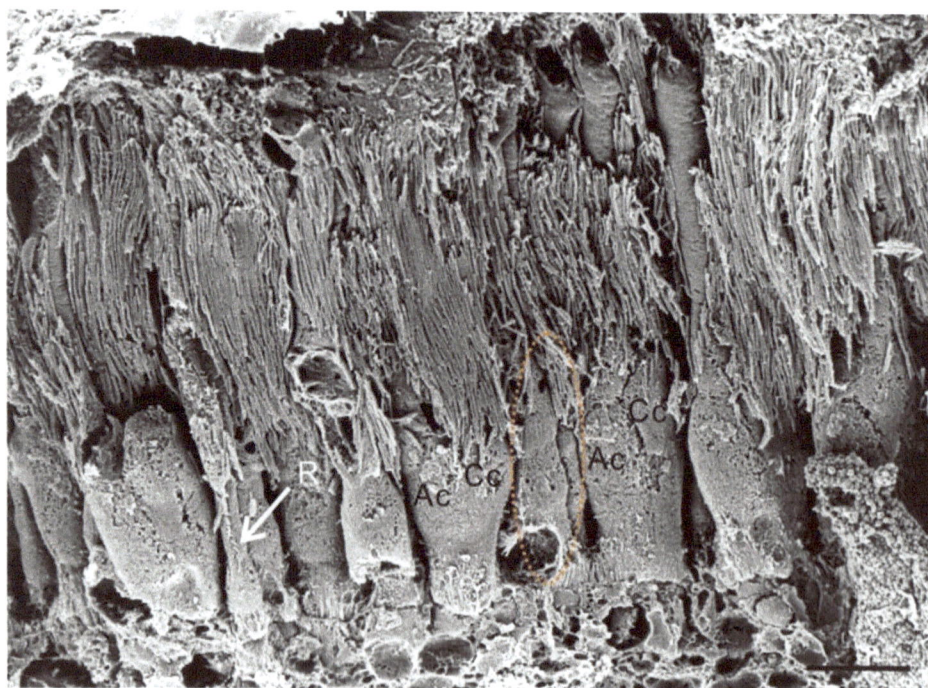

Figure 1.16k.

Two large pairs of double cones, with the accessory cones (Ac) and chief cones (Cc) are labelled. There is also a pair of what are possibly slender double cone (circle). On the left, a rod cell (R) is noted. Bar = 10 μm.

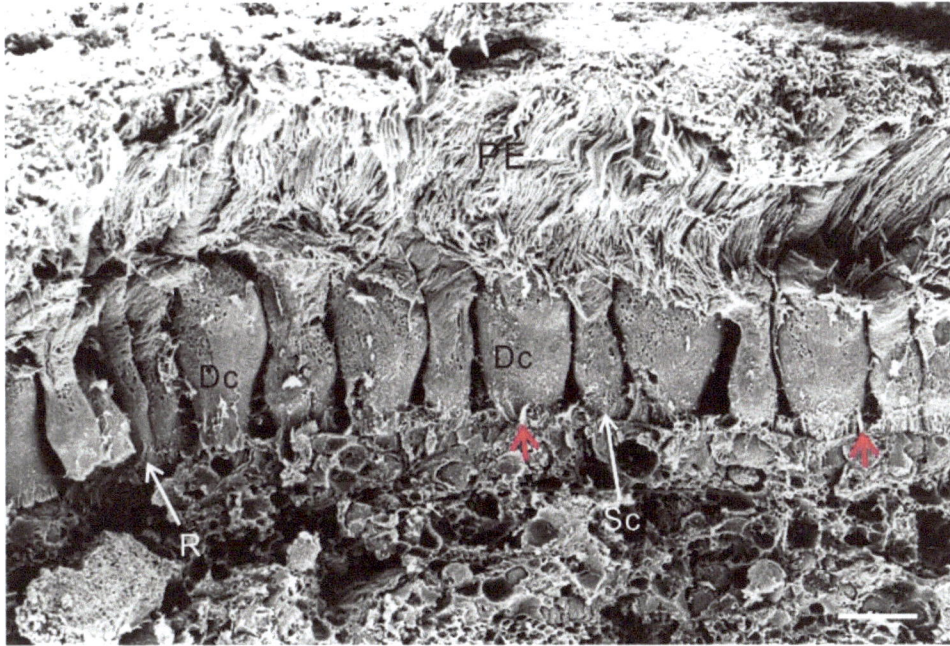

Figure 1.16l.

A layer of visual cells containing double cones (Dc), single cones (Sc) and a rod (R) are shown. Covering the visual cells is the pigment epithelial layer (PE). In the golden gecko, fewer Müller cell processes (red arrows) are noted around the inner segments. Bar = 10 μm.

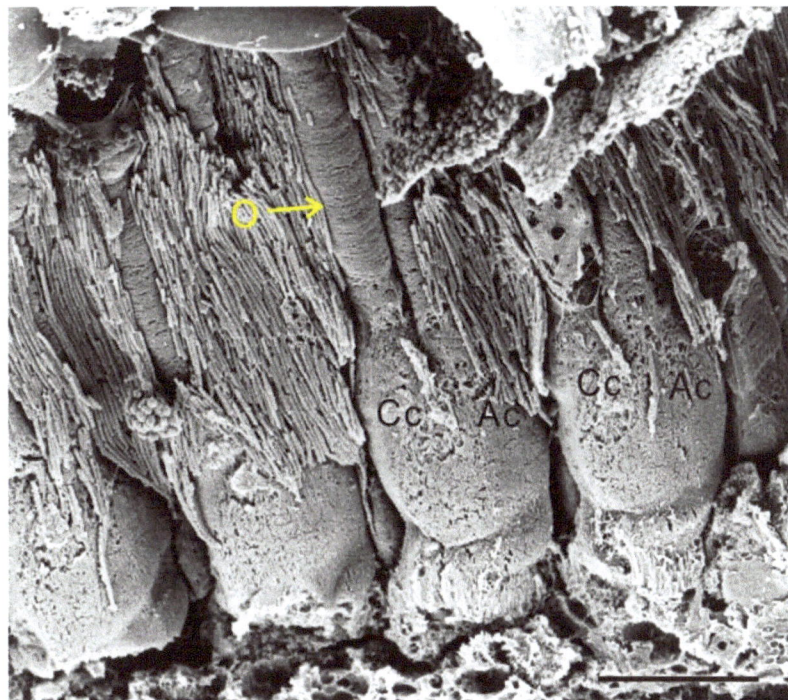

Figure 1.16m.

Two pairs of double cones with accessory cones (Ac) and chief cones (Cc) are shown. Note that in the case of golden gecko, the size of the accessory cone and chief cone are not so different. The outer segment (O) of a chief cone with its stacks of membranes are clearly illustrated. Bar = 10 μm.

17. SOFTSHELL TURTLE

The softshell turtle which naturally lives in muddy areas of freshwater has a retina which consists of 1 to 2 layers of outer nuclear layer. This thin outer nuclear layer is consistently seen in other reptile species. The inner nuclear layer of this animal is about 5 layers thick with loosely packed cells. The ganglion cell layer has quite a number of ganglion cells. Moreover, a thick nerve fiber layer is also observed. The visual cells of this animal lack the typical outer segments; only tiny outer segment like protrusions are noted. However, there are many oil droplets present in the visual cells.

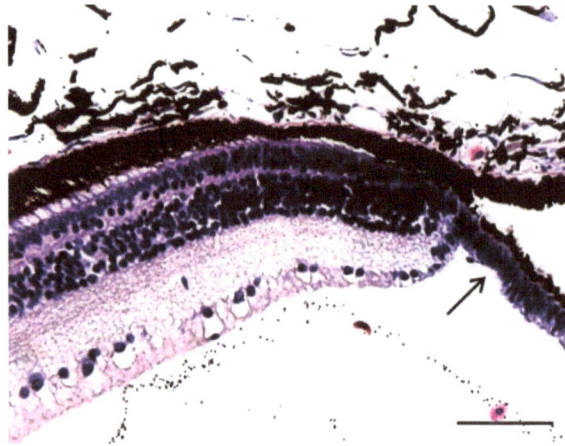

Figure 1.17a. *Anterior retina, near ora serrata.*

This figure shows the transitional region from the anterior retina to the ora serrata of a soft-shell turtle. There are no visual cells in the ora serrata (arrow). Bar = 50 μm.

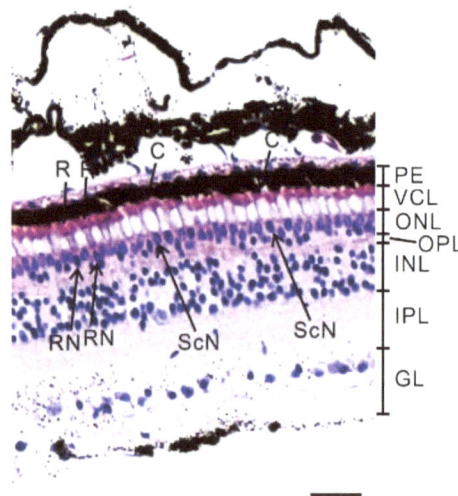

Figure 1.17b. *Peripheral retina.*

The clear oval structures shown in this figure are the proximal inner segments of the visual cells. The distal inner segments are highly stained with eosin, appearing deep pink in color. Among the different types of visual cells are cones (C) and rods (R). The rods have cylindrical inner segments whereas the cones appear more spherical in shape. In the outer nuclear layer, the cell nuclei of the cones (ScN) and rods (RN) can be distinguished by their different positions. Bar = 30 μm.

(GL - Ganglion cell layer; INL - Inner nuclear layer; IPL - Inner plexiform layer; ONL - Outer nuclear layer; OPL - Outer plexiform layer; PE - Pigment epithelium; VCL - Visual cell layer).

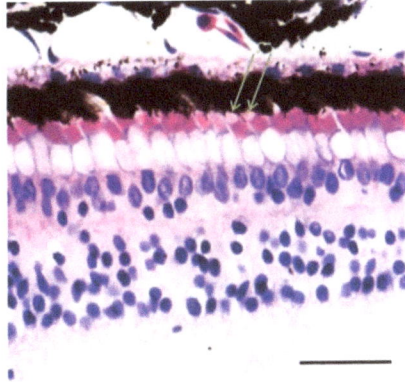

Figure 1.17c. *Peripheral retina.*

Oil droplets (yellow arrows) are noted in the distal inner segments of some cone cells. Bar = 30 μm.

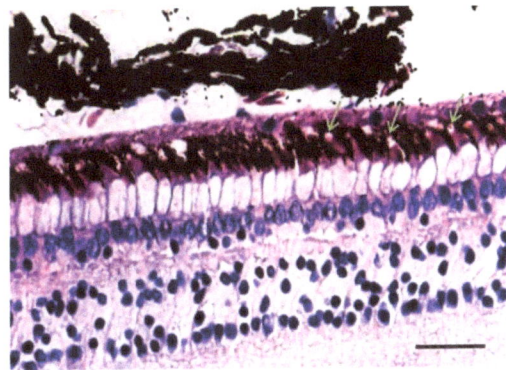

Figure 1.17d. *Central retina.*

Visual cells are more highly packed in the central region. Oil droplets (green arrows) are still present. Bar = 30 μm.

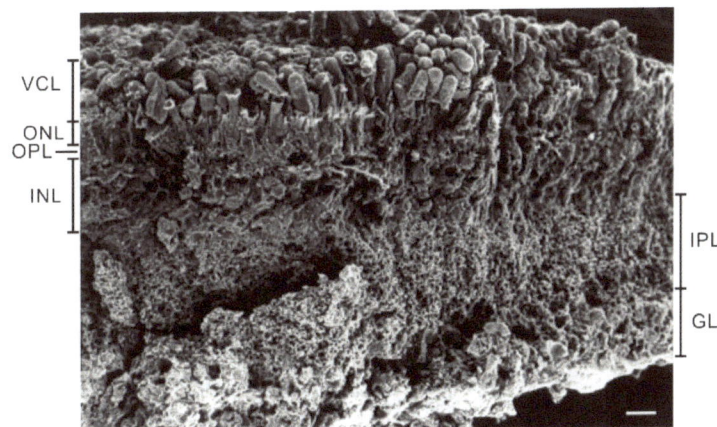

Figure 1.17e.

A scanning electron micrograph showing the retinal layers of a soft-shell turtle. The visual cell layer (VCL) contains small and short photoreceptors. Both the outer (ONL) and inner nuclear layers (INL) are comparatively thinner than the inner plexiform layer (IPL). Bar = 10 μm.

(GL - Ganglion cell layer; INl - Inner nuclear layer; IPL - Inner plexiform layer; ONL - Outer nuclear layer; OPL - Outer plexiform layer; VCL - Visual cell layer).

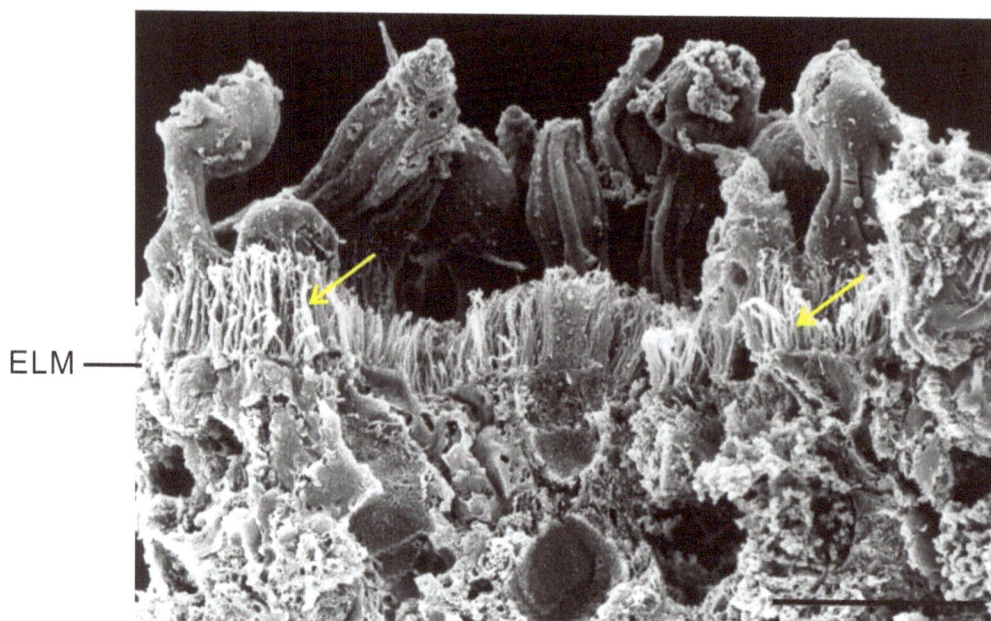

Figure 1.17f.

In the anterior retina, small visual cells with atypical morphologies are noted. The contour of the inner segments is irregular and rough. Extending from the external limiting membrane (ELM) are many long microvilli (yellow arrows) that surround the basal part of the visual cells. Bar = 10 μm.

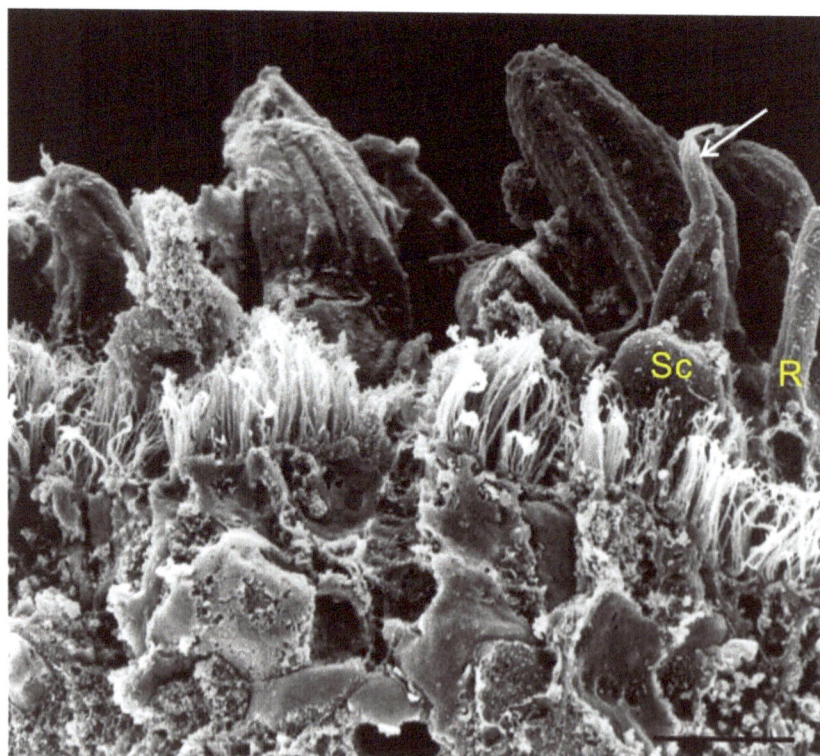

Figure 1.17g.

A single cone (Sc) with a growing cilium (white arrow) is noted in the anterior retina. On the side, there is a cylindrical rod (R). Bar = 5 μm.

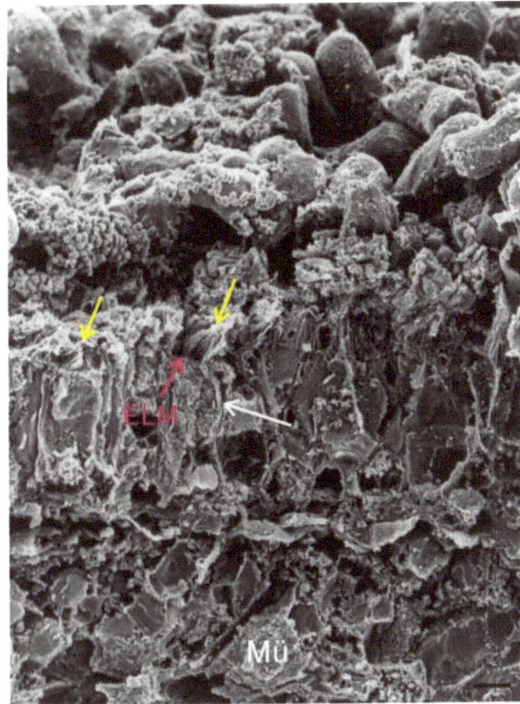

Figure 1.17h.

Müller cells (Mü) have large cell bodies and extensive processes (white arrow). A highly dense group of microvilli (yellow arrows) forming the external limiting membrane (ELM) is also noted. Bar = 10 μm.

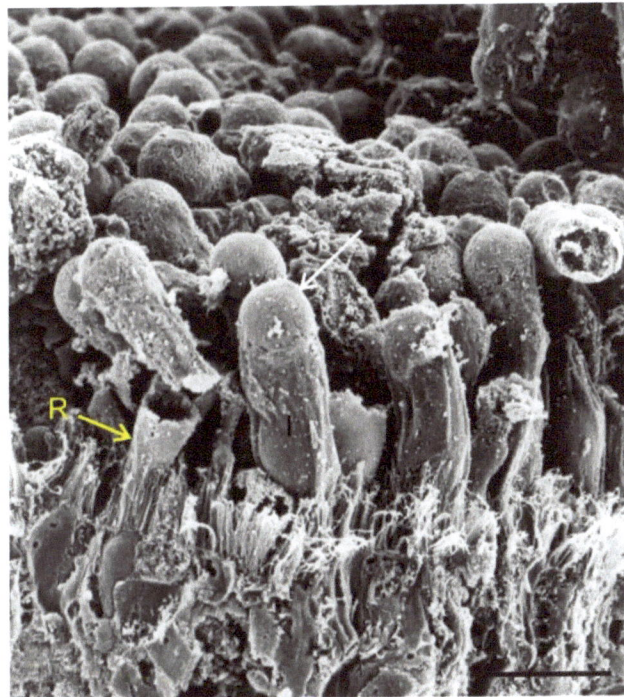

Figure 1.17i.

Cones of this animal have a round oil droplet (white arrow) and a short inner segment (I). A possible rod (R) is also seen, with an inverted cone shaped inner segment. Bar = 10 μm.

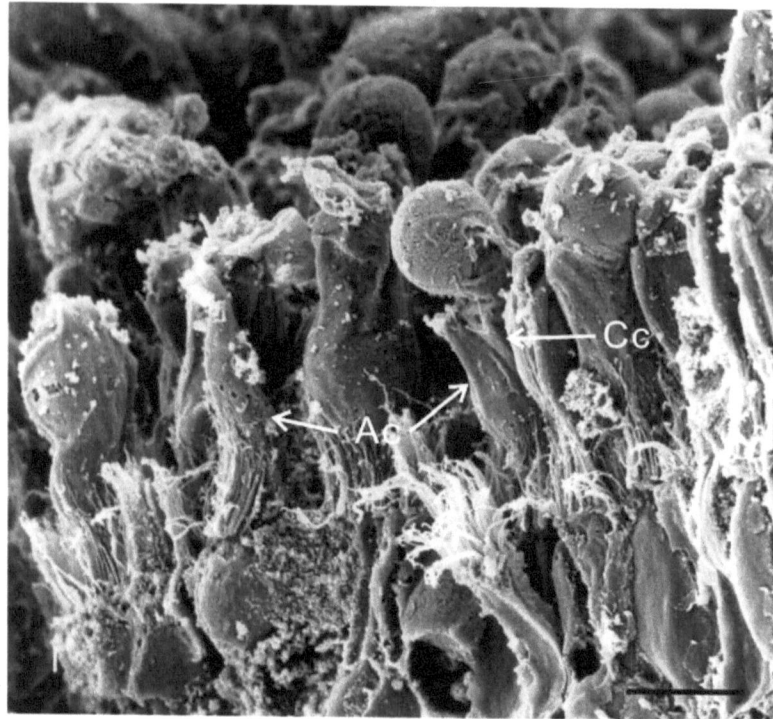

Figure 1.17j.

The two components of the double cone is noted. An oil droplet is seen in the chief cone. Bar = 5 μm.

(Cc - Chief cone; Ac - Accessory cone).

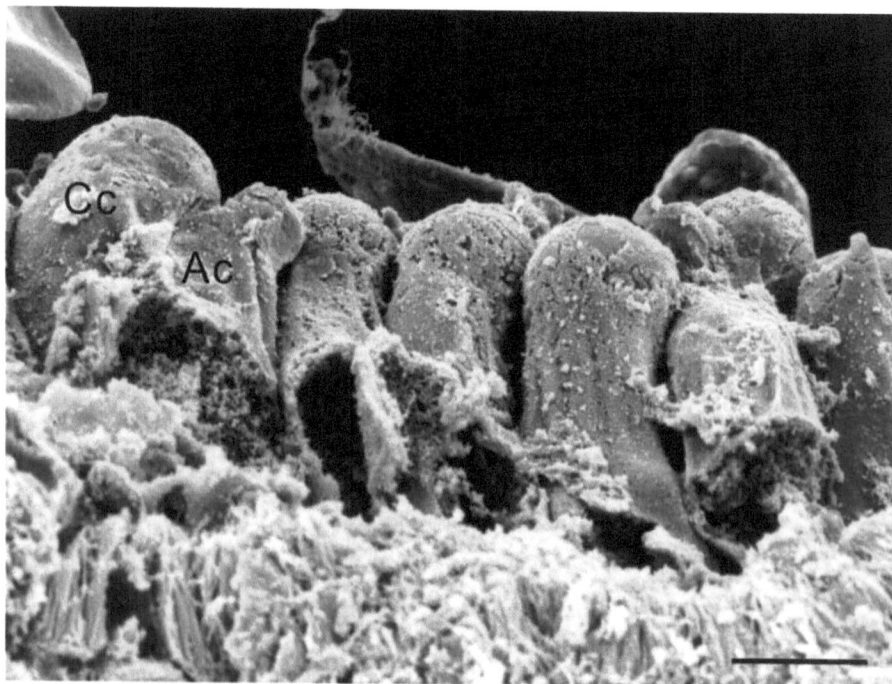

Figure 1.17k.

Inferior and frontal view of the chief (Cc) and accessory (Ac) components of a double cone is shown. Bar = 5 μm.

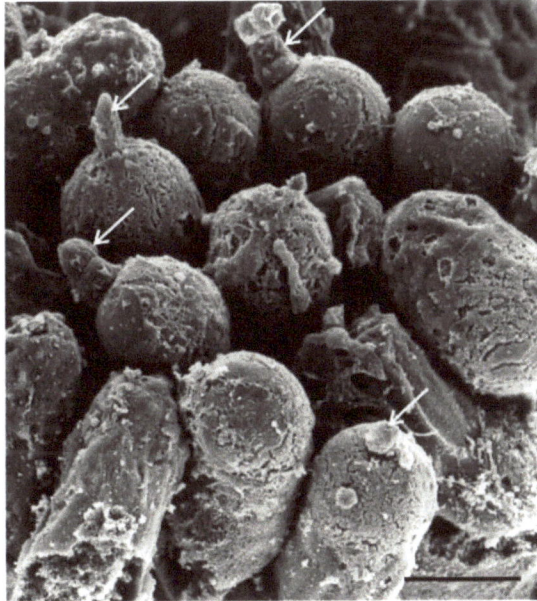

Figure 1.17l.

In this animal, typical outer segments are not observed, but small protrusions (white arrows) are seen to grow from some distal inner segments. Bar = 5 μm.

18. DOMESTIC DUCK

In both the domestic ducks and Chinese francolin, the Müller cells are very obvious even under the common haematoxylin and eosin staining. In the duck, the outer nuclear layer is not thick (usually 2 to 3 layers) whilst the inner nuclear layer is about 7 to 8 layers thick. There is also a very thick inner plexiform and nerve fiber layers. Oil droplets are present in the some of the visual cells.

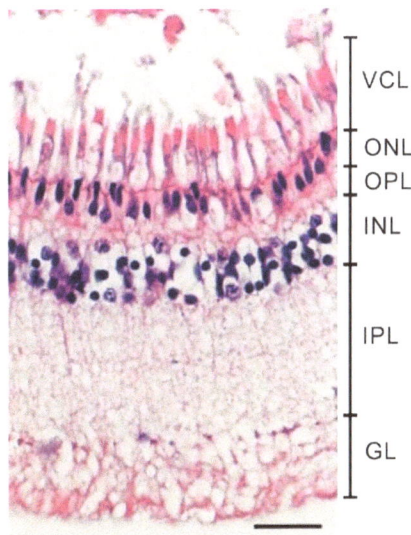

Figure 1.18a. *Anterior retina.*

The different layers of the domestic duck retina are shown. Bar = 50 μm.

(GL - Ganglion cell layer; INL - Inner nuclear layer; IPL - Inner plexiform layer; ONL - Outer nuclear layer; OPL - Outer plexiform layer; VCL - Visual cell layer).

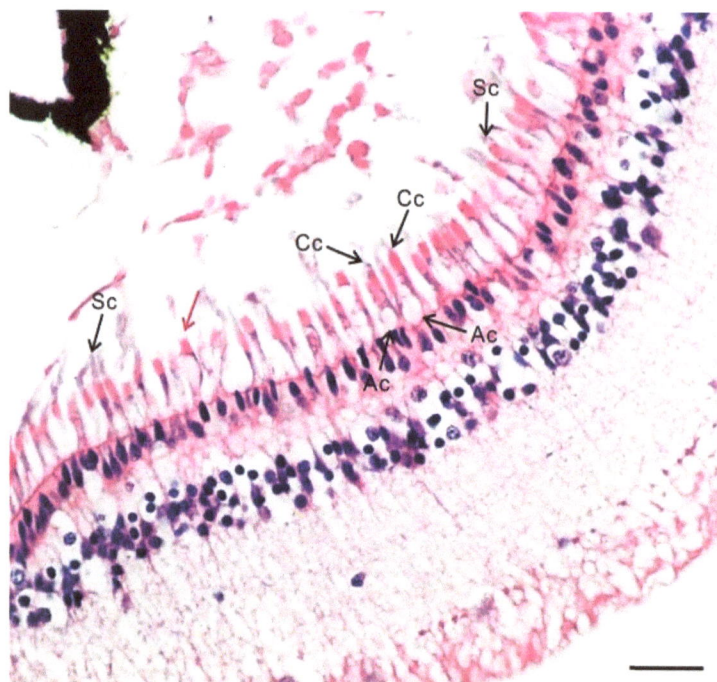

Figure 1.18b. *Anterior retina.*

The different types of cones in the anterior retina of the domestic duck are shown. The tall chief cone (Cc) has an oil droplet whereas the short accessory cone (Ac) does not. The chief and accessory cones form the double cones of this species. "Sc" denotes a single cone with an oil droplet in the inner segment as well. The red arrow indicates the oil droplet of the chief cone. Bar = 50 μm.

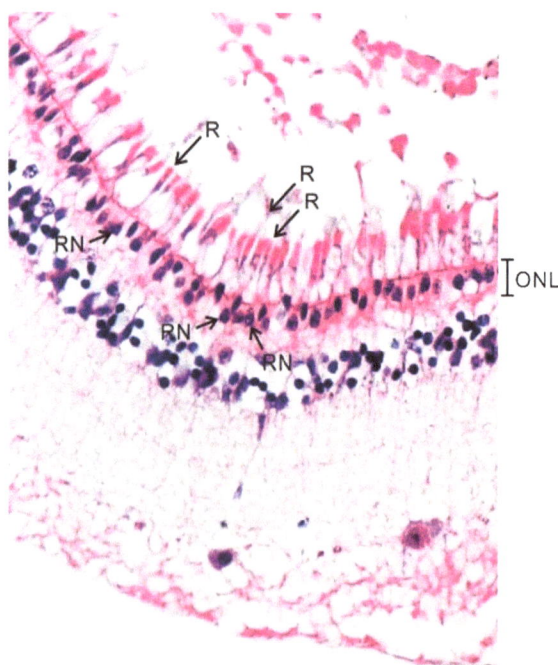

Figure 1.18c. *Anterior retina.*

The anterior retina of the duck illustrates the presence of rods (R) among the various cones. The nuclei of the rods (RN) are identified in lower position of the outer nuclear layer (ONL). Bar = 50 μm.

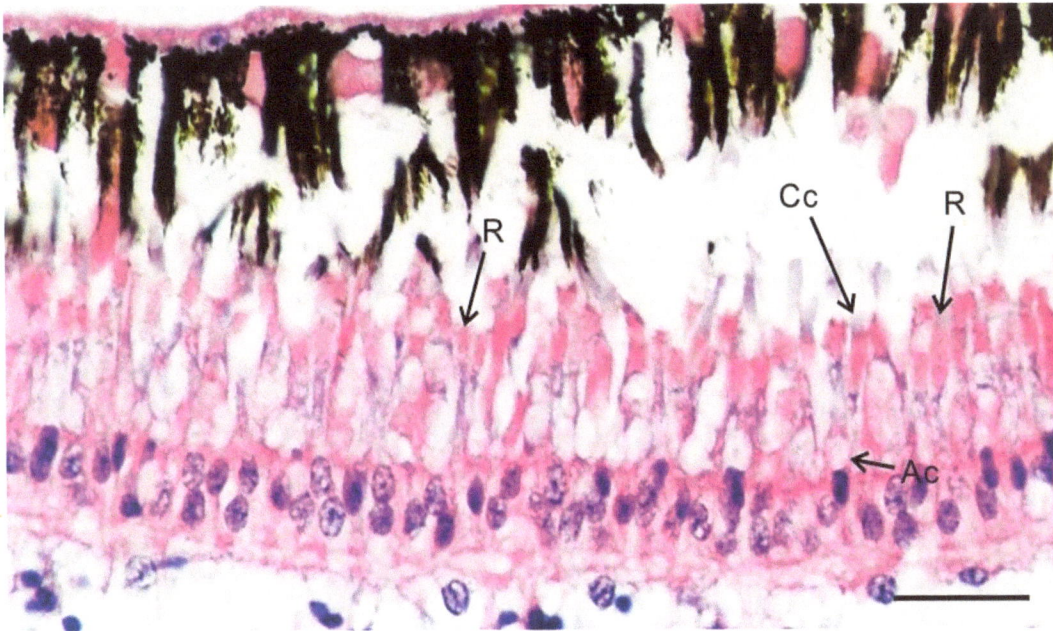

Figure 1.18d. *Peripheral retina.*

The peripheral retina still contains a lot of cones and they are highly packed. Some chief cones (Cc), accessory cones (Ac), and rods (R) are identified. Bar = 50 μm.

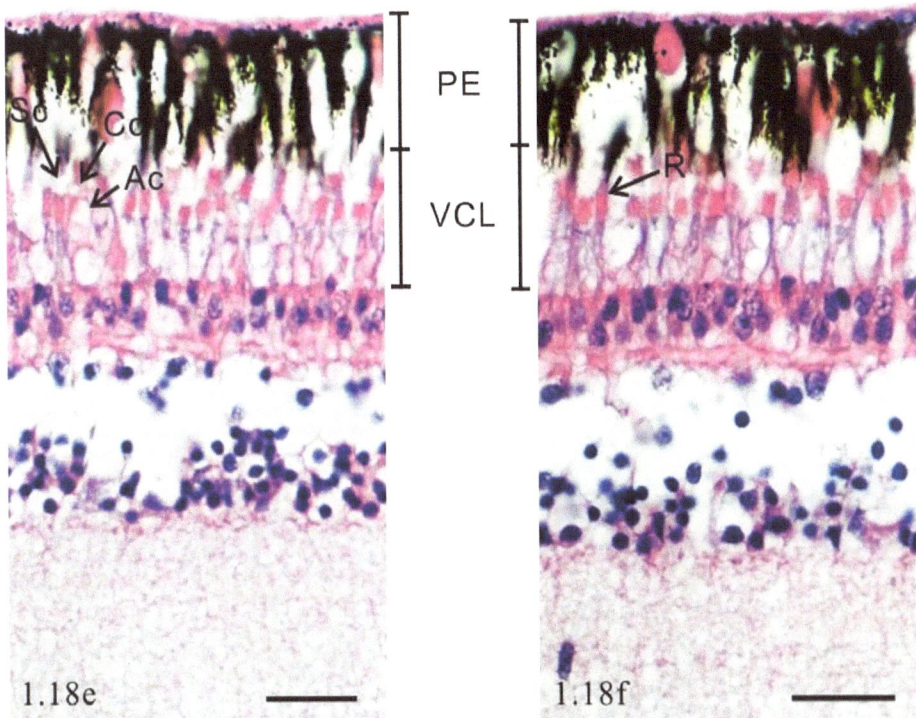

Figures 1.18e & 1.18f. *Peripheral retina.*

Peripheral retina with a pigment epithelium (PE) covering the visual cell layer (VCL). Another chief cone (Cc), accessory cone (Ac), single cone (Sc), and rod (R) are illustrated. Single and chief cones display oil droplets in the distal inner segments. Bar = 50 μm.

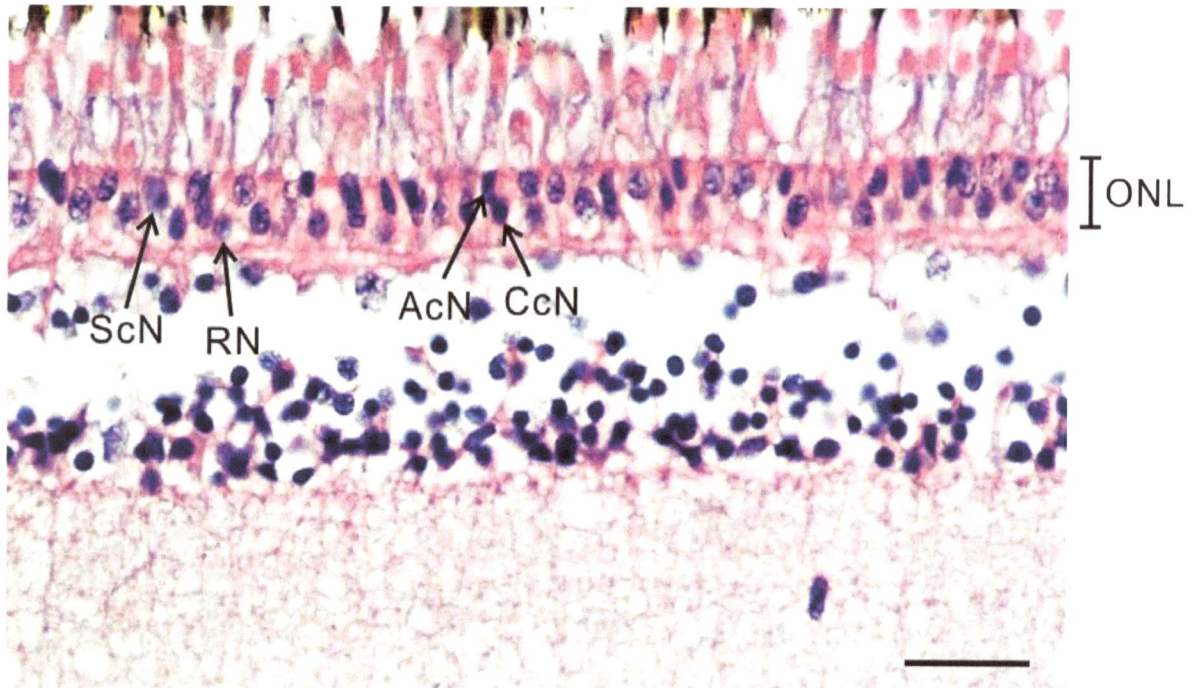

Figure 1.18g. *Peripheral retina.*

The nuclei of the chief cone (CcN), accessory cone (AcN), single cone (ScN), and rods (RN) are distributed at different levels of the outer nuclear layer (ONL). Bar = 50 μm.

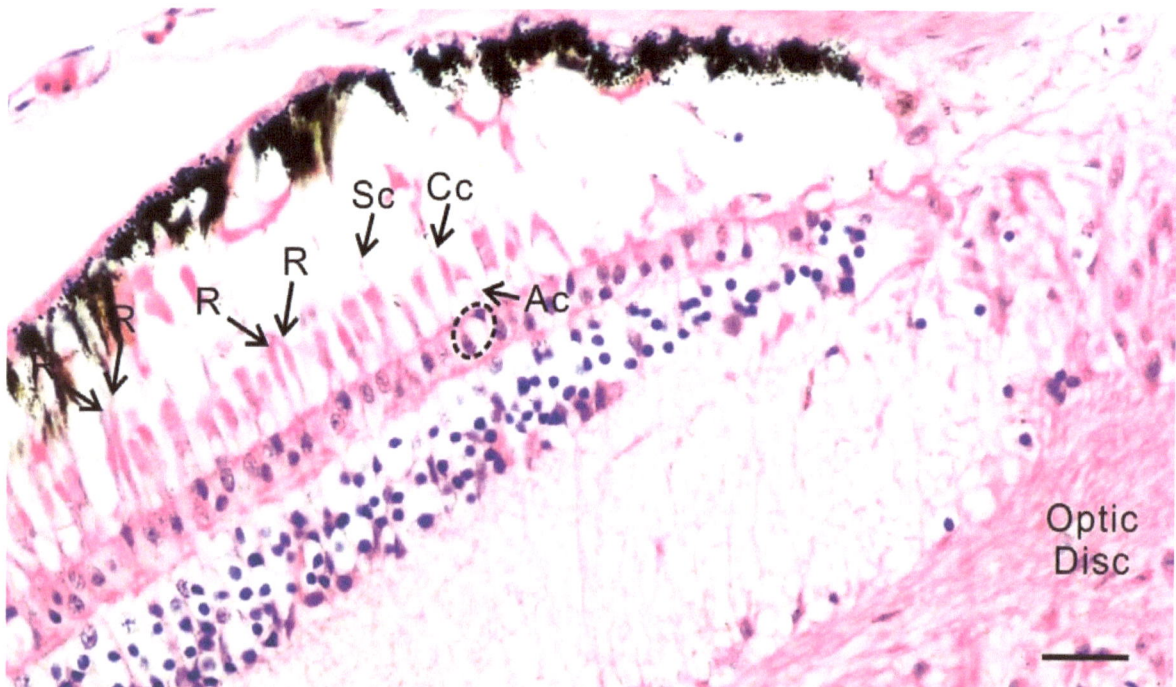

Figure 1.18h. *Posterior central retina, near optic nerve.*

The retina at this region has a low density of visual cells. However the typical visual cell types - chief cones (Cc), accessory cones (Ac), single cones (Sc) and rods (R) are observed. Double cones have 2 nuclei (circle) - the higher one belongs to the accessory cone and the lower one belongs to the chief cone. Bar = 50 μm.

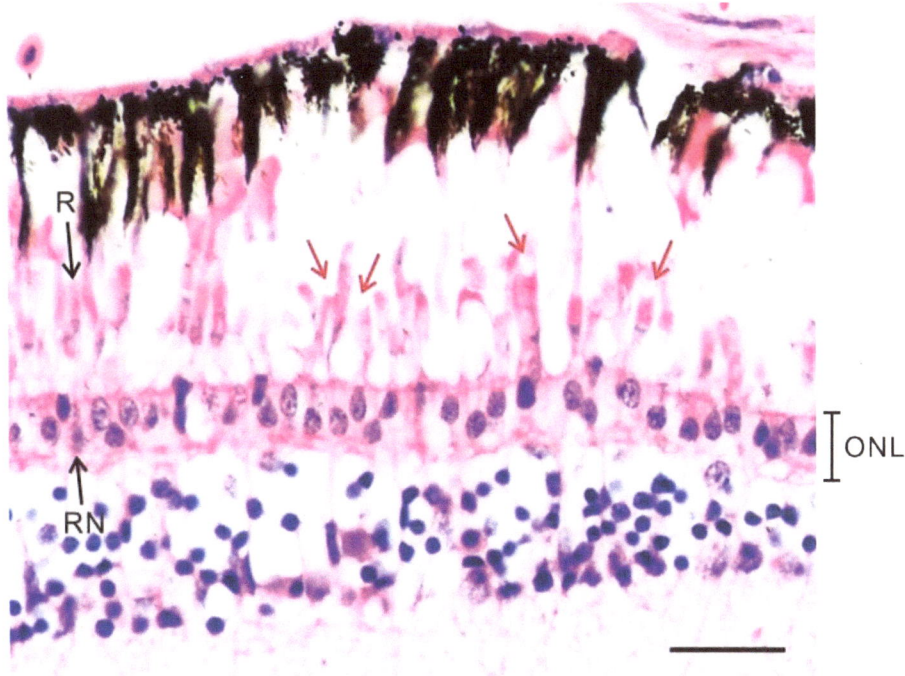

Figure 1.18i. *Posterior central retina, near optic nerve.*

A magnified photo of the retina near the optic nerve. Oil droplets (red arrows) are clearly displayed in some of the cone cells. A rod (R) without an oil droplet is shown on the left. Its nucleus (RN) is located in the lowest level of the outer nuclear layer (ONL). Bar = 50 μm.

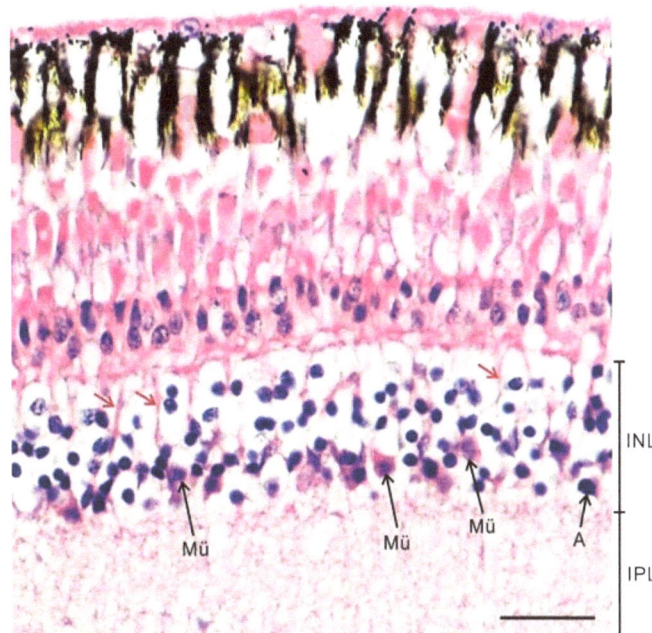

Figure 1.18j. *Central retina.*

The visual cells in this region are more highly packed. There are still many double cones with the occasional rod. Müller cells (Mü) with many of their processes (red arrows) are clearly shown in the inner nuclear layer (INL). More amacrine cells (A) are also noted close to the inner plexiform layer (IPL). Bar = 50 μm.

19. CHINESE FRANCOLIN

The Chinese francolin retina is very similar to that of the domestic duck in structural arrangement. Oil droplets are also present in the visual cells of this animal. In both the domestic duck and the Chinese francolin, the nuclei of the outer nuclear layer are more elongated in shape. The nerve fiber layer of the Chinese francolin is not as thick as the domestic duck.

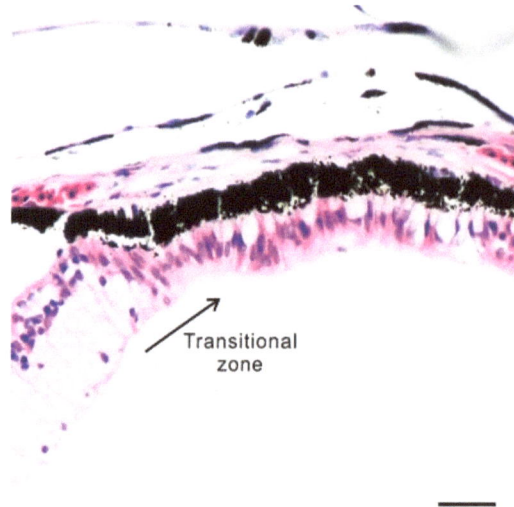

Figure 1.19a. *Ora serrata.*

A slow and gradual transition (arrow) into the ora serrata. Bar = 50 μm.

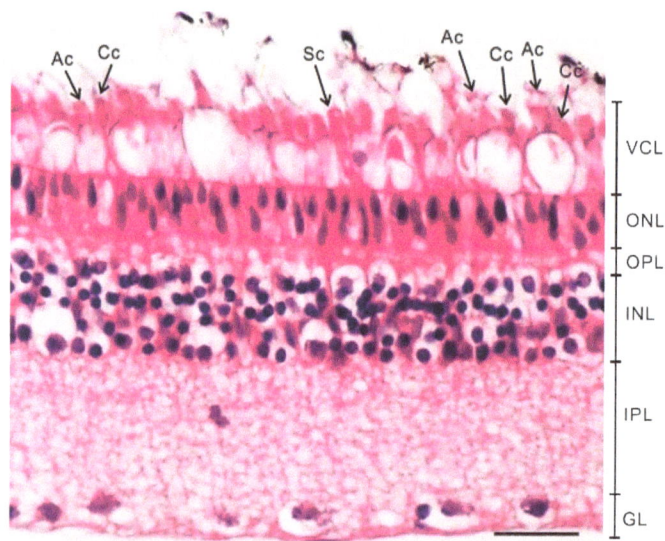

Figure 1.19b. *Anterior retina.*

In the anterior region of the retina, many double cones are seen. The double cones are characterized by having a large and oval shaped accessory cone (Ac) and a slender chief cone (Cc). A type of single cone (Sc) is noted in the middle of this figure. Bar = 50 μm.

(GL - Ganglion cell layer; INL - Inner nuclear layer; IPL - Inner plexiform layer; ONL - Outer nuclear layer; OPL - Outer plexiform layer; VCL - Visual cell layer).

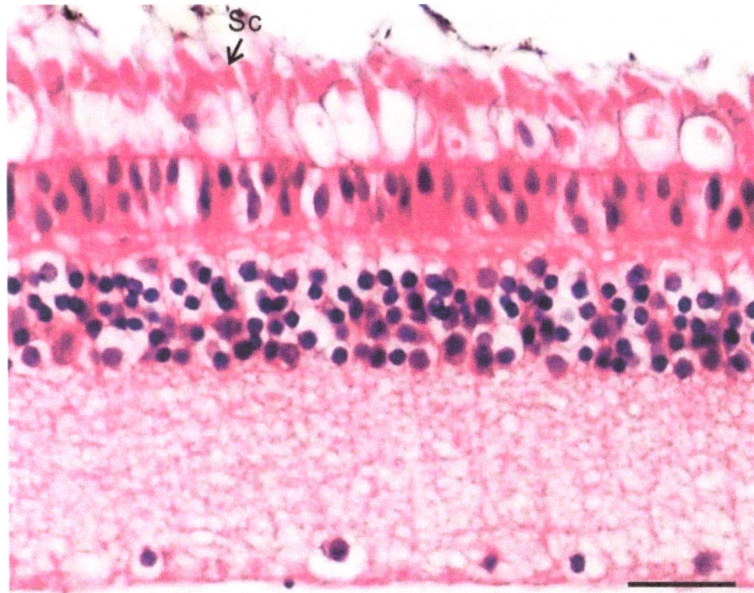

Figure 1.19c. *Anterior retina.*

Another type of single cone (Sc) is seen in the anterior retina. Bar = 50 μm.

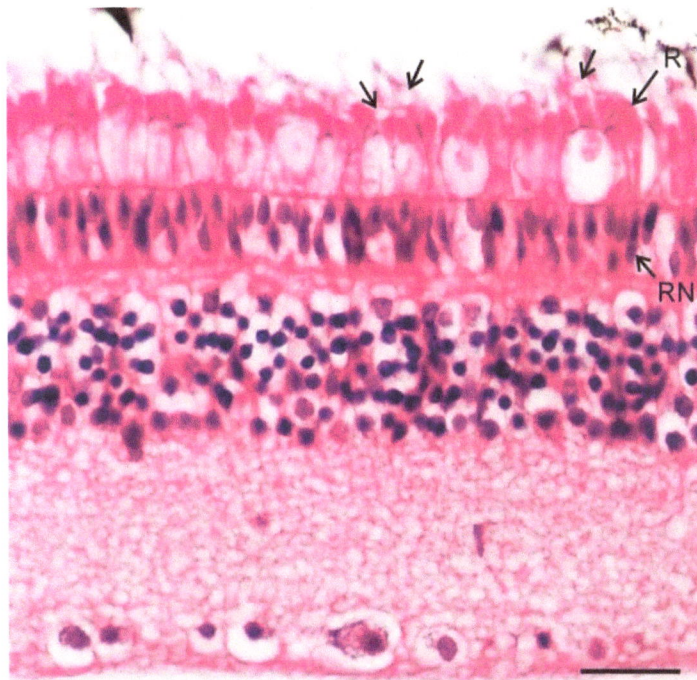

Figure 1.19d. *Peripheral retina.*

Oil droplets are found in many of the cone cells (arrows). A slender rod (R) without any oil droplet is noted in this figure. It comes out from a more elongated nucleus (RN). Bar = 50 μm.

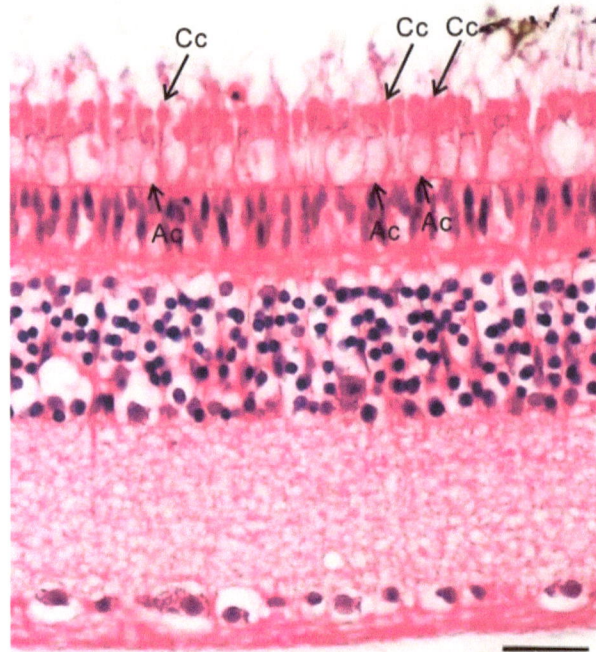

Figure 1.19e. *Peripheral retina.*

Many chief cones (Cc) and accessory cones (Ac) are also present in the peripheral visual layer. The accessory cones are still having enlarged inner segments which are structurally distinct from other visual cells. Bar = 50 μm.

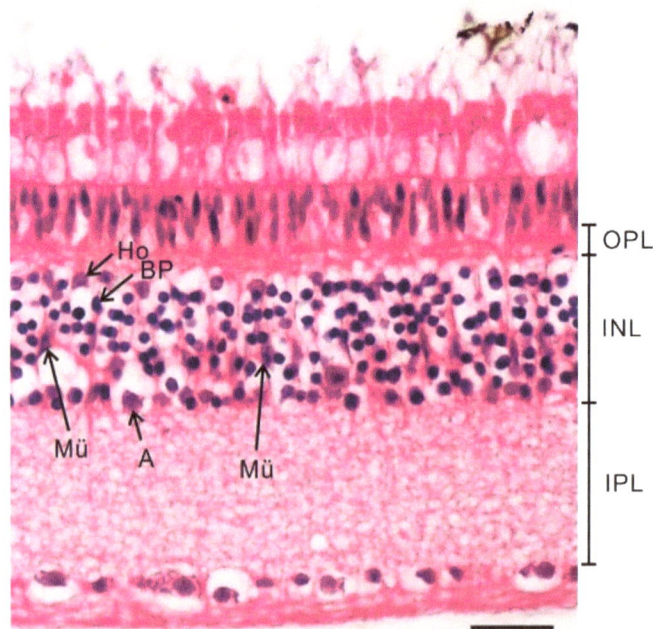

Figure 1.19f. *Peripheral retina.*

Different cell types are noted in the inner nuclear layer (INL). "Ho" denotes a horizontal cell close to the outer plexiform layer (OPL). "BP" is a bipolar cell and "Mü" is a Müller cell with its extensive processes. "A" is an amacrine cell located near to the inner plexiform layer (IPL). Bar = 50 μm.

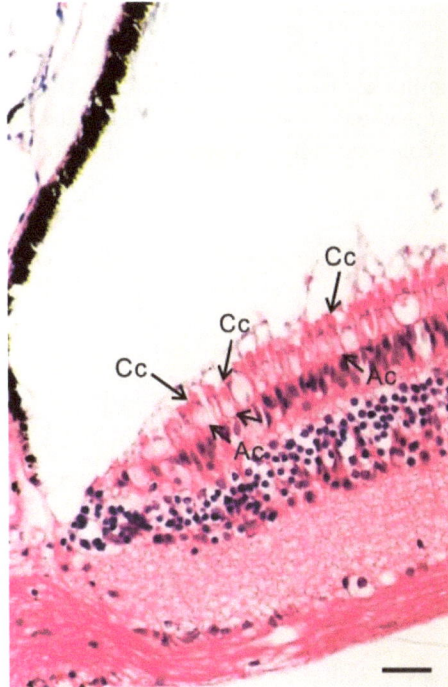

Figure 1.19g. *Central retina.*

The central retina also contains many double cone complexes - chief cones (Cc) and accessory cones (Ac). Bar = 50 μm.

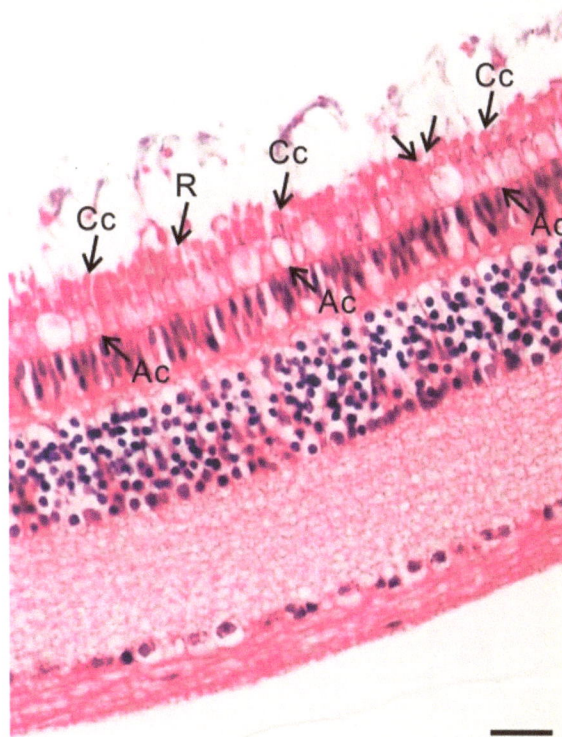

Figure 1.19h. *Central retina.*

An occasional rod cell (R) is observed along with different chief cones (Cc) and accessory cones (Ac). Oil droplets are also present in the cone cells (arrows). Bar = 50 μm.

20. DOMESTIC CHICKEN

The retina of the domestic chicken has evolved to contain with many different cone cells particularly the double cones. All accessory components of the double cones consist of a paraboloid. Oil droplets are also numerous in this animal and they appear in different colors including red, green, and yellow.

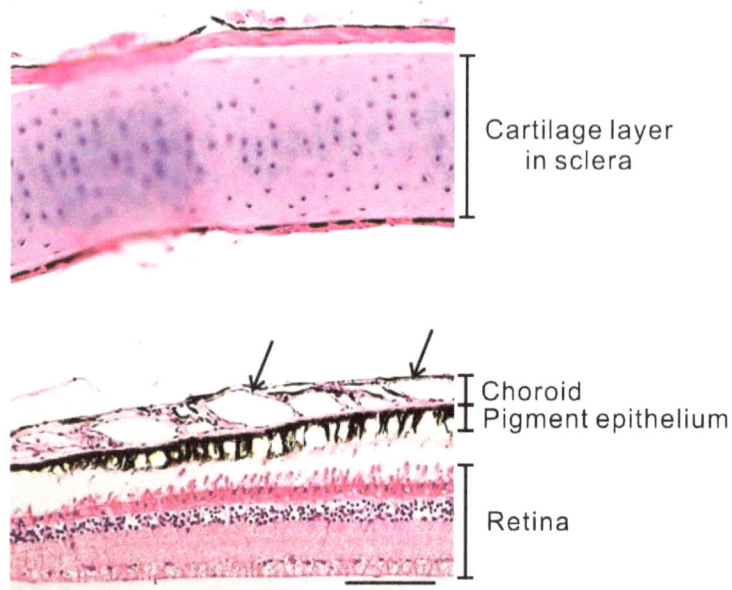

Figure 1.20a. *Anterior retina.*

A low power view of the anterior retina of the chicken with a thick layer of cartilage exterior it to. Arrows indicate the blood vessels in the choroid layer. Bar = 50 μm.

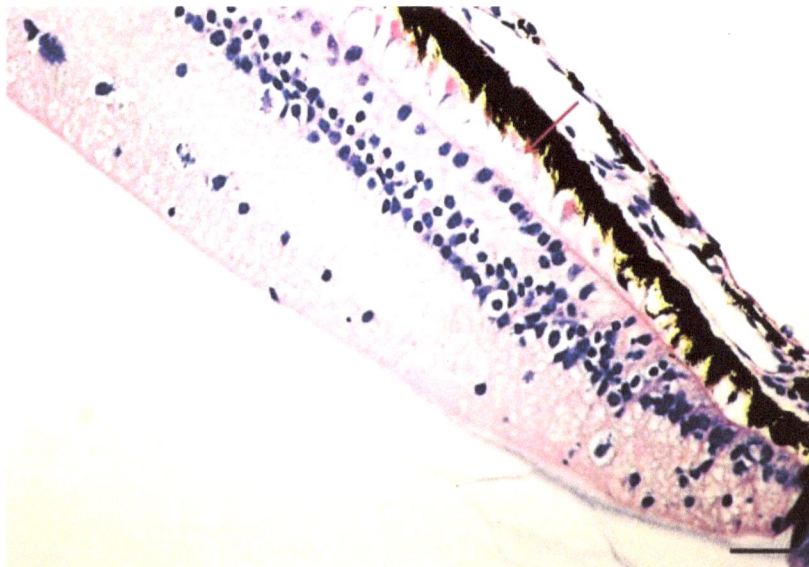

Figure 1.20b. *Anterior retina, near ora serrata.*

The number of visual cells (red arrow) and the number of retinal layers decrease towards the anterior region of the retina. Bar = 50 μm.

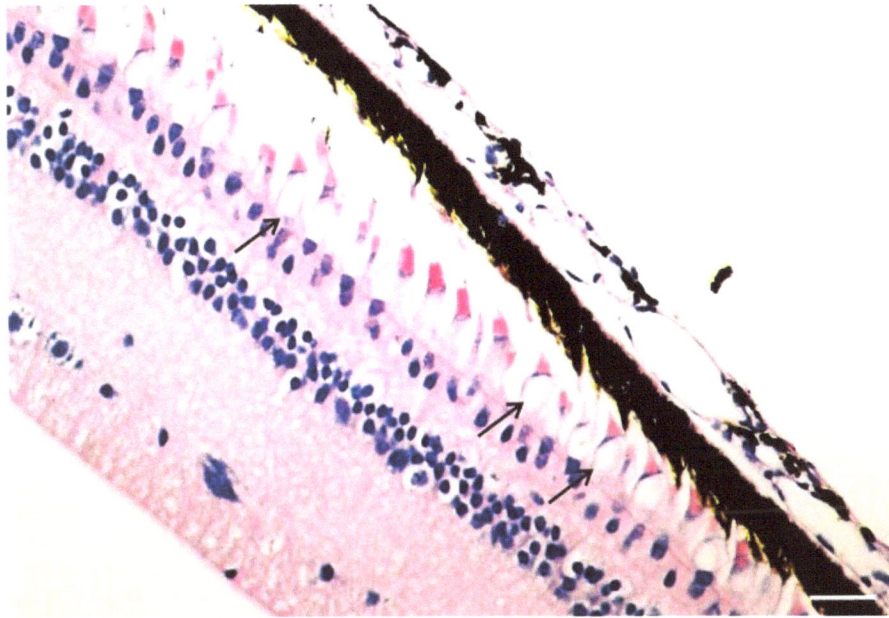

Figure 1.20c. *Anterior retina.*

There are many cone cells in the anterior retina of the chicken. Similar to the Chinese francolin, many cone cells consist of large oval inner segments (arrows) with clear internal contents. Bar = 50 μm.

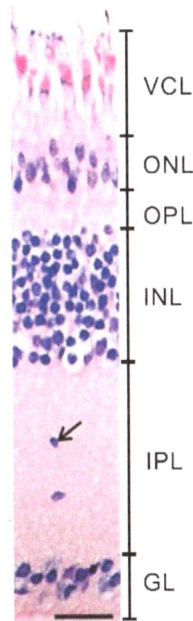

Figure 1.20d. *Anterior retina.*

Layers of the chicken retina are identified. Note that the inner nuclear layer is thicker than the outer nuclear layer. There are only about three layers of cell nuclei in the outer nuclear layer while about ten layers of cells are found in the inner nuclear layer. The inner plexiform layer of this animal is also thick with some displaced cells (arrow) occasionally found. Bar = 50 μm.

(GL - Ganglion cell layer; INL - Inner nuclear layer; IPL - Inner plexiform layer; ONL - Outer nuclear layer; OPL - Outer plexiform layer; VCL - Visual cell layer).

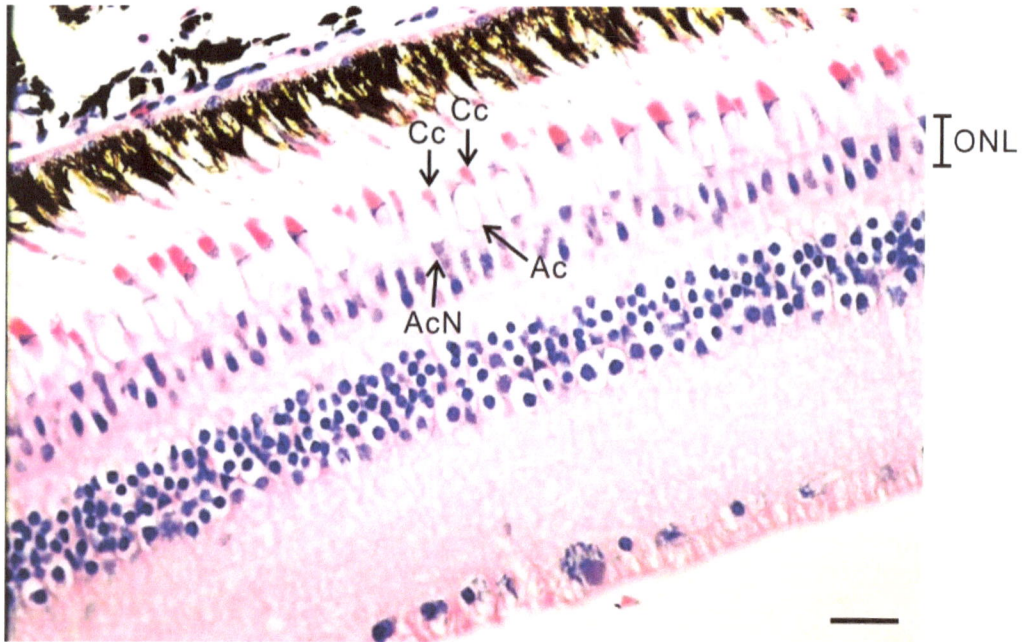

Figure 1.20e. *Anterior retina.*

Double cones are seen in the anterior retina. The chief cones (Cc) of the double cones appear taller and have thin inner segments. The accessory cones which are closely adhered to the side the chief cones have larger and oval shaped inner segments. The nuclei of the accessory cones (AcN) are located in the uppermost level of the outer nuclear layer (ONL) and close to their inner segments. "AC" denotes the accessory cone. Bar = 50 μm.

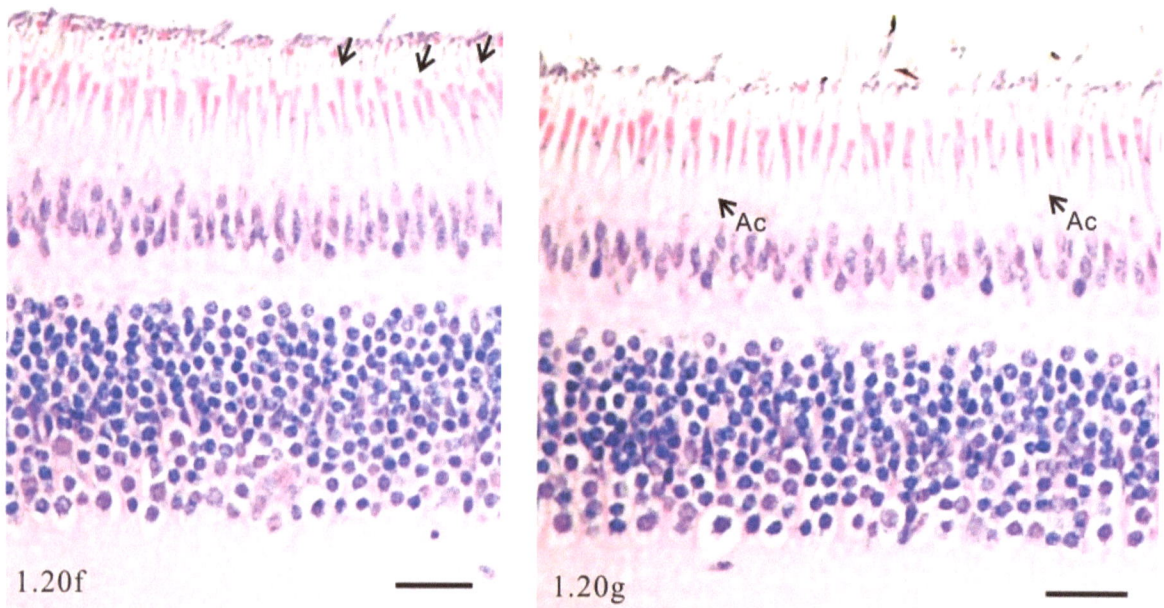

Figures 1.20f & 1.20g. *Peripheral retina.*

A higher density of visual cells is noted in the peripheral region of the retina. The visual cells appear slimmer in shape than those seen in the anterior retina. Double cones are also noted. Although the accessory cones (Ac) still have oval shaped inner segments, they do not appear as clear structures. Many colorless ball shaped structures which are oil droplets (arrows) are noted in the distal end of the visual cell inner segments. Bar = 50 μm.

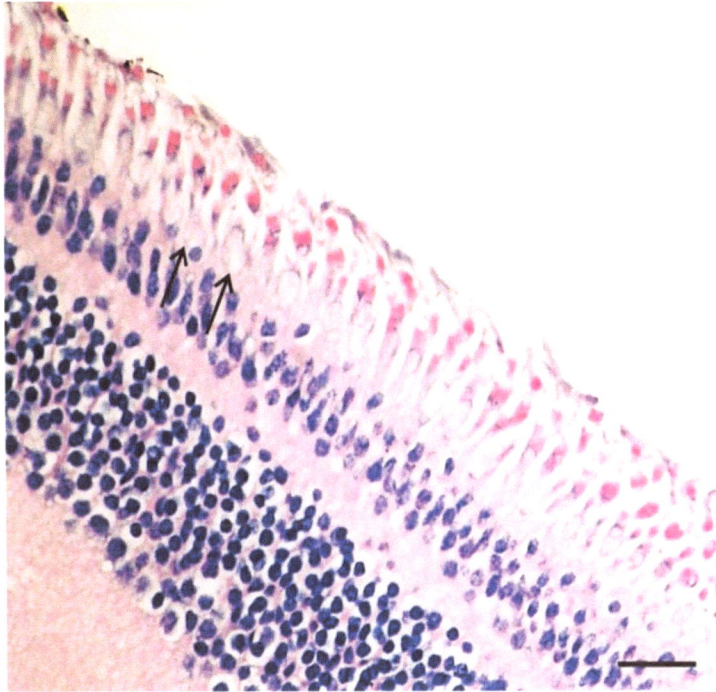

Figure 1.20h. *Central retina.*

There are also many cone cells including the double cones in the central retina. The arrows show the accessory components of the double cones. Bar = 50 μm.

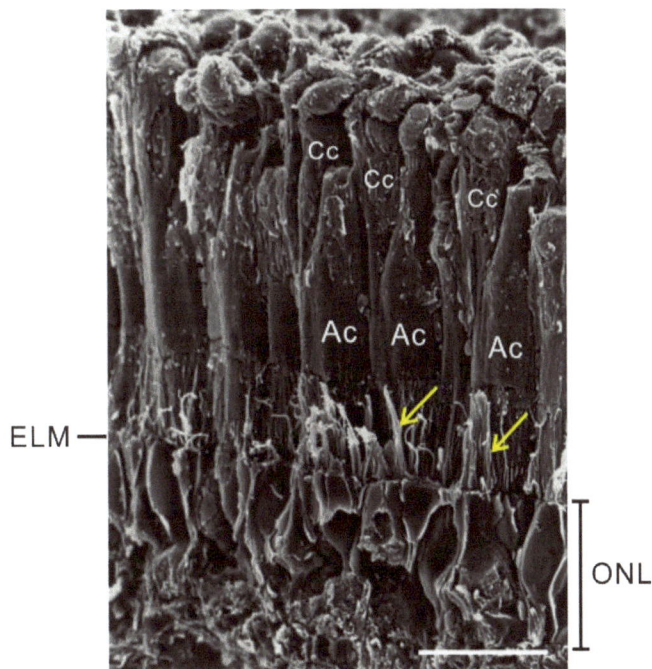

Figure 1.20i.

This electron scanning micrograph shows a series of double cones in the chicken retina. "Cc" denotes the chief cones and "Ac" denotes the accessory cones. Surrounding the proximal inner segments of the visual cells are microvilli (yellow arrows) extending from the external limiting membrane (ELM). Bar = 10 μm.

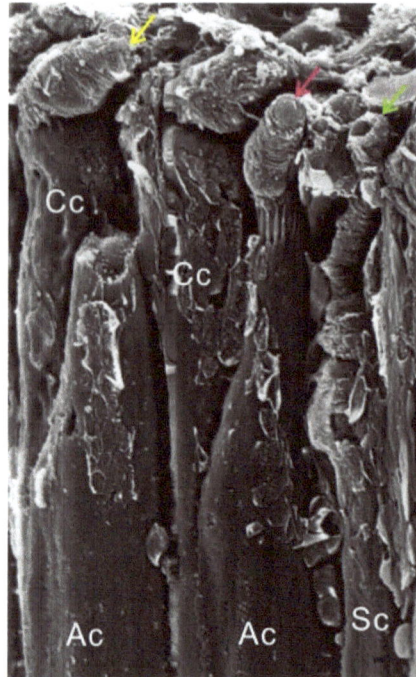

Figure 1.20j.

A higher magnification of figure 1.20i showing two double cones and a single cone (Sc). The outer segments of the chief cone (yellow arrow) appear thicker in diameter than the accessory cone (red arrow). However, both outer segments of the double cones are shorter in length when compared to the single cone's outer segment (green arrow) located on the right of this figure. Bar = 1 μm.

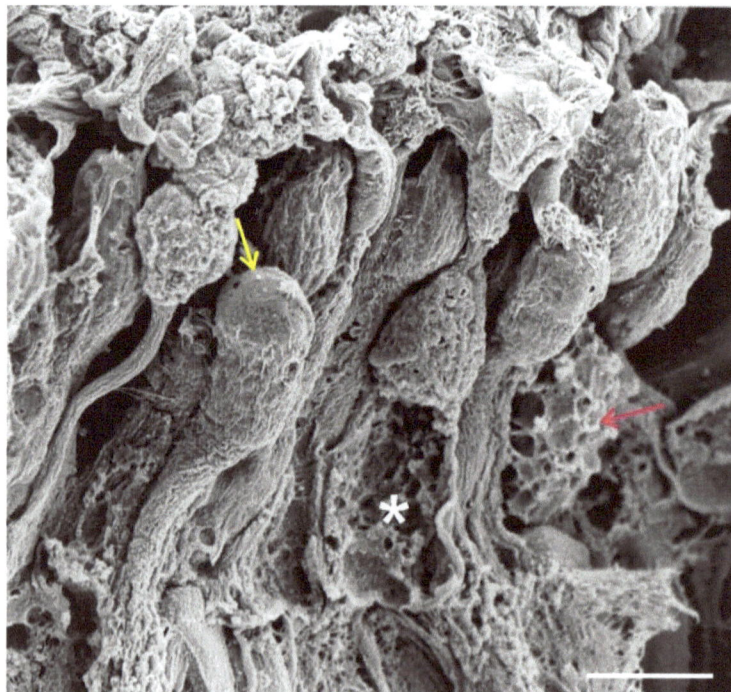

Figure 1.20k.

An empty space (asterisk) that is shown in an accessory cone in this figure was originally occupied by a glycogen body called paraboloid. Paraboloid can be seen in the accessory cones of the chicken. An exposed paraboloid with irregular surface (red arrow) is also shown on the right of this figure. The yellow arrow indicates an oil droplet inside a single cone. Bar = 5 μm.

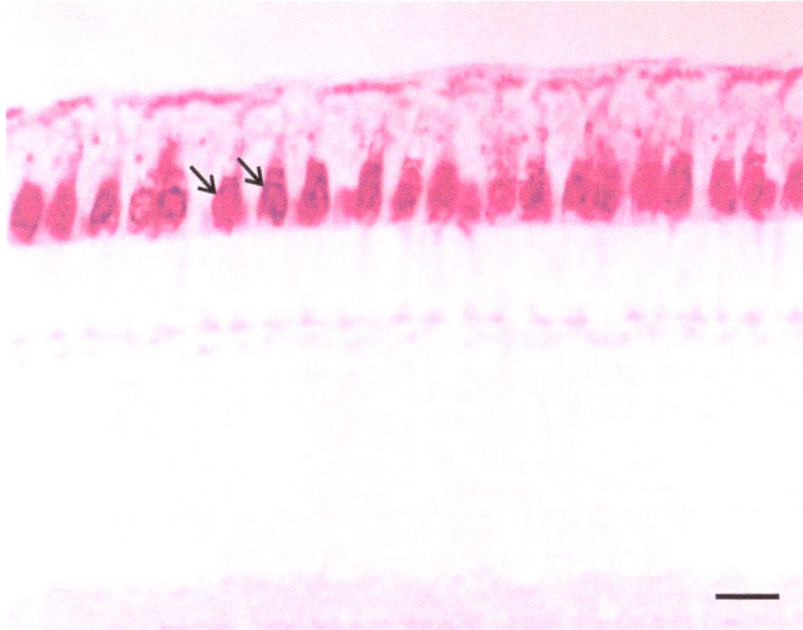

Figure 1.20l.

The paraboloids (arrows) inside the inner segments of the accessory cones are stained dark pink by Periodic acid Schiff reagent. Bar = 50 μm.

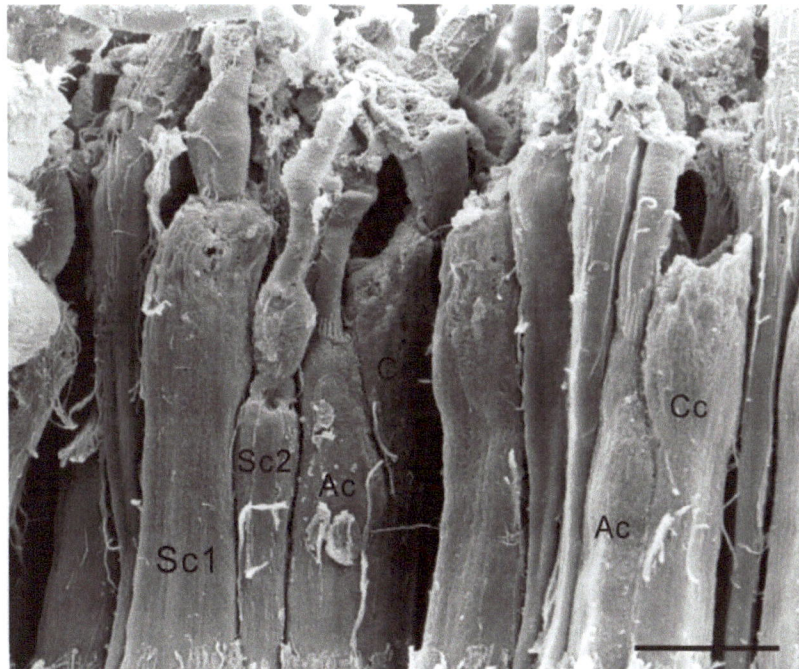

Figure 1.20m.

More than one type of single cones (Sc1 and Sc2) are observed in this animal. The single cones labeled as "Sc1" have relatively longer and broader inner segments whereas "Sc2" have shorter and thinner inner segments. Moreover, the outer segments of the two types of single cones are also different in length. "Sc2" have longer outer segments than "Sc1". Two double cones are also noted in this figure; each composed of two components with different morphologies. Bar = 5 μm.

(Ac- Accessory cone; Cc - Chief cone).

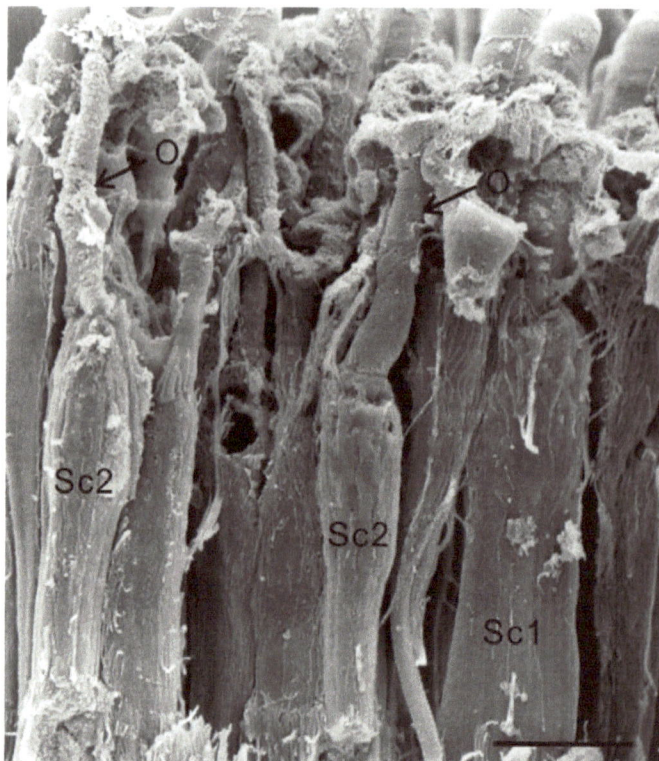

Figure 1.20n.

This figure shows more "Sc1" and "Sc2" single cones in the outer part of the retina. Note the tapered outer segments (O) of the "Sc2" single cone. Bar = 5 μm.

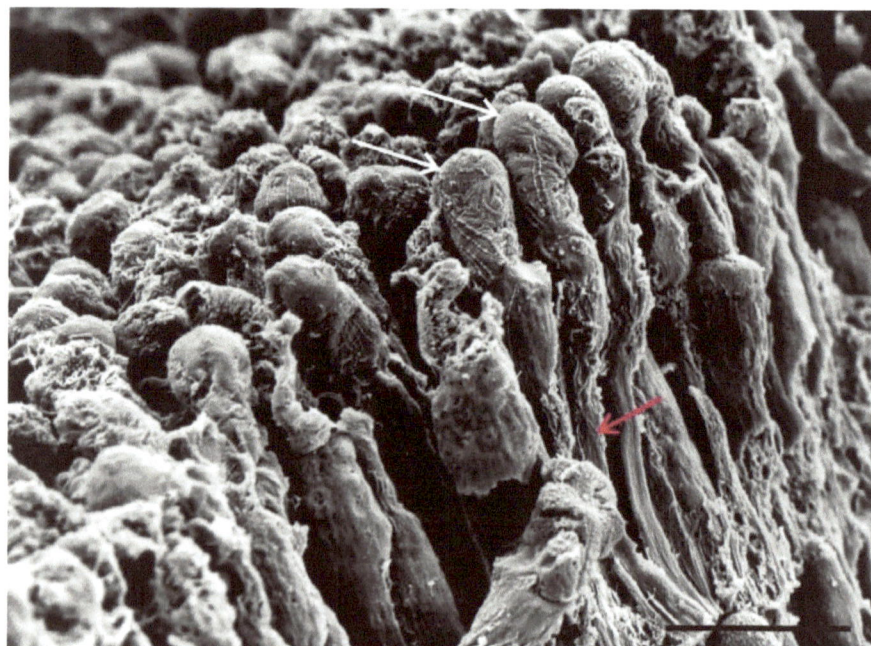

Figure 1.20o.

Another type of cone cells with glove-like outer segments are illustrated (white arrows). This type of cone cells consist of thin and longer proximal inner segments (red arrow). The distal part of the inner segments is dilated. Bar = 10 μm.

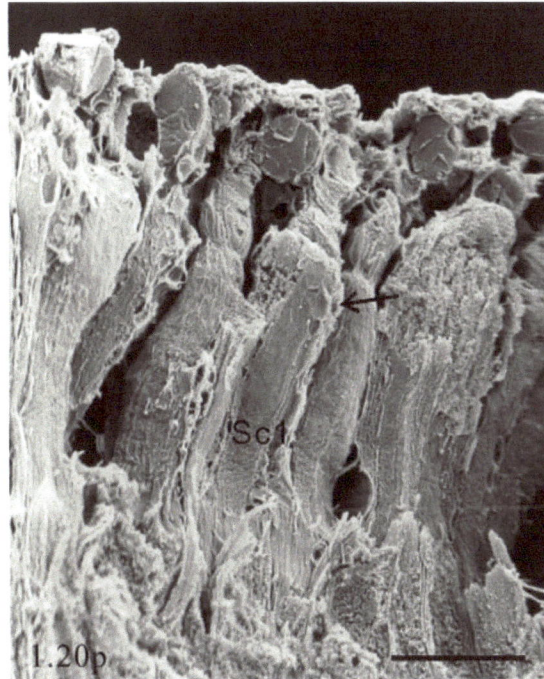

Figure 1.20p.

This figure shows a "Sc1" single cone. Note the bulging part of its distal inner segment (arrow). It contains an oil droplet inside. Bar = 5 μm.

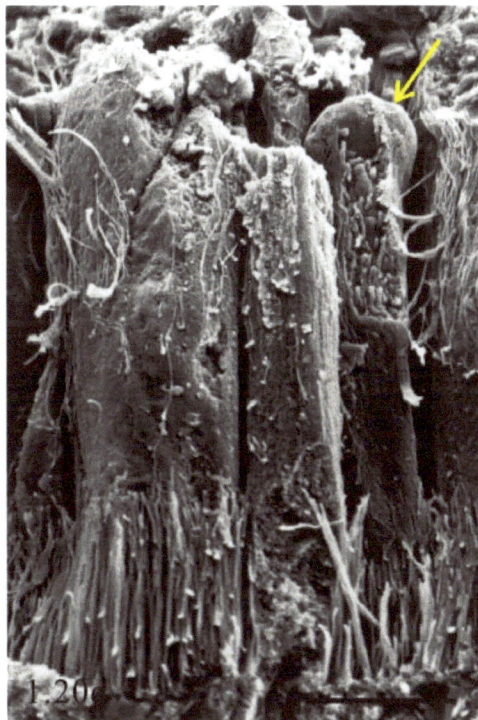

Figure 1.20q.

One single cone in this figure has a broken inner segment with an oil droplet inside (arrow). Bar = 5 μm.

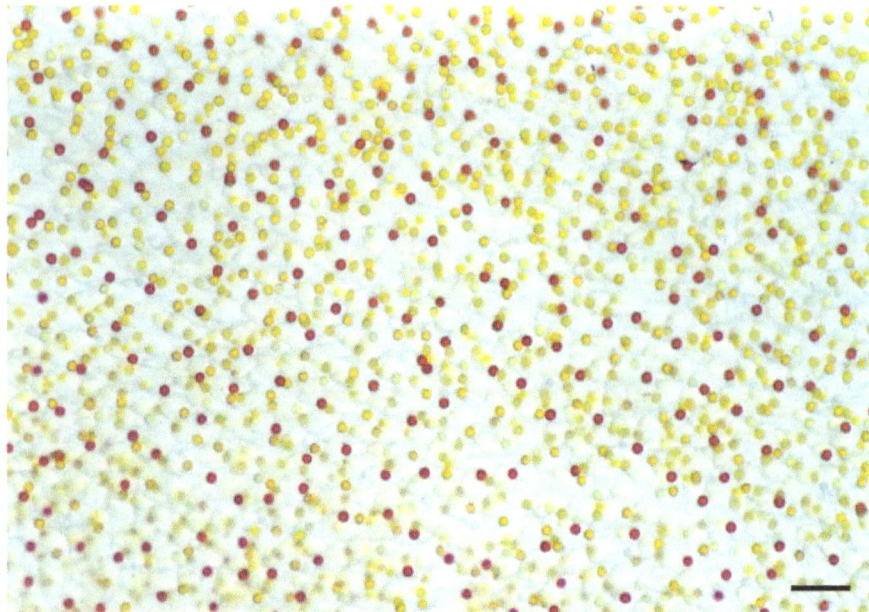

Figure 1.20r.

This figure shows the oil droplets in the cones of the chicken retina. They are in various different colors such as red, green and yellow. Bar = 50 μm.

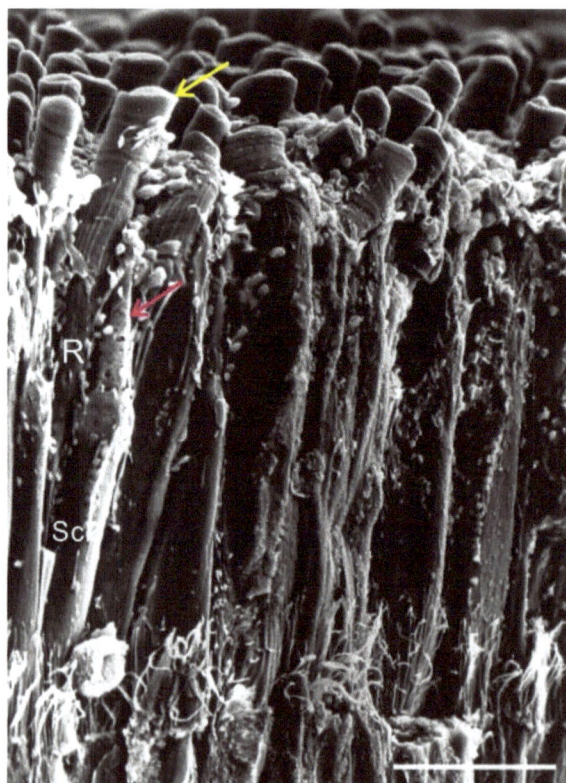

Figure 1.20s.

A rod (R) with a cylindrical outer segment (yellow arrow) is shown. On its right is a "Sc2" type single cone with a tapered outer segment (red arrow). Bar = 10 μm.

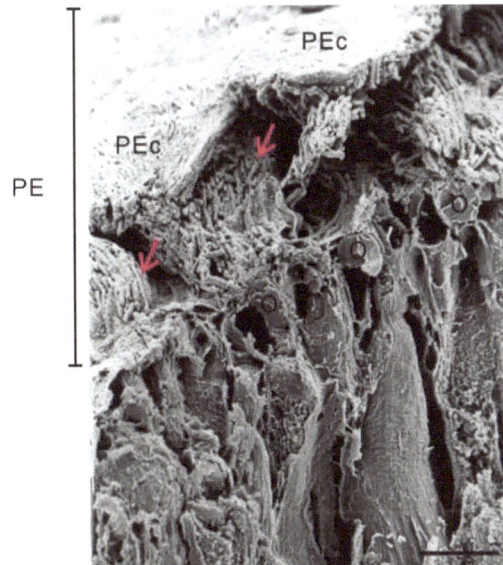

Figure 1.20t.

This figure clearly shows a layer of pigment epithelium (PE) covering the visual cell layer. Note the hexagonal shape of the epithelial cells (PEc) and their processes (red arrows) which intermingle with the outer segments (O) of the visual cells. Bar = 5 μm.

21. COW

Like all other mammals, the cow has a retina composed of thick outer nuclear layer (about 6 layers) and thin inner nuclear layer (about 3 layers). The cell nuclei of the outer nuclear layer are relatively large in size. Like those in the lower vertebrates, double cones are consistently observed. Sometimes multiple cone complexes (containing many cones are also demonstrable.

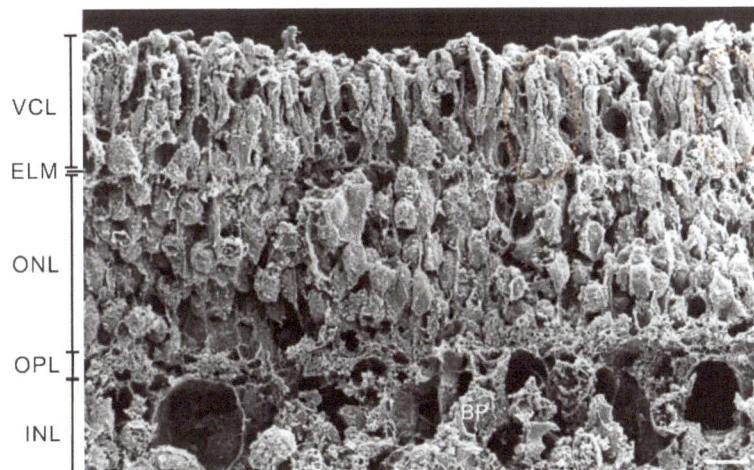

Figure 1.21a.

The retina of the cow revealed by electron scanning microscopy shows two cone complexes (circles). The one on the left is a double cone consisting of chief and accessory cones. The one on the right is a multiple cone. The outer nuclear layer (ONL) is thick and has at least five layers. A bipolar cell (BP) is shown in the inner nuclear layer. Bar = 5 μm.

(ELM - External limiting membrane; INL - Inner nuclear layer; ONL - Outer nuclear layer; OPL - Outer plexiform layer; VCL - Visual cell layer).

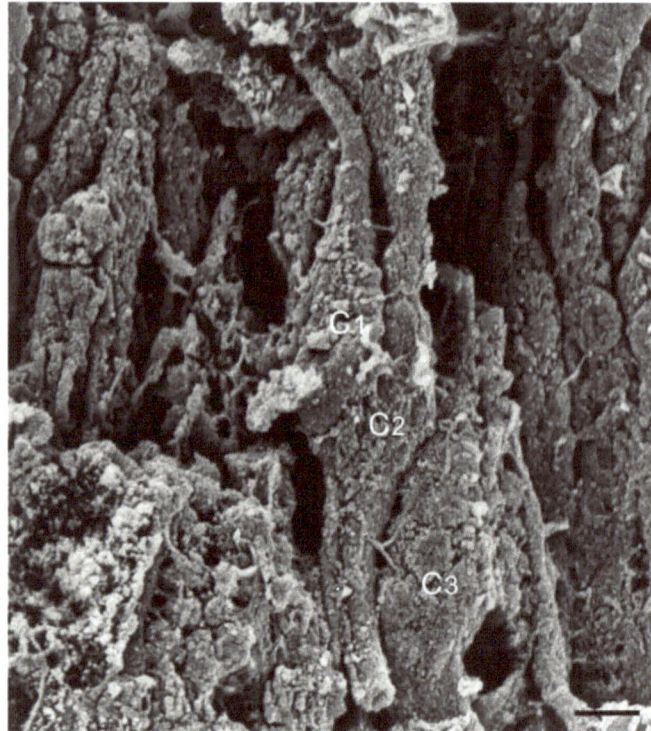

Figure 1.21b.

Enlarged multiple cones from figure 1.21a. Three cones (C1, C2 and C3) of different shapes and sizes are adhered with each other. Bar = 1 µm.

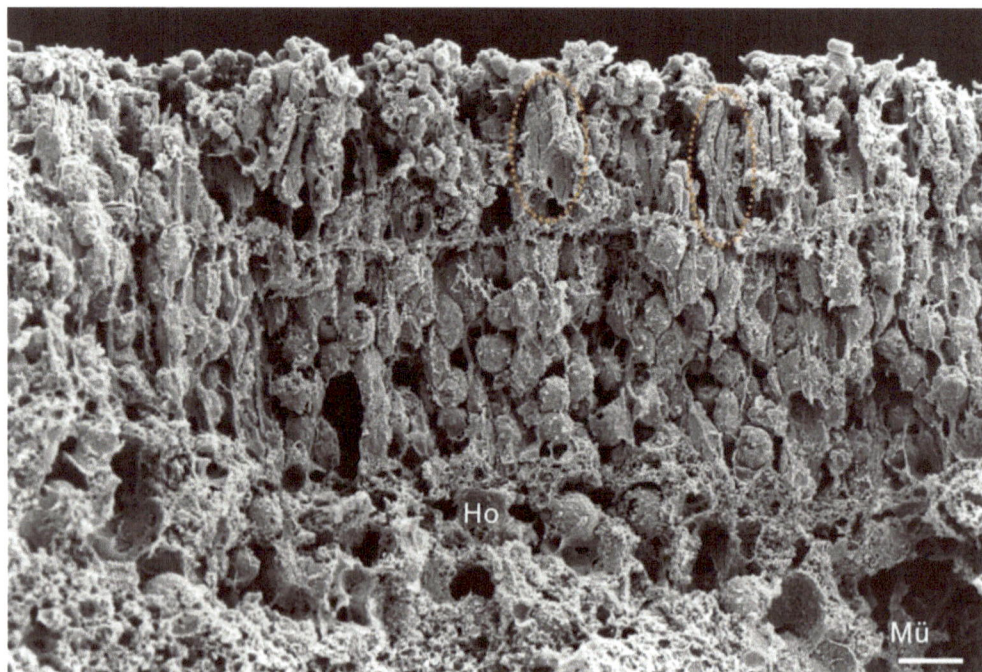

Figure 1.21c.

Multiple cone systems with many cones joined together are seen (circles). "Ho" denotes a horizontal cell and "Mü" indicates a Müller cell, both are located in the inner nuclear layer. Bar = 5 µm.

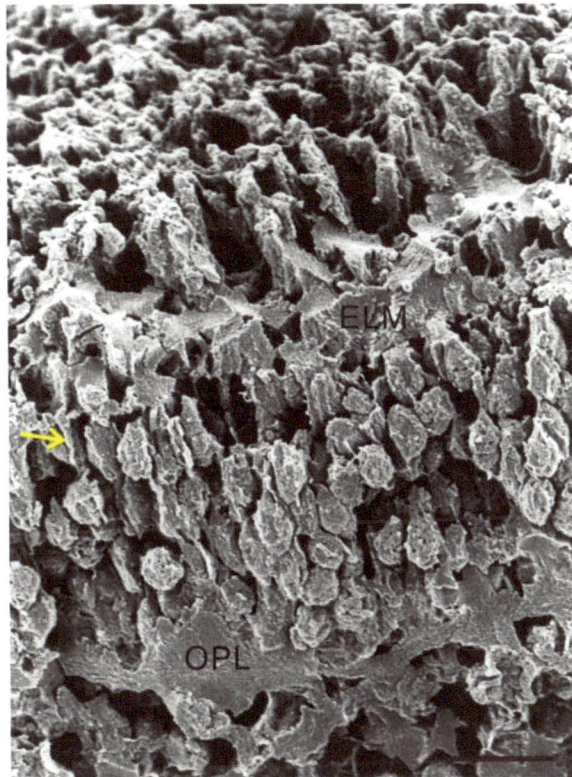

Figure 1.21d.

Large branches of the Müller cells (yellow arrow) intervene in the outer plexiform layer (OPL) and the external limiting membrane (ELM). Bar = 10 μm.

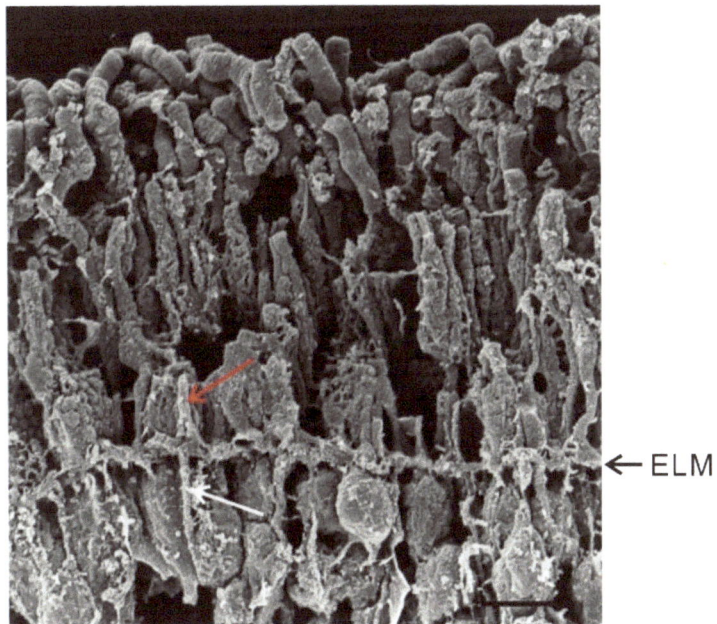

Figure 1.21e.

Note the Müller fibers (white arrow) projecting through the external limiting membrane (ELM) with very long microvilli (red arrow). Bar = 5 μm.

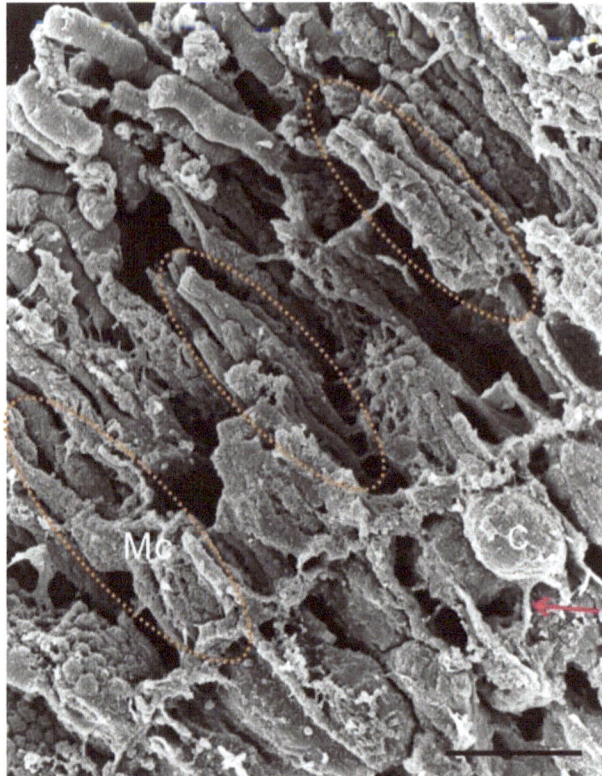

Figure 1.21f.

A few double cones are shown (circles). A cone cell body (C) with a branch ending on the cell body of another cell (red arrow) is also shown. Bar = 5 μm.

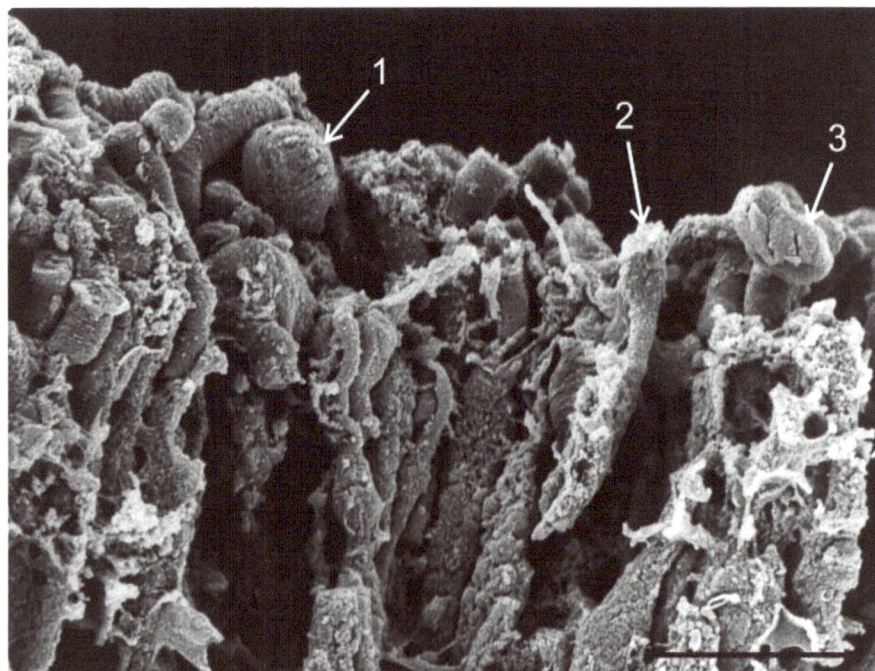

Figure 1.21g.

Note the shedding of ball-like outer segments (1, 2 and 3) of different sizes. Bar = 5 mm.

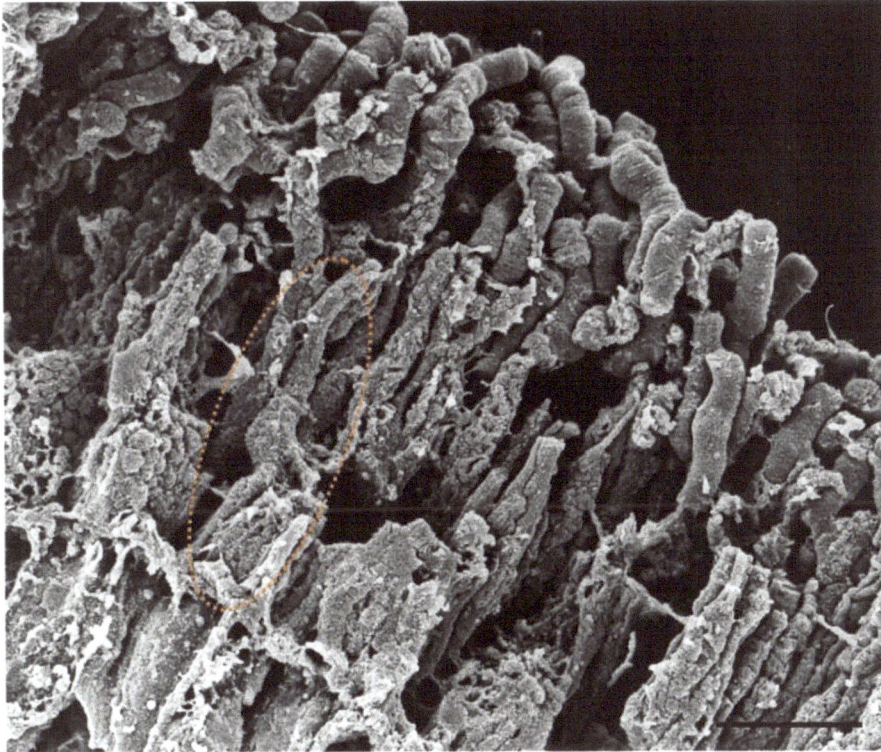

Figure 1.21h.

Circle of a multiple cone consisting of slender cones. Bar = 5 μm.

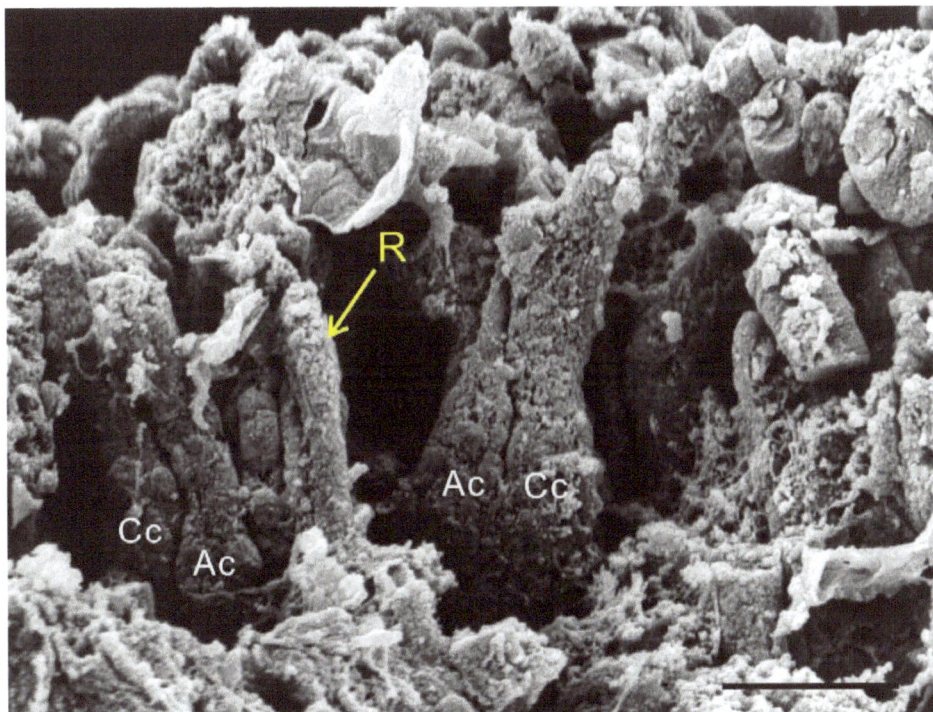

Figure 1.21i.

Accessory (Ac) and chief (Cc) cones of the double cone complex are shown. "R" indicates a rod cell. Bar = 5 μm.

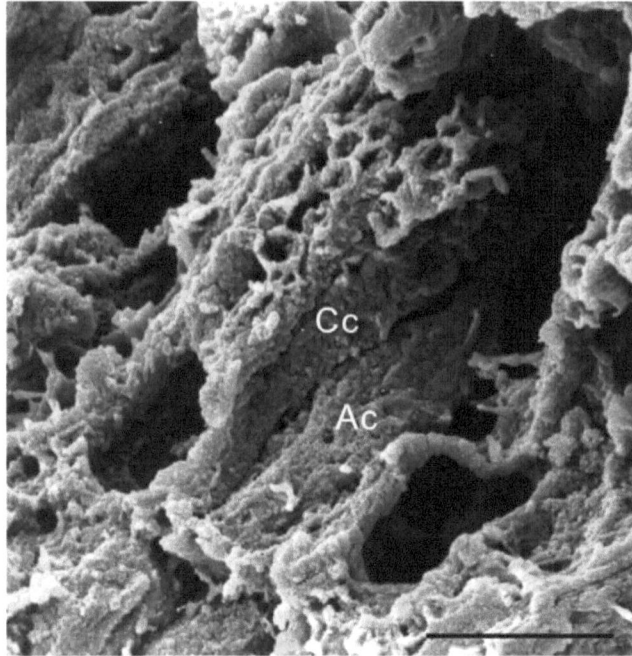

Figure 1.21j.

The proximal inner segments of a double cone. "Cc" denotes a chief cone and "Ac" denotes an accessory cone. Bar = 3 μm.

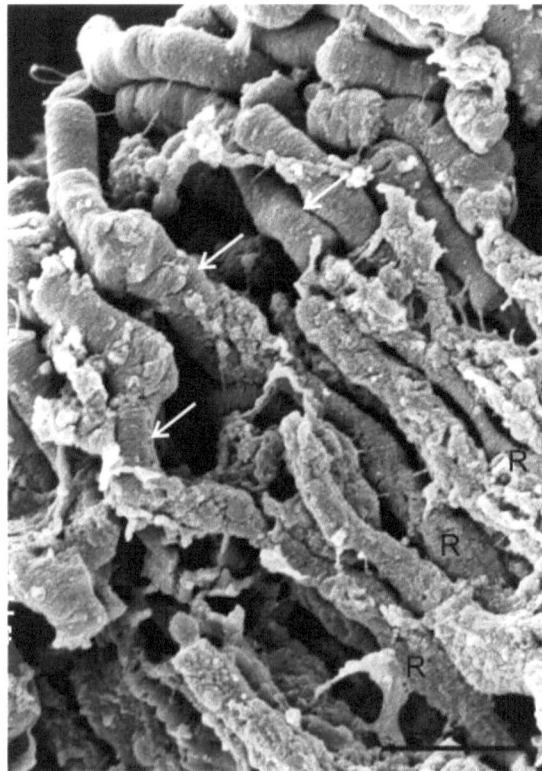

Figure 1.21k.

It is generally observed that the rod cells (R) have longer outer segments (white arrows). Bar = 3 μm.

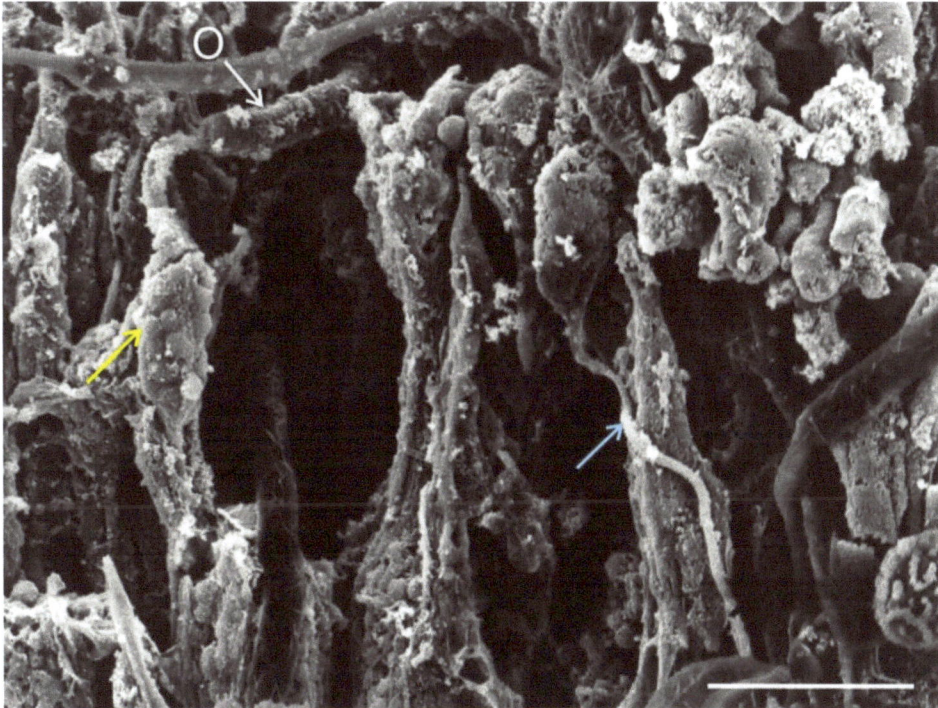

Figure 1.21l.

A type of cone cell consisting of a very long and thin inner segment with an enlarged distal end is noted (light blue arrow). On the left, there is a visual cell (yellow arrow) with a long and rod-like outer segment (O), suggesting it is a rod cell. Bar = 5 μm.

22. ARABIAN CAMEL

The retina of the arabian camal displays very large and obvious ganglion cells with conspicuous axons. The outer nuclear layer is thicker than the inner nuclear layer. The retina is mixed with rods and cones.

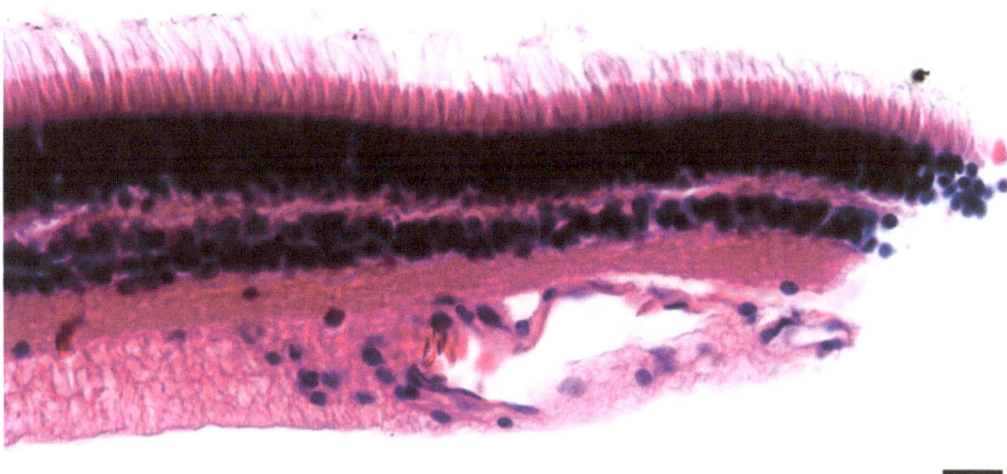

Figure 1.22a. *Anterior retina.*

This figure shows the anterior region of a camel retina. Like most of the animals, the visual cells in this region are shorter in height. However, there is no change in terms of cell density. Bar = 30 μm.

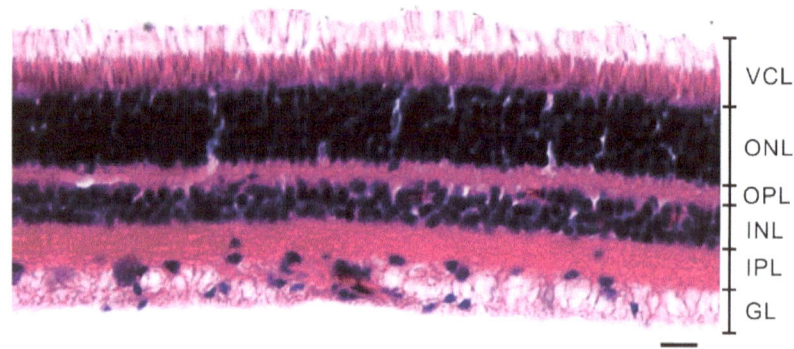

Figure 1.22b. *Peripheral retina.*

Different retinal layers are illustrated. Note the thick outer nuclear layer which is made up of about 5 to 6 layers of cell nuclei. The inner nuclear layer is thinner and consists of fewer cells compared to the outer nuclear layer. Bar = 30 μm.

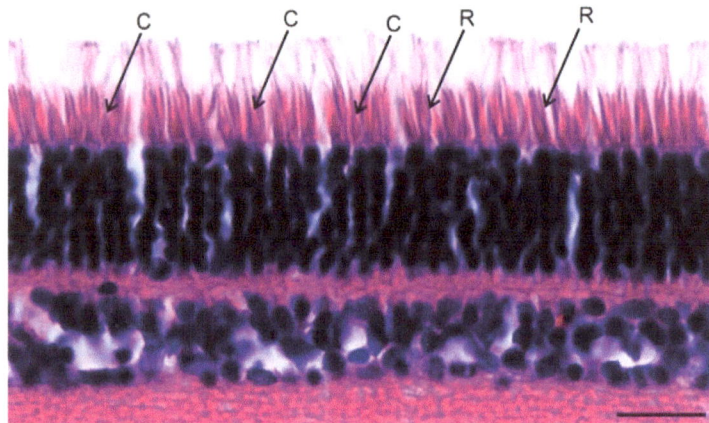

Figure 1.22c. *Peripheral retina.*

In this animal, two major types of visual cells are noted, cone (C) cells and rod cells (R). The cones appear as flask-shaped whereas the rods are long and cylindrical in shape. Bar = 20 μm.

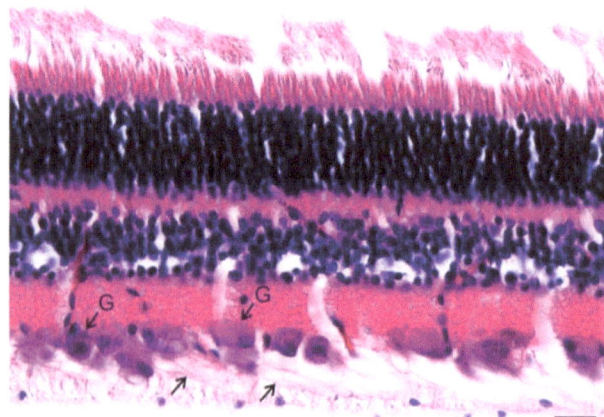

Figure 1.22d. *Central retina.*

The density of visual cells does not change obviously in the peripheral and central region of the retina. In this figure, large ganglion cells (G) and their axons are clearly illustrated (arrows). Bar =20 μm.

23. DOG

The dog's retina is similar to those of the pig in that the inner nuclear layer is only one third the thickness of the outer nuclear layer. There are, however, more ganglion cells than those of the pig. In the visual cells, some outer segments are shaped like boxer gloves and the cilia linking inner and outer segments are usually long and thick. Double cones are also observed in this species.

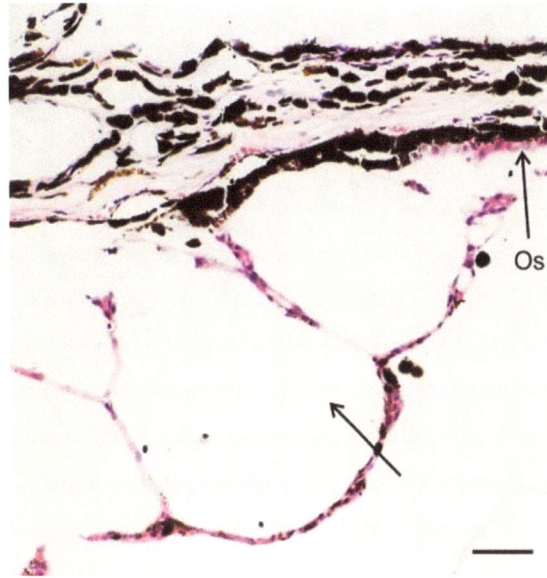

Figure 1.23a. *Ora serrata.*

Beyond the ora serrata (Os) of the dog retina, there are large spaces (arrow). Bar = 50 μm.

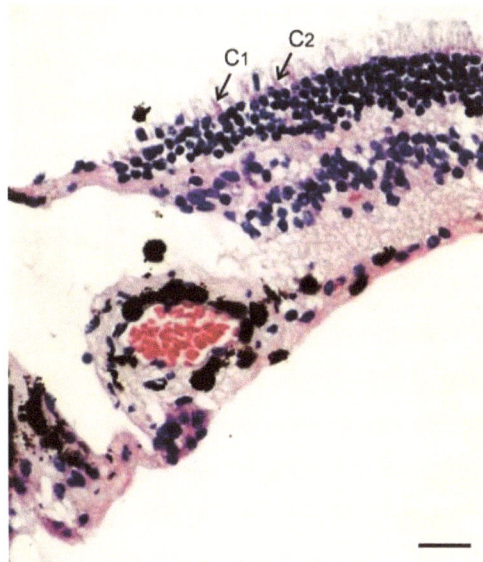

Figure 1.23b. *Near ora serrata.*

The area near the ora serrata shows few number of visual cells. Some are cone cells of different types (C1 and C2). Bar = 50 μm.

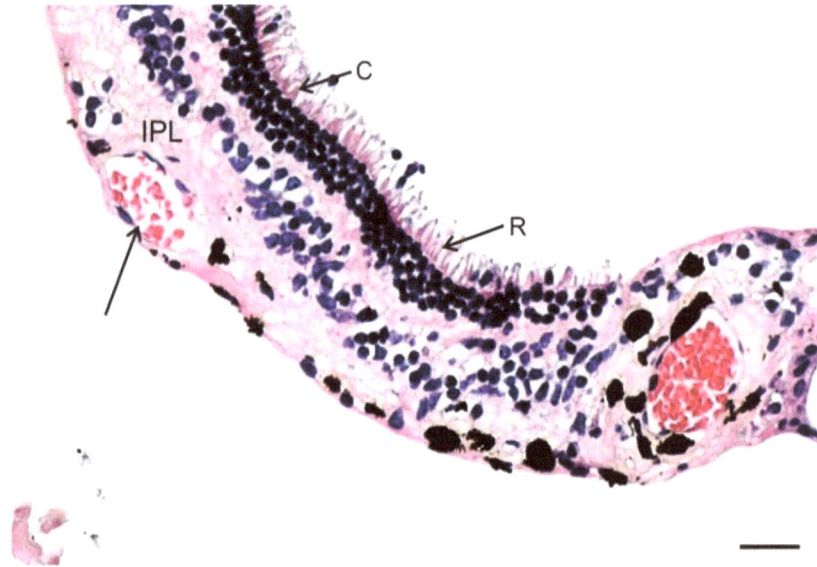

Figure 1.23c. *Anterior retina.*

There is a gradual decrease in the number of visual cells in the anterior retina towards the ora serrata. Some rod (R) cells with elongated inner segments and some cone (C) cells with pear shaped inner segments are noted. The arrow indicates a vessel in the inner plexiform layer (IPL). Bar = 50 μm.

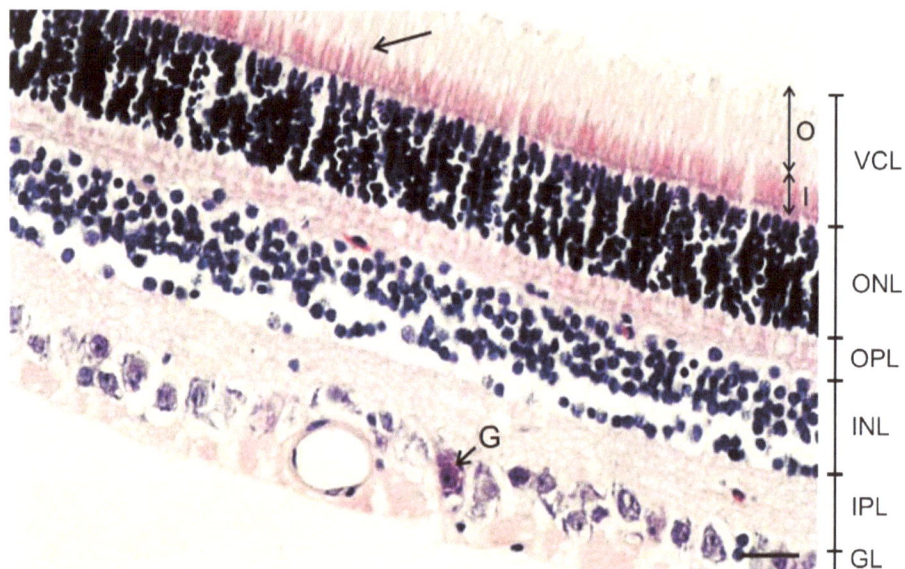

Figure 1.23d. *Peripheral retina.*

The peripheral retina of the dog shows a dense layer of visual cells (VCL). Some rods (arrow) are noted amongst the different visual cells. In this animal, the visual cell outer (O) and inner (I) segments can be clearly identified even under light microscope. The ganglion cells (G) in the innermost layer are large with prominent nucleoli, and they are densely situated. Bar = 50 μm.

(GL - Ganglion cell layer; INL - Inner nuclear layer; IPL - Inner plexiform layer; ONL - Outer nuclear layer; OPL - Outer plexiform layer; VCL - Visual cell layer).

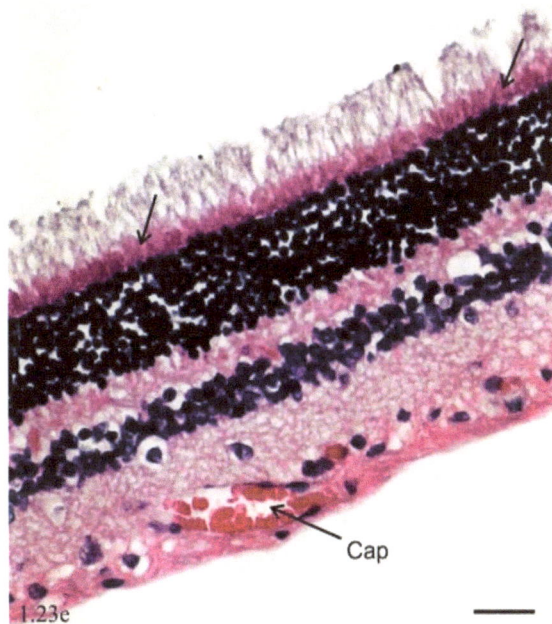

Figures 1.23e and 1.23f. *Central retina.*

The central retina shows a lot of cone cells (arrow) with pear shaped inner segments. Prominent small blood vessels (Cap) are seen in both inner nuclear and ganglion cell nerve fiber layers. Bar = 50 μm.

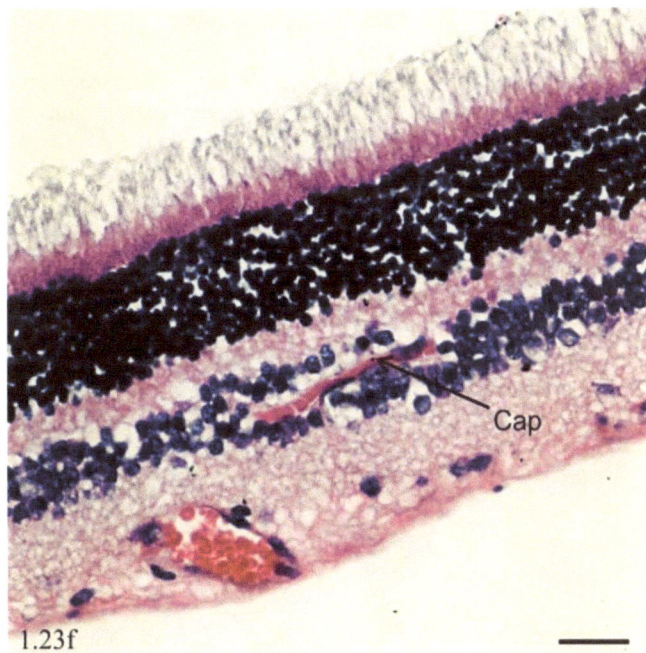

Figure 1.23g.

Under scanning electron microscopy, two kinds of rod cells (R1 and R2) in the retina of the dog are noted. Moreover, this micrograph illustrates their outer segments (green arrows) at different stages of maturation and/or shedding. Bar = 5 μm.

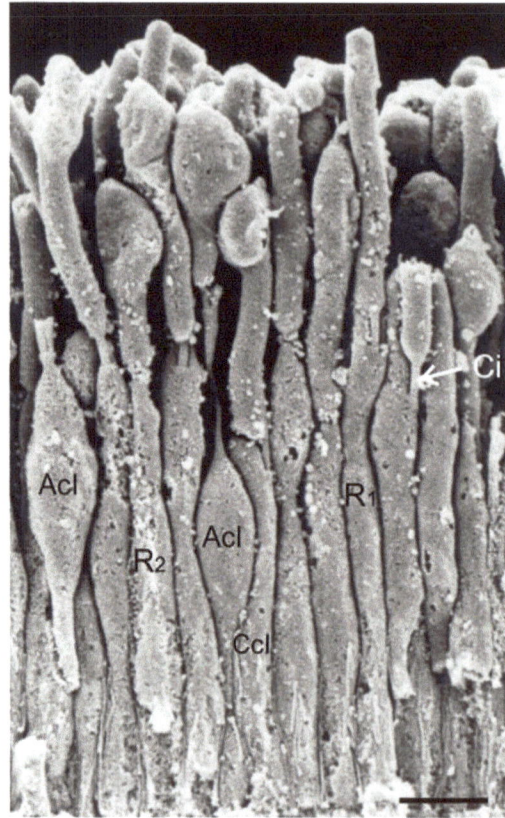

Figure 1.23h.

The retina of the dog shows numerous rods (R1 and R2) and cones. The accessory cones (AcI) have torch-shaped inner segments. "CcI" is the chief cone inner segment. "Ci" denotes the cilium. Bar = 5 μm.

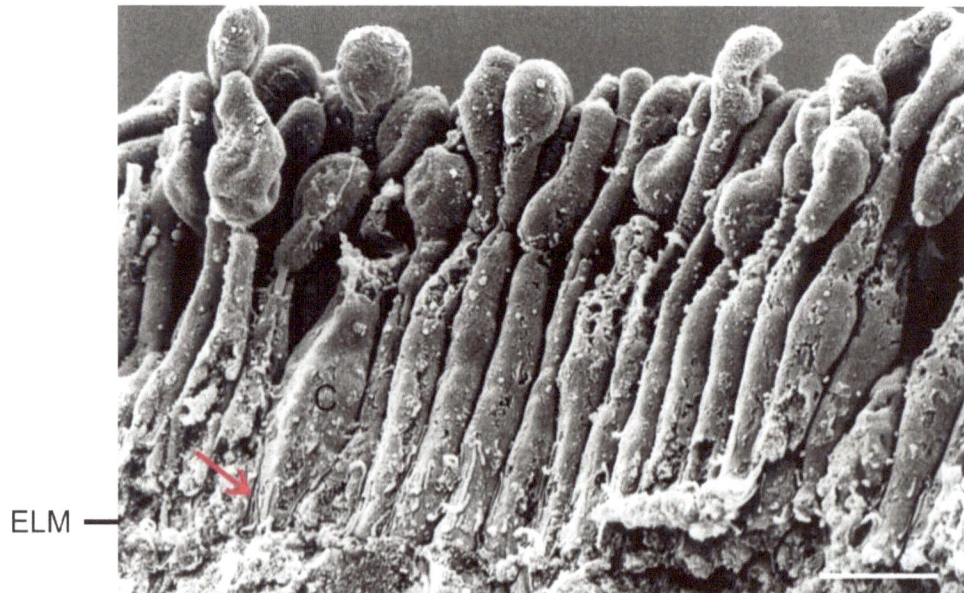

Figure 1.23i.

Yet another cone (C) of the dog with a rhomboid shaped inner segment is shown. There are fewer microvilli (red arrow) from the external limiting membrane (ELM) in this animal. Bar = 3 μm.

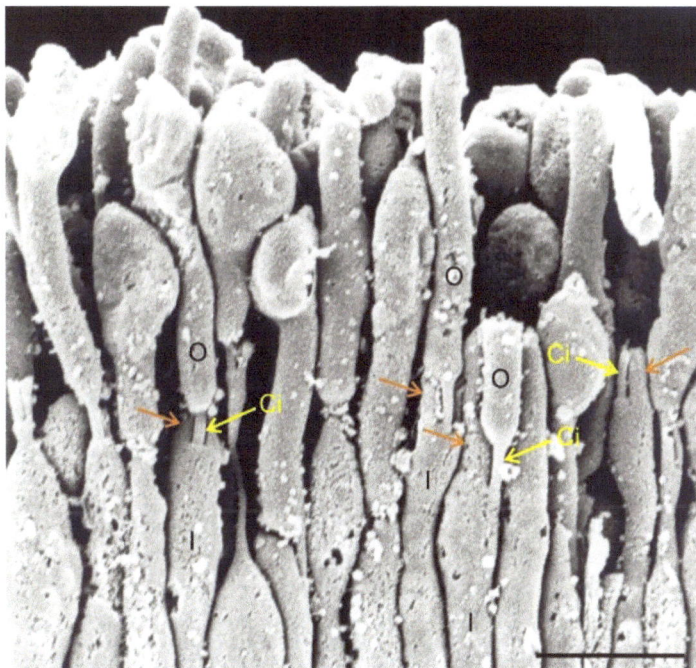

Figure 1.23j.

Visual cells of the dog's retina showing outer segment (O), inner segment (I) and calyce (orange arrows). Calyce is a flap of tissue on the side of the photoreceptor. "Ci" denotesthe cilia growing from the inner segments. Bar = 3 μm.

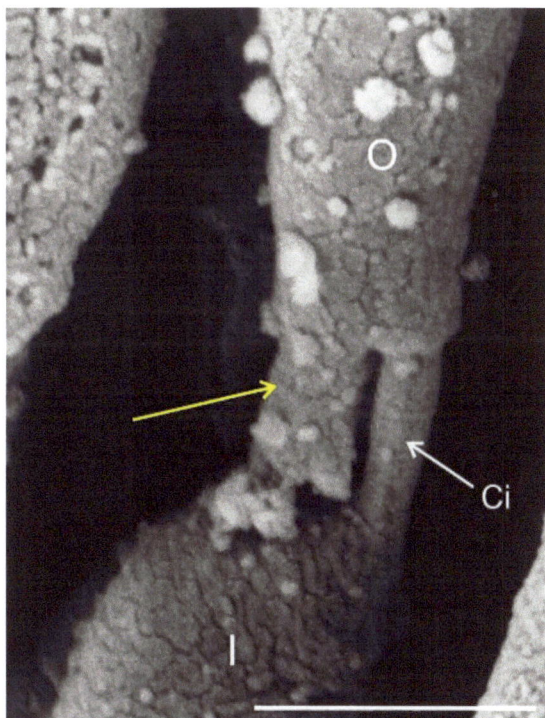

Figure 1.23k.

A high power view of the previous diagram showing the outer segment (O), inner segment (I), calyce (yellow arrow), and cilium (Ci). Bar = 1 μm.

24. CAT

The retina of the cat has conspicuous Müller cells. The outer nuclear layer is again about three times thicker than the inner nuclear layer. The nuclei of the outer nuclear layer are large and oriented longitudinally. There are many types of visual cells including double cone, single cone, and rod.

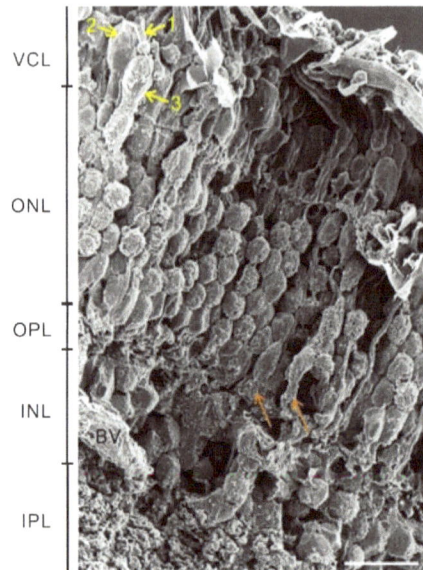

Figure 1.24a.

A double cone in the retina of the cat with components 1 and 2 while a single cone cell 3 is in front. Arrows point to the spherules of the synapses of rod. The outer plexiform layer (OPL) is thin while the inner plexform layer (IPL) is thick. Huge blood vessels (BV) traverse the inner nuclear layer (INL) and the inner plexiform layer (IPL).Bar = 10 μm.

(INL - Inner nuclear layer; IPL - Inner plexiform layer; ONL - Outer nuclear layer; OPL - Outer plexiform layer; VCL - Visual cell layer).

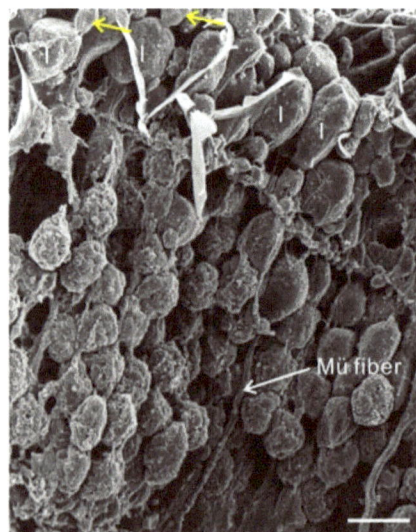

Figure 1.24b.

Note the small round to oval shapes of the inner segments (I) of cones in the cat. They have small outer segments (yellow arrows). "Mü" denotes a Müller cell fiber in the outer nuclear layer. Bar = 5 μm.

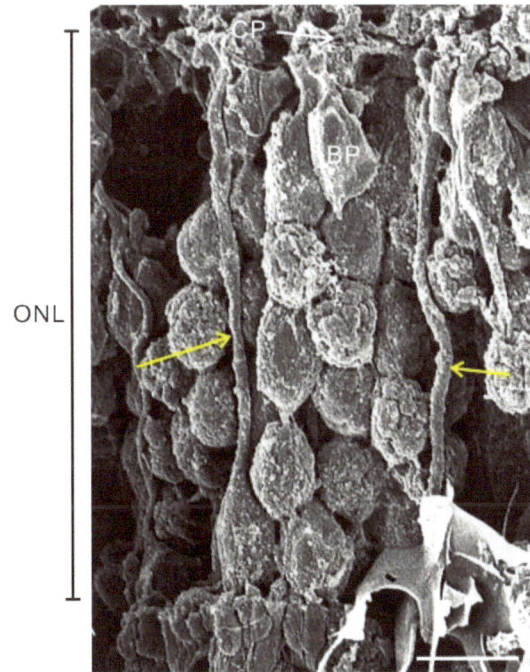

Figure 1.24c.

This figure shows the outer nuclear layer (ONL). The Müller cell processes are long and thick as indicated (yellow arrows). "Mü" indicates Müller cell bodies. "BP" indicates a bipolar with processes going to a cone pedicle (CP). Bar = 5 μm.

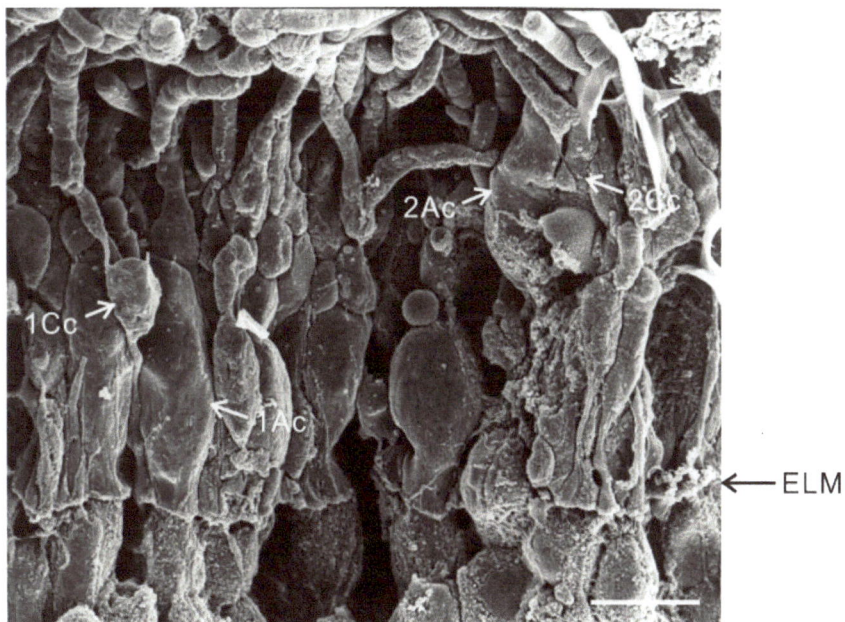

Figure 1.24d.

The cat has keen vision and thus morphologically there may be different types of double cones. "1Ac" is an accessory cone and "1Cc" is a chief cone, comprising type 1 double cones. "2Ac" and "2Cc" belong to an accessory cone and a chief cone comprising type 2 double cones. Most chief cones have long stalks. Bar = 10 μm.

(ELM - External limiting membrane).

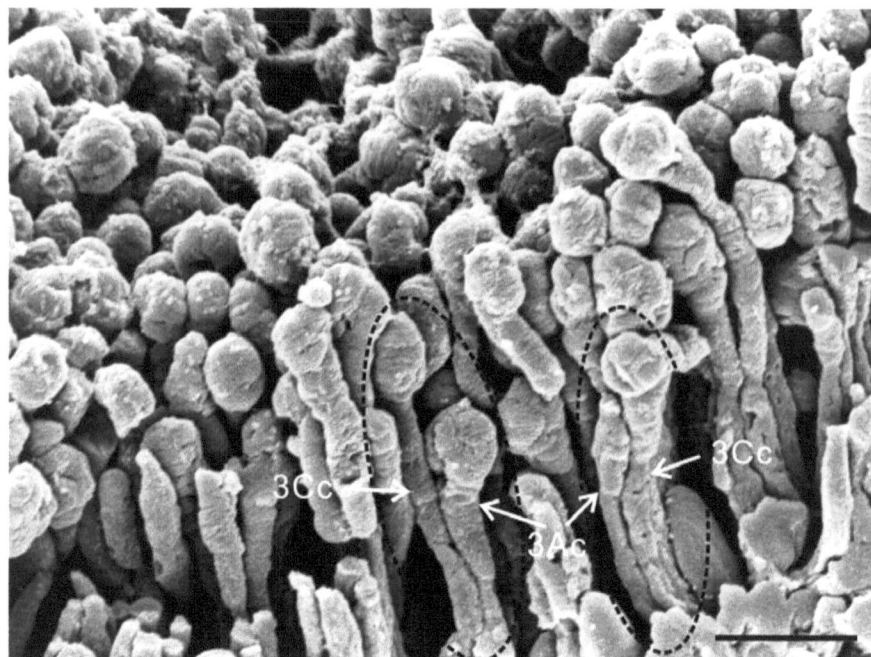

Figure 1.24e.

Type 3 chief cones (3Cc) and accessory cones (3Ac) are both slender. Two are circled in this figure. Bar = 10 μm.

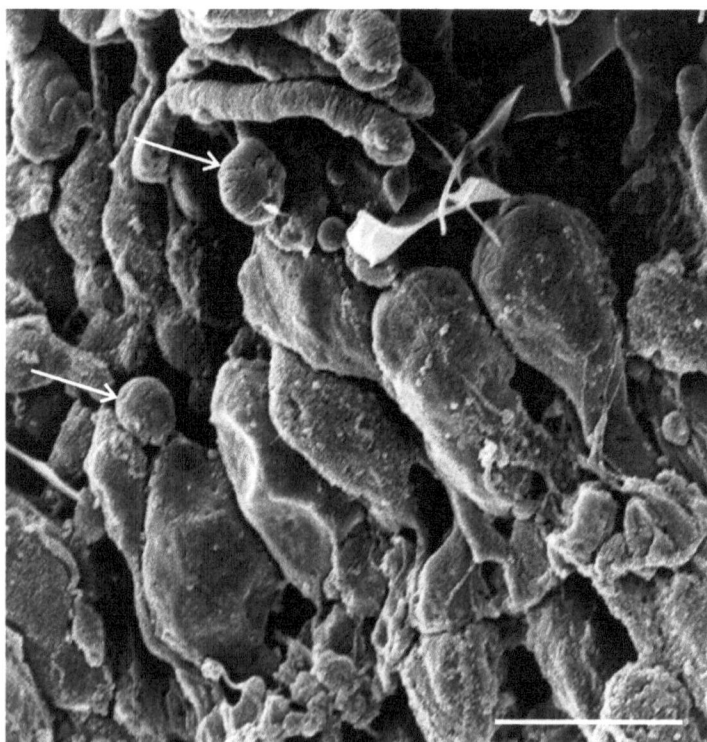

Figure 1.24f.

Some cones have ball-like outer segments (white arrows). Bar = 5 μm.

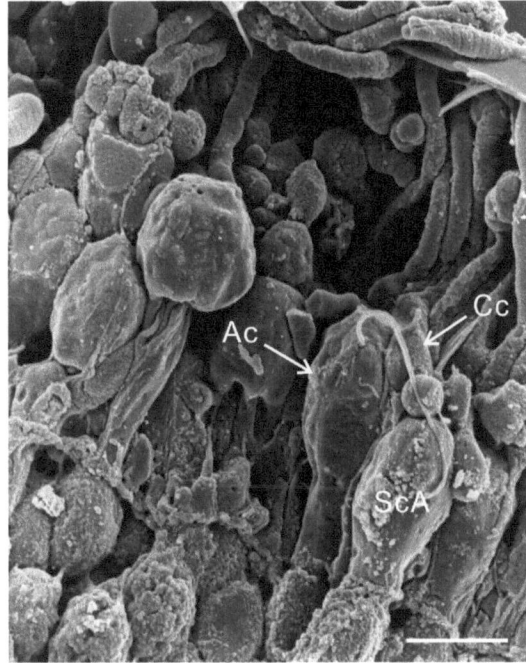

Figure 1.24g.

The type A single cone (ScA) in this figure has ball-like outer segment. A double cone is located lateral to the type A single cone. "Ac" denotes the accessory cone component and "Cc" denotes the chief cone component. Bar = 5 μm.

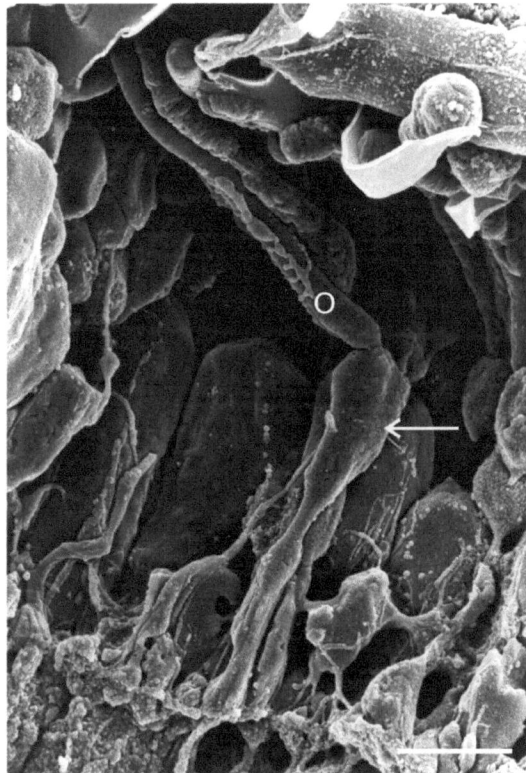

Figure 1.24h.

A rod (white arrow) with long outer segment (O) is seen. Bar = 3 μm.

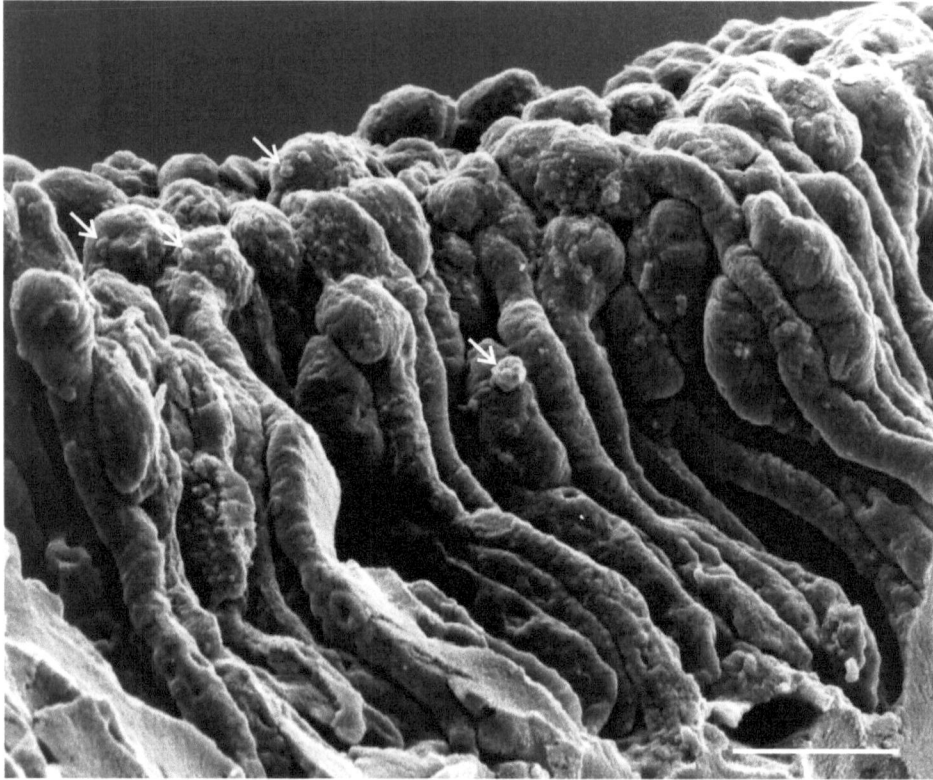

Figure 1.24i.

Many protrusions of various sizes can be observed on the surface of the dilated tip of the outer segments (white arrows). Bar = 3 μm.

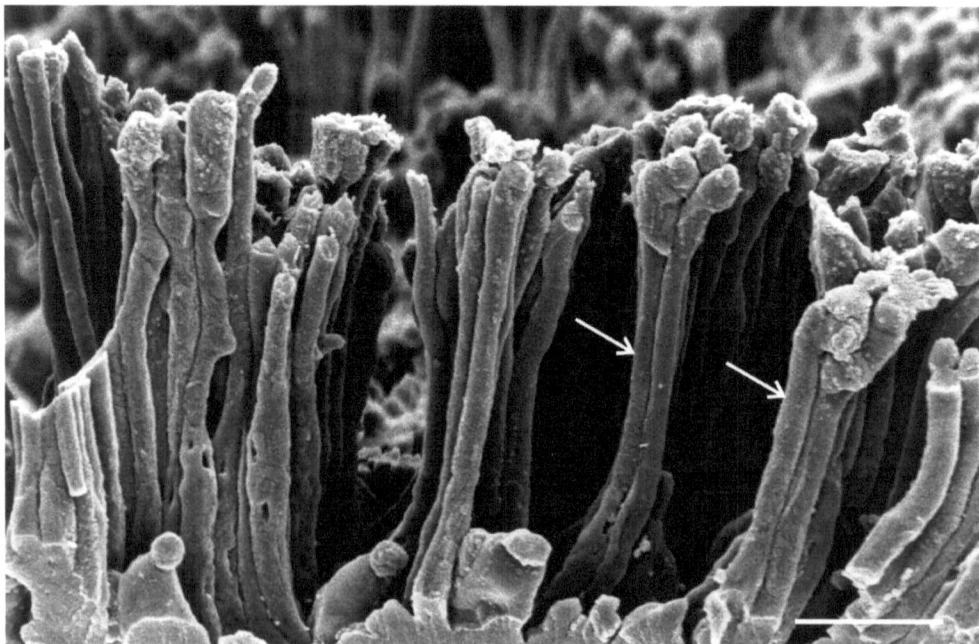

Figure 1.24j.

Two groups of duplex rod cells adhere tightly together (white arrows). Are these the remnant of twin rods in the lower species? Bar = 5 μm.

25. MONKEY

Monkey has retina consisting of more rods than cones. The outer nuclear layer is thicker (about 6 to7 rows of cells) than the inner nuclear layer. Several types of cones are observable as that of the lower species.

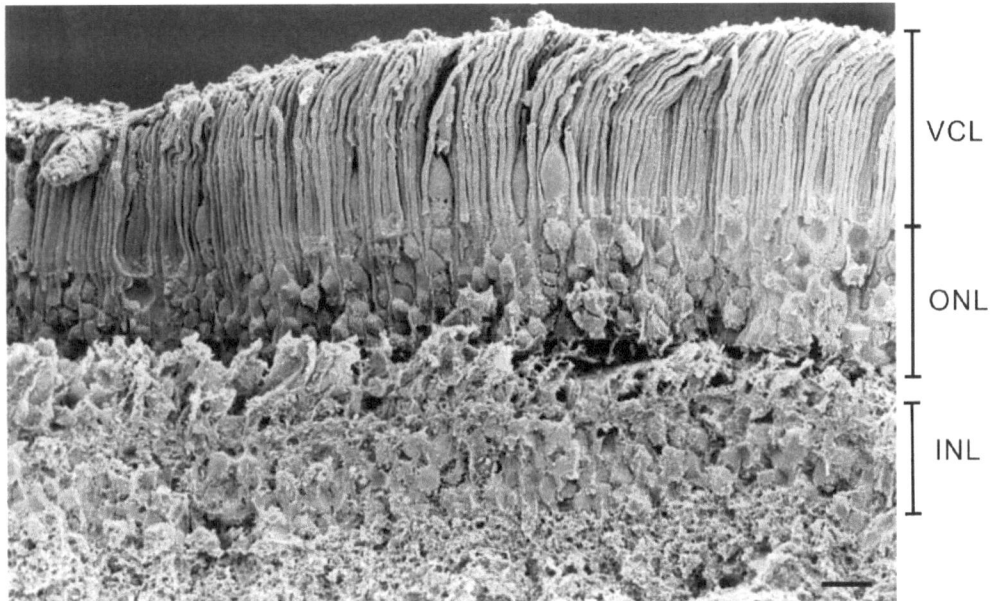

Figure 1.25a.

Scanning electron microscopy shows the retina of a monkey at the mid-peripheral region. The visual cell layer (VCL) is highly packed with different types of photoreceptors. There are about 6 rows of cell bodies in the outer nuclear layer (ONL) and 4 rows of cell bodies in the inner nuclear layer (INL). Bar = 10μm.

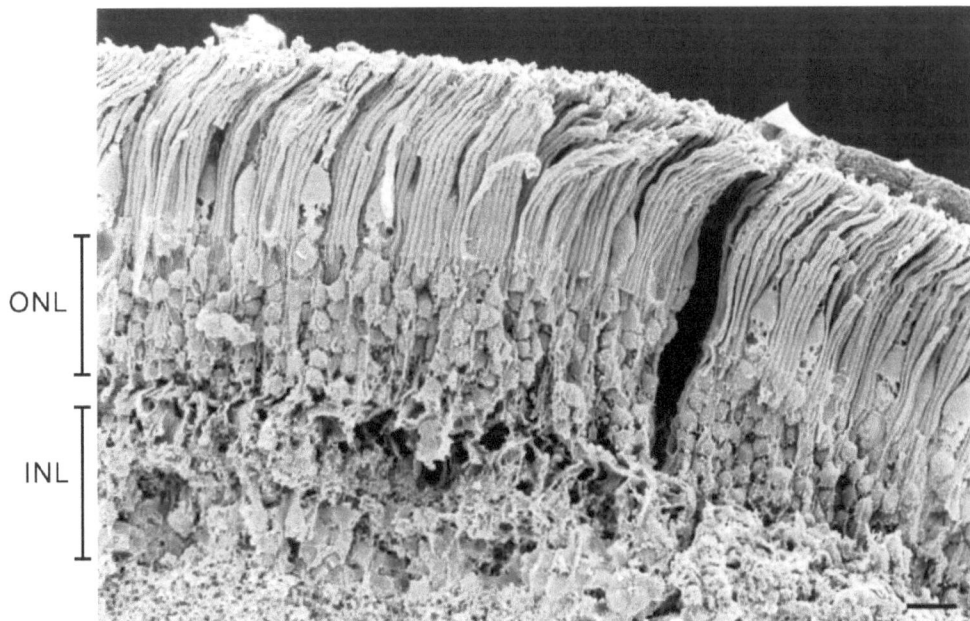

Figure 1.25b.

The central retina of the monkey has 7 layers of cell bodies in the outer nuclear layer (ONL) and 6 layers of cell bodies in the inner nuclear layer (INL). Bar = 10 μm.

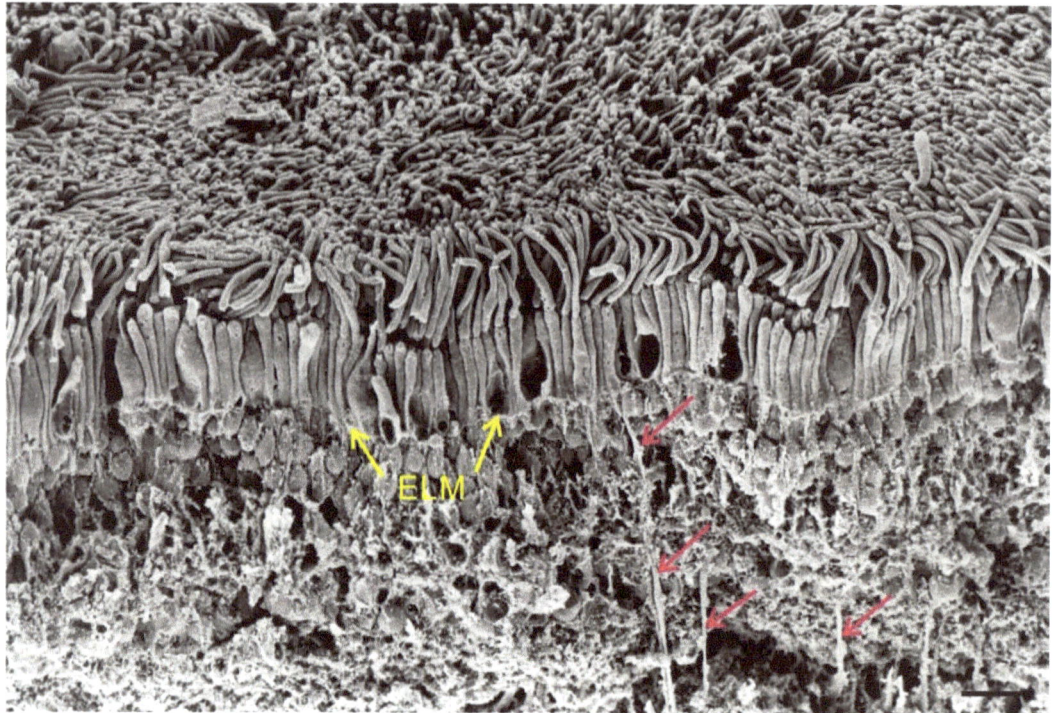

Figure 1.25c.

The monkey retina shows ascending fibers of glial cells (Müller cells) (red arrows) going to form the external limiting membrane (ELM). Bar = 10 μm.

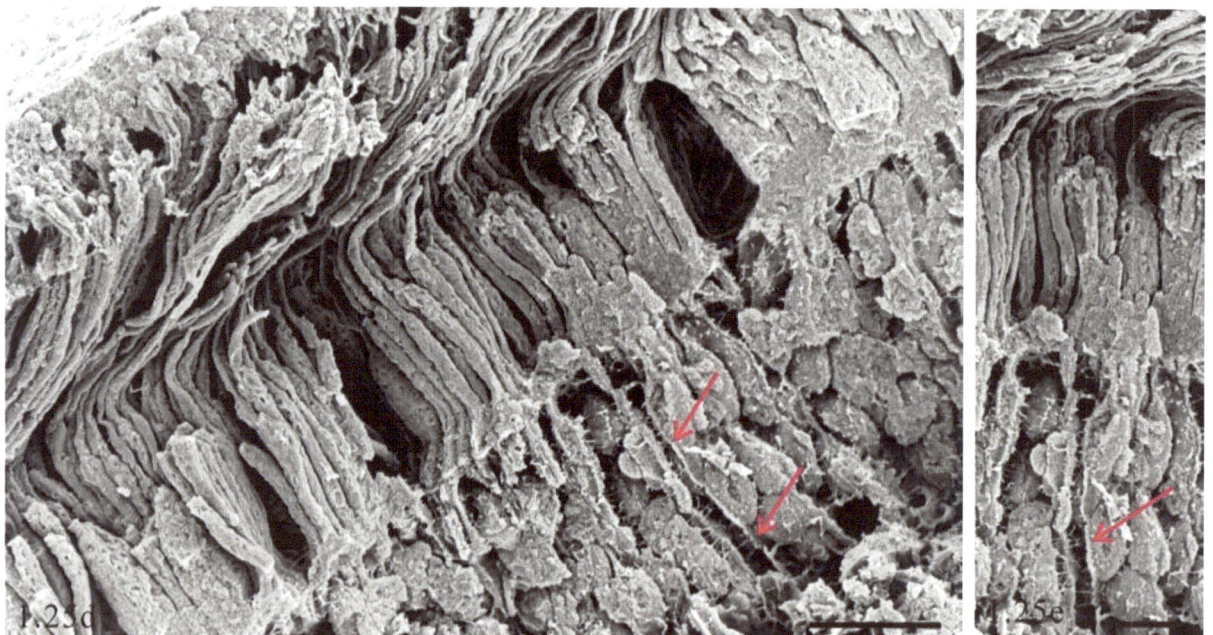

Figures 1.25d and 1.25e.

The Müller cell bodies in the inner nuclear layer are leaf-like in morphology in the monkey retina. The red arrows indicate the long fibers of the Müller cells. Note the spiny processes on the surface of those fibers. Bar = 10 μm.

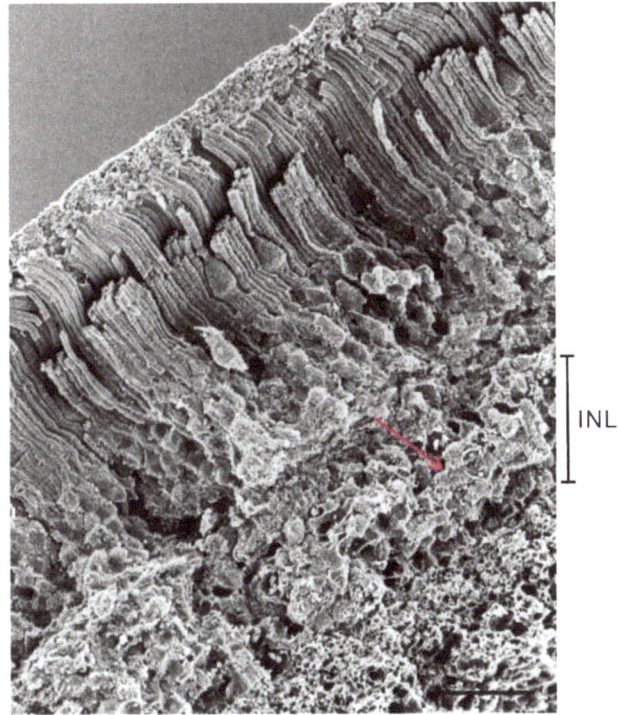

Figure 1.25f.

Müller cell bodies in the inner nuclear layer (INL) are leaf-like (red arrow). Bar = 20 μm.

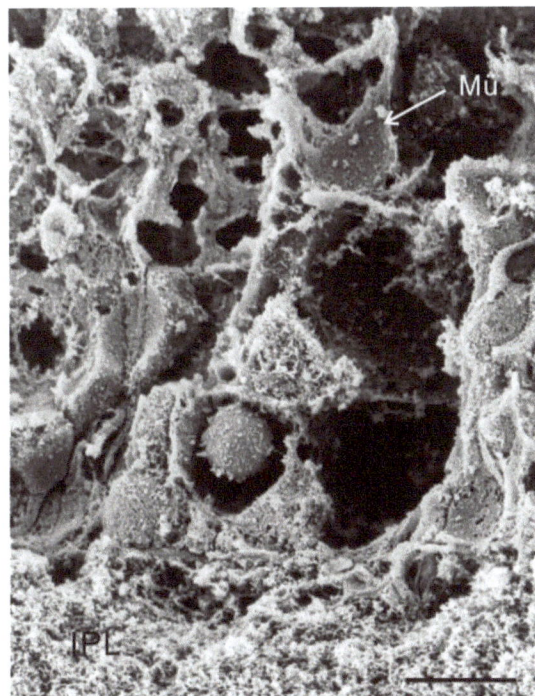

Figure 1.25g.

A higher power shows the leaf-like morphology of the cell body of the Müller cell (Mü). Bar = 5 μm.

(IPL - Inner plexiform layer).

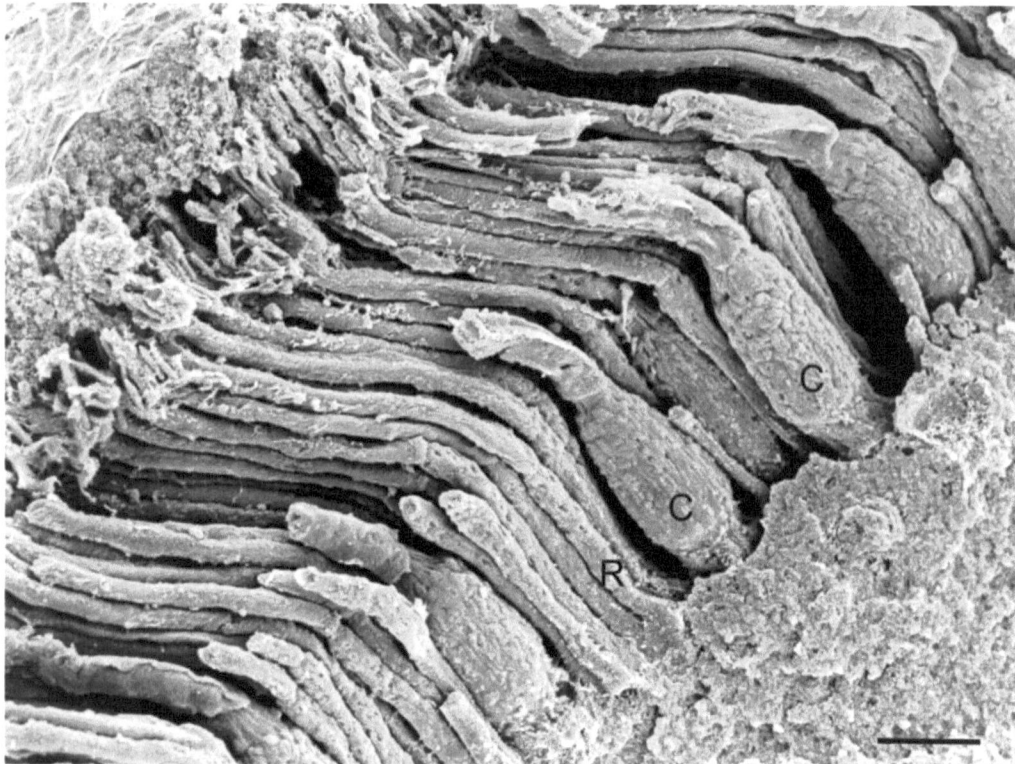

Figure 1.25h.

Note the presence of the cones (C) and rods (R) in the monkey. Bar = 5 μm.

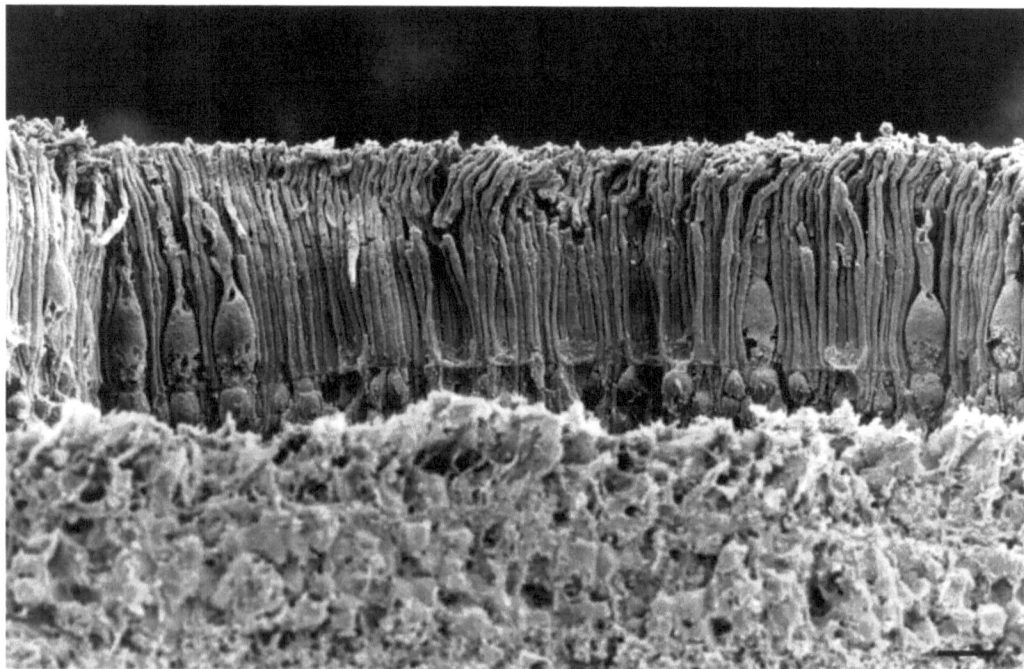

Figure 1.25i.

At a lower magnification, the variation between the number of cones and rods is apparent. More rods than cones are present. Bar = 10 μm.

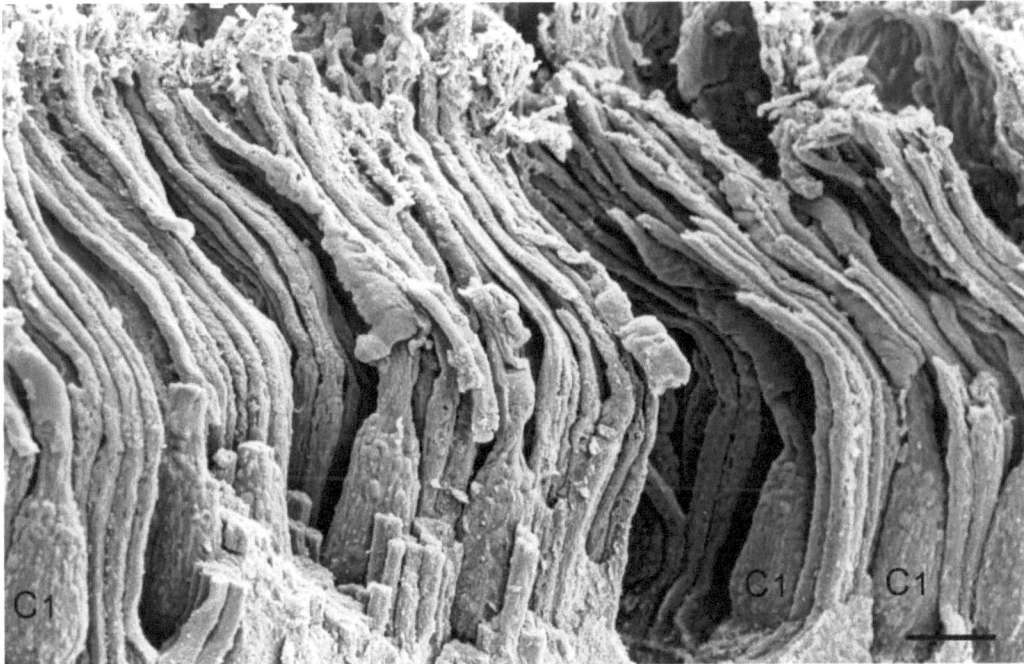

Figure 1.25j.

One type of cones here are labeled as "C1" (type 1 single cone) with an elongated body and a slender outer segment. Bar = 5 μm.

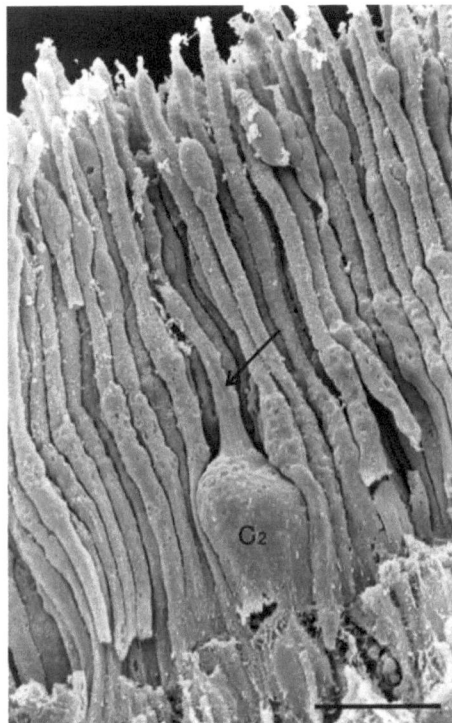

Figure 1.25k.

This figure shows a "C2" (type 2 single cone) with a more spherical cell body and a thin long outer segment (arrow). Bar = 10 μm.

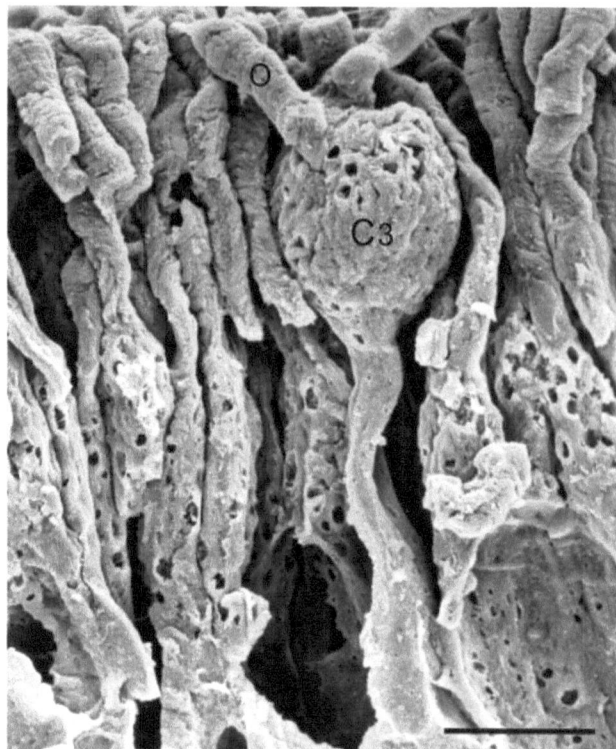

Figure 1.25l.

This figure shows a "C3" (type 3 single cone) with elongated part of the inner segment and an average sized outer segment (O). Note the large dilation on distal inner segment. Bar = 5 μm.

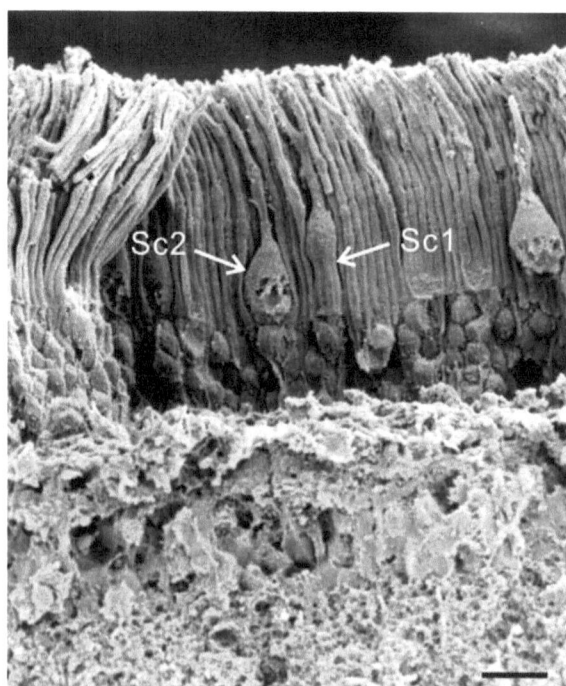

Figure 1.25m.

Both type 1 (Sc1) and type 2 (Sc2) single cones are present in this region of the monkey retina. Bar = 10 μm.

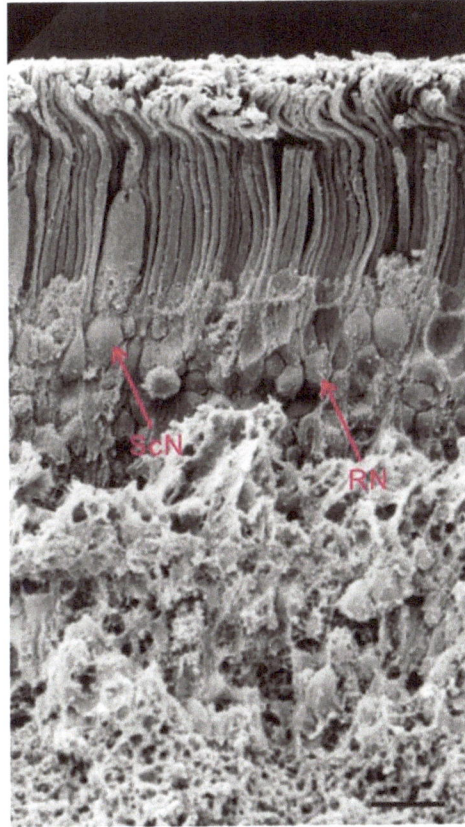

Figure 1.25n.

This figure shows the cell nuclei of a single cone (ScN) and a rod (RN) inside the outer nuclear layer. Bar = 10 μm.

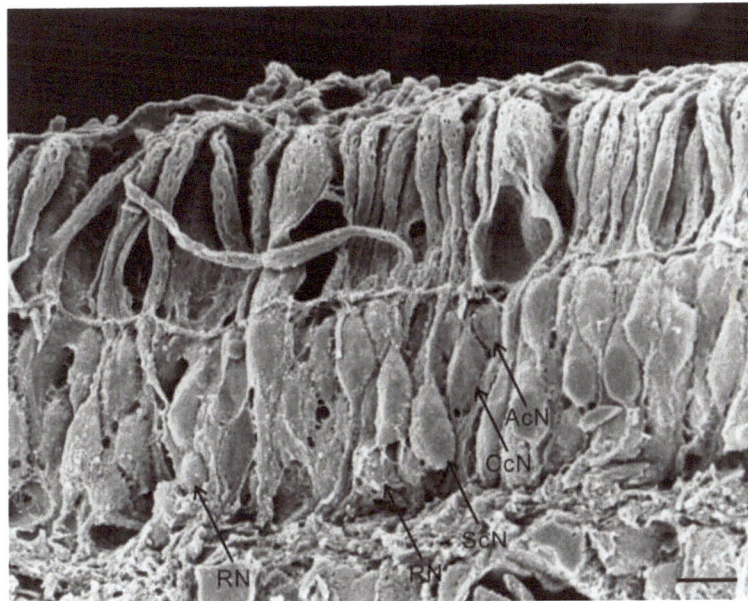

Figure 1.25o.

Nuclei positions of the rods (RN), single cones (ScN), accessory cone (AcN) and chief cone (CcN) are shown. Bar = 5 μm.

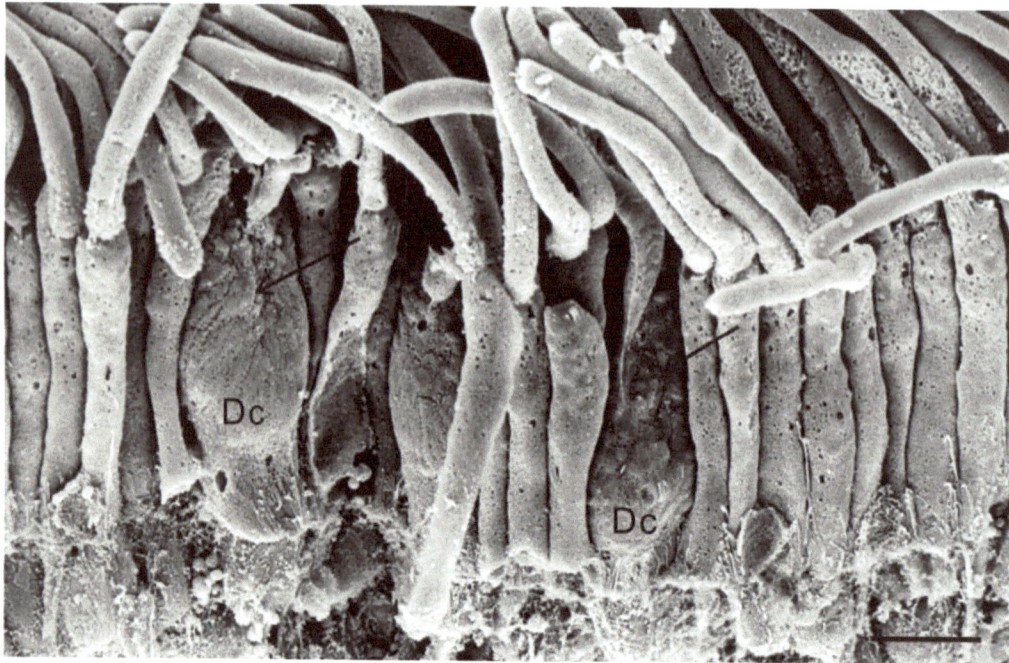

Figure 1.25p.

Double cone cells (Dc) in the periphery of the monkey retina. Note the boundary between the two components (yellow arrows). Bar = 5 μm.

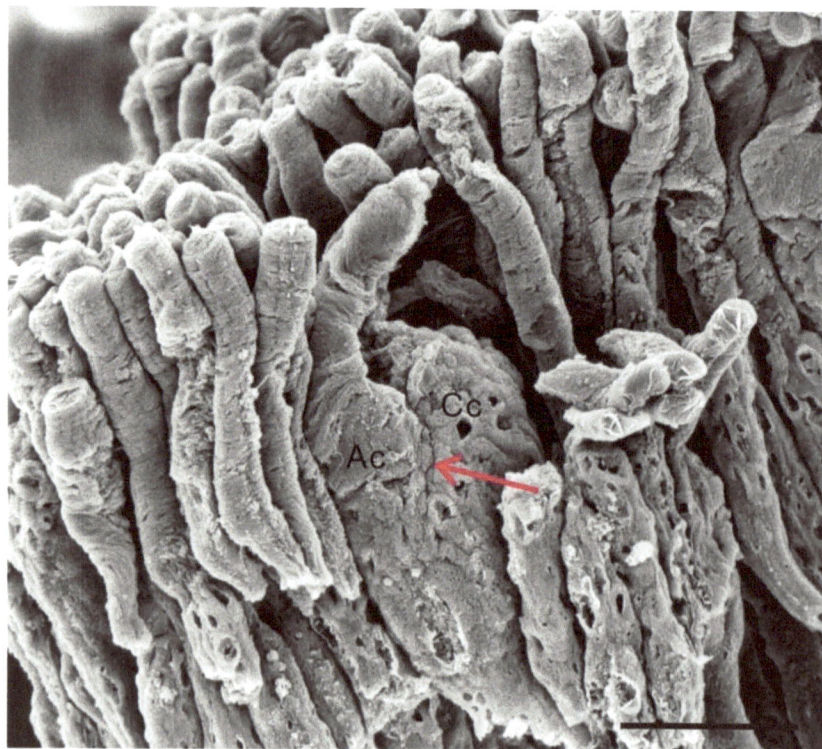

Figure 1.25q.

One type of double cone has a slightly longer chief cone inner segment (Cc) than the other component (i.e. accessory cone; Ac). A red arrow shows the boundary in between the two cells. Bar = 5 μm.

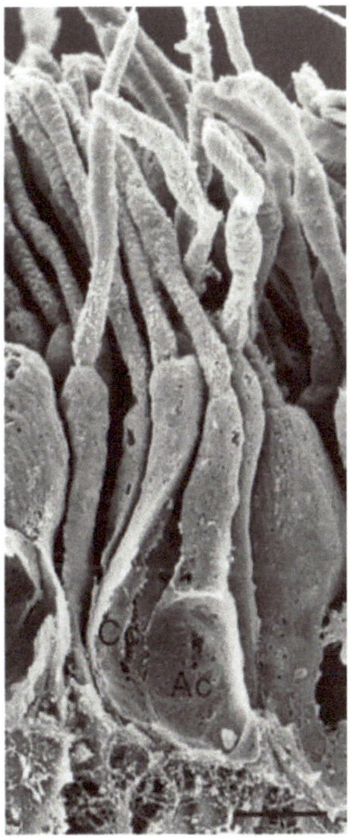

Figure 1.25r.

A fractured and opened double cone cell revealing a chief cone (Cc) and an accessory cone (Ac) in the central retina of the monkey. The presence of double cones in the primate retina has not been revealed before. Bar = 10 μm.

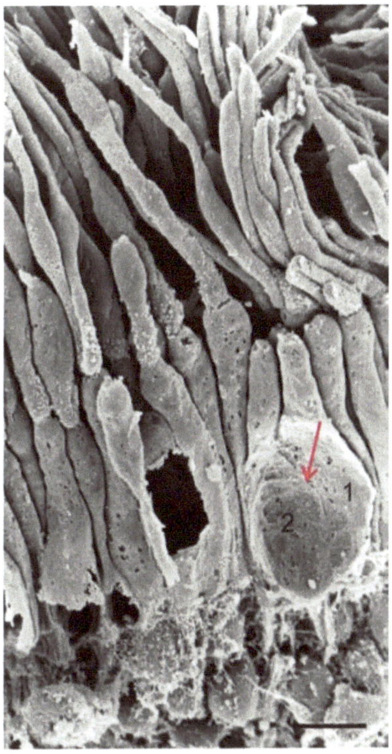

Figure 1.25s.

Another double cone has two components (1 and 2) with an inner segment almost similar in sizes. A red arrow shows the boundary in between. Would this be evolved from twin cone? Bar = 5 μm.

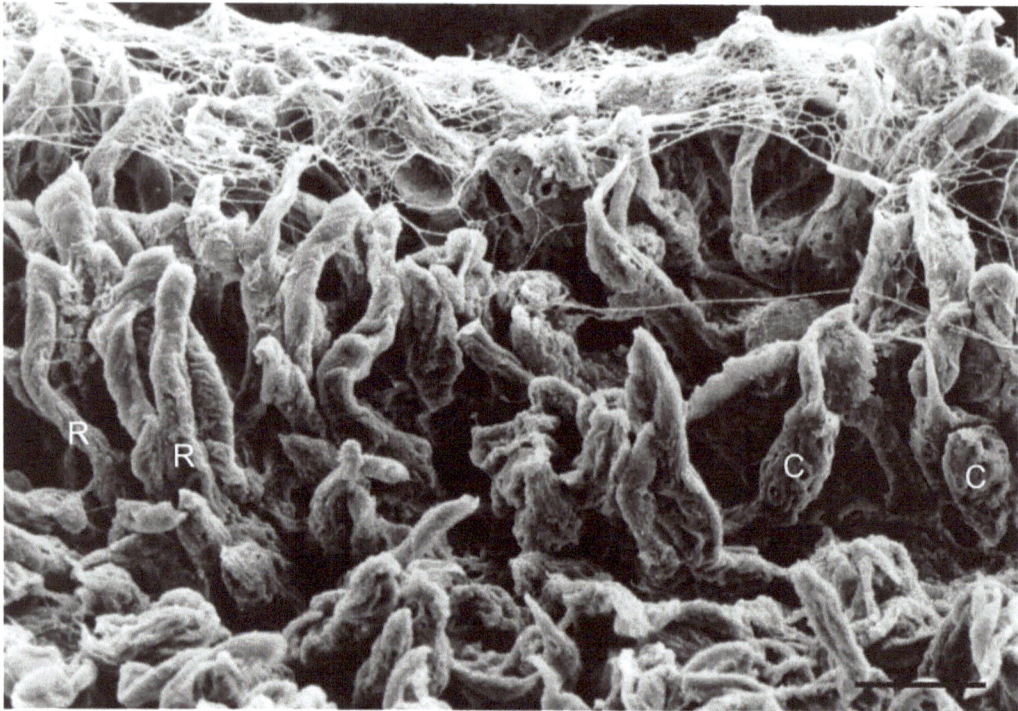

Figure 1.25t.

At the region near to anterior retina, rods (R) and small cone (C) like structures are noted. Bar = 5 μm.

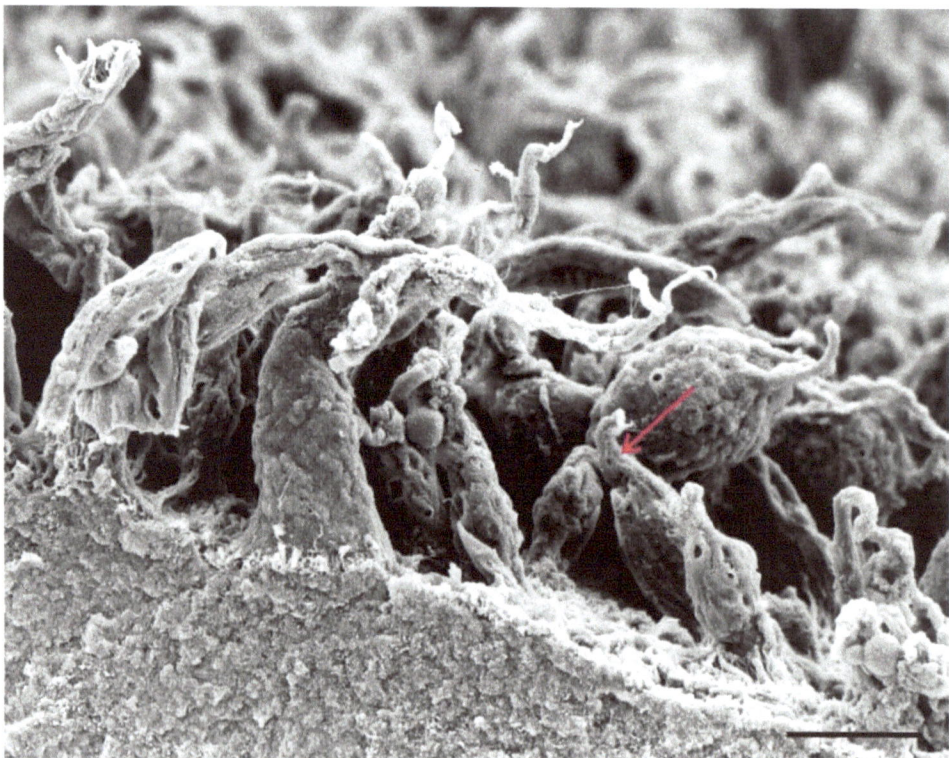

Figure 1.25u.

Near the ora serrata, the cone cells are small and have short pointed outer segments (red arrow). Bar = 5 μm.

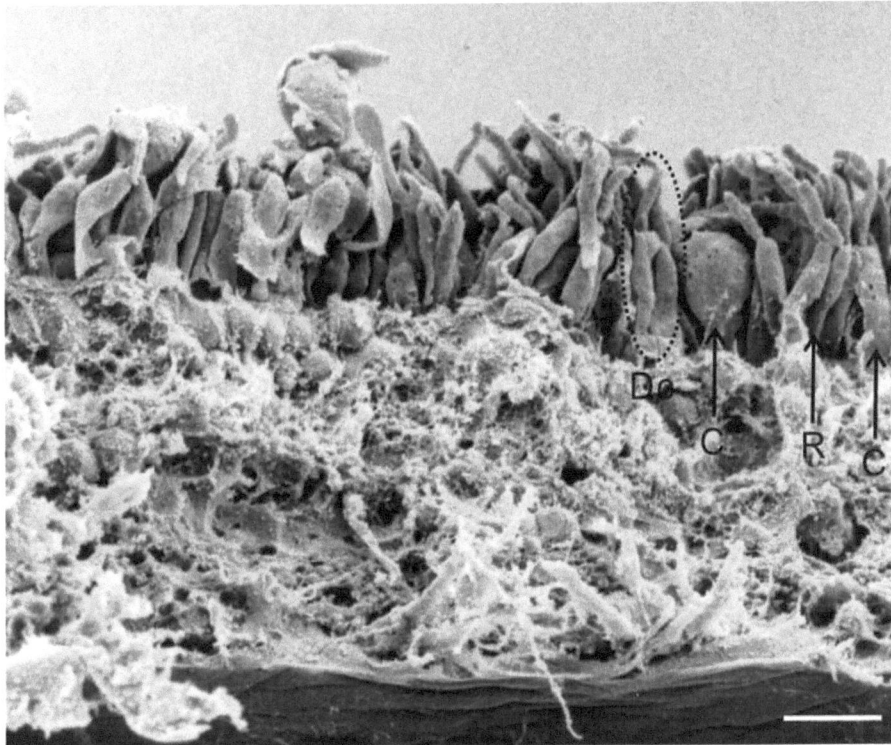

Figure 1.25v.

The anterior retina of the monkey near ora serrata reveals both cones (C) and rods (R) of different sizes and morphologies. A double cone (Dc; circle) is also noted. Bar = 10 μm.

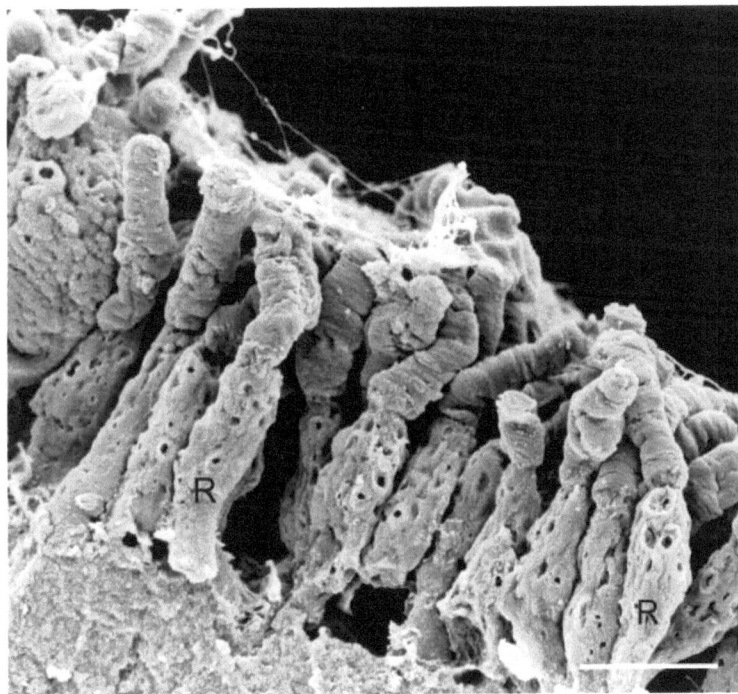

Figure 1.25w.

Small rods (R) with short inner and outer segments in the periphery of the retina. Bar = 5 μm.

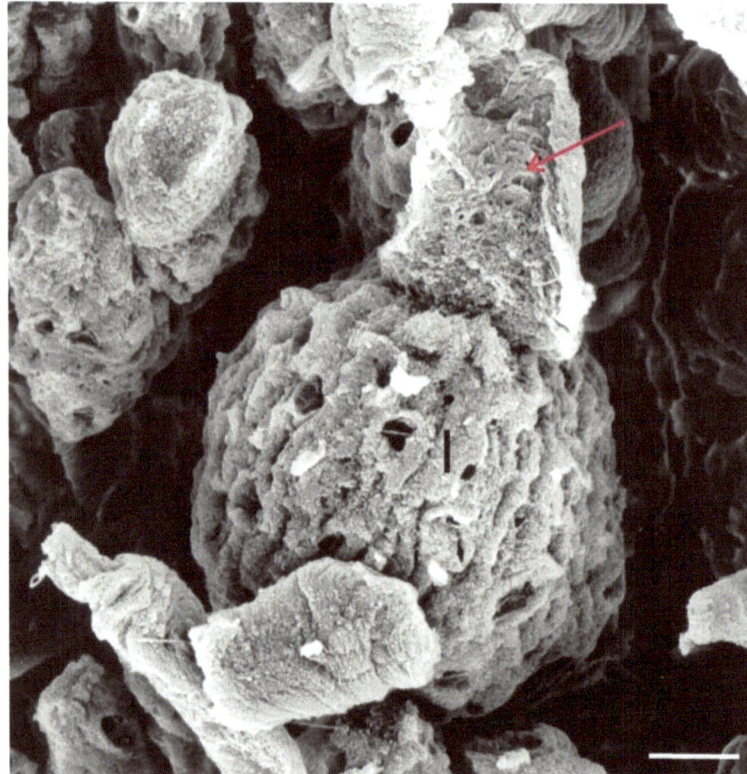

Figure 1.25x.

A type C3 single cone showing part of the inner segment (I) and stacks of the outer segment (red arrow). Bar = 1 μm.

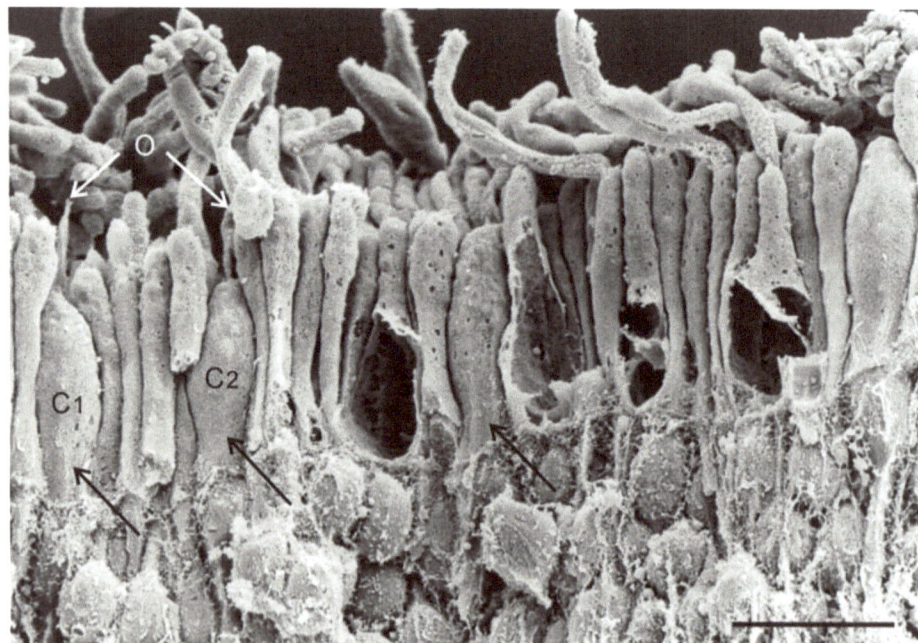

Figure 1.25y.

More elongated cone cells (arrows) in the periphery of the monkey retina. Size and shape are different from that of the previous figure (e.g. figure 1.25x). Note C1 and C2 have very fine outer segments (O). Bar = 10 μm.

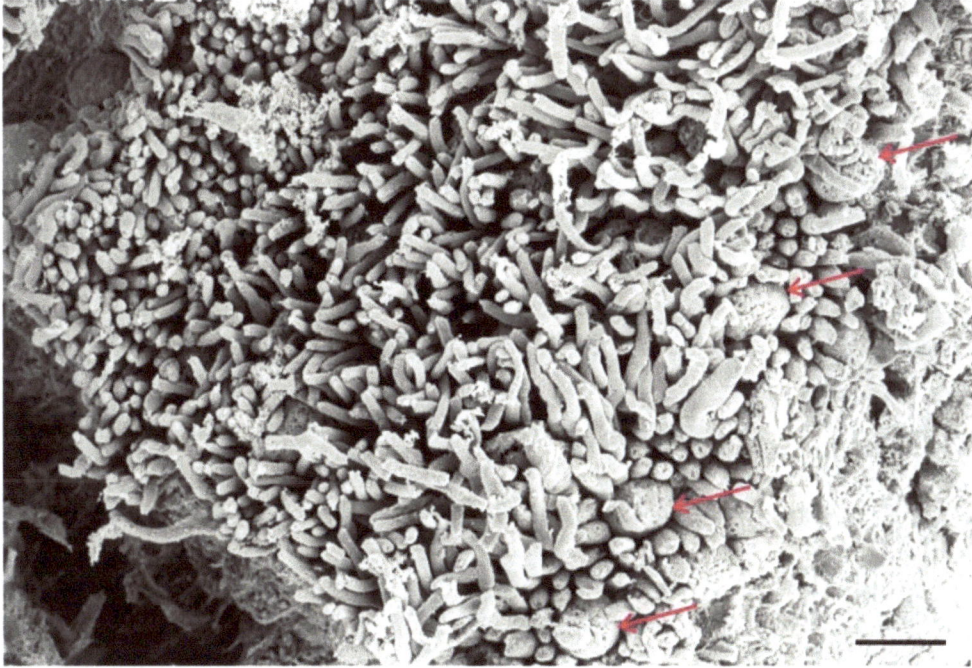

Figure 1.25z.

An overhead view of the mid-peripheral region of the visual cells reveals a few large cone cells with round inner segments (red arrows). Bar = 10 μm.

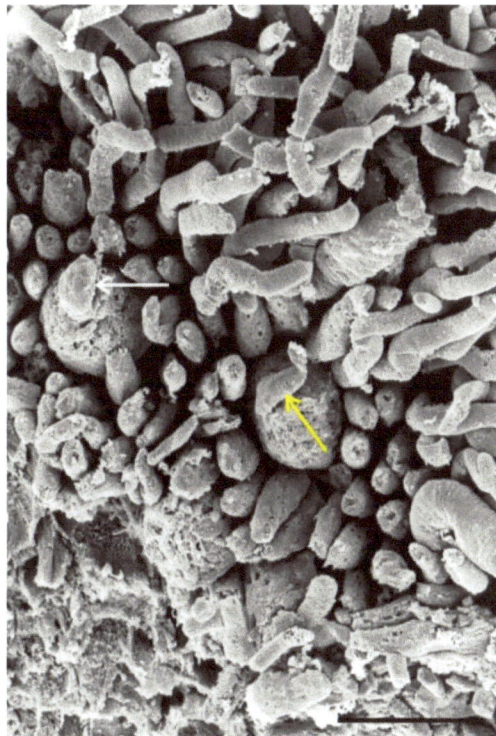

Figure 1.25aa.

A leaf-like outer segment from a cone (yellow arrow) and a more dilated outer segment from another cone (white arrow). Bar = 10 μm.

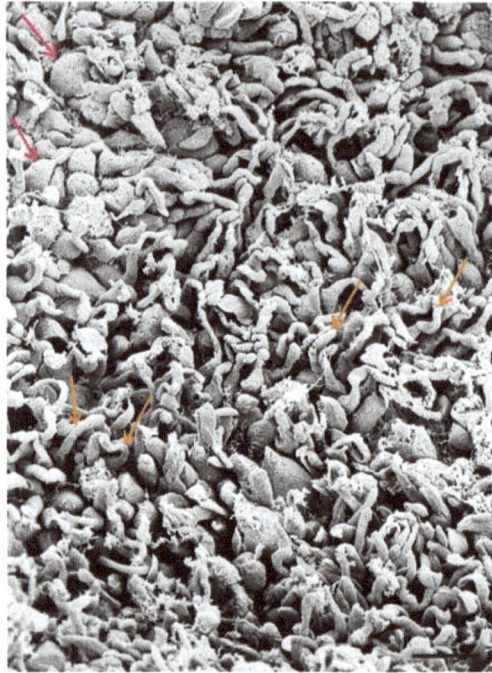

Figure 1.25ab.

In another region of the mid-peripheral retina, visual cells at different growing stages are observed. The ones indicated by the red arrows are at an early stage of development. The outer segments are still not yet formed. Others, which are indicated by the orange arrows, are at a more advanced stage, bearing worm-like outer segments. Bar = 10 μm.

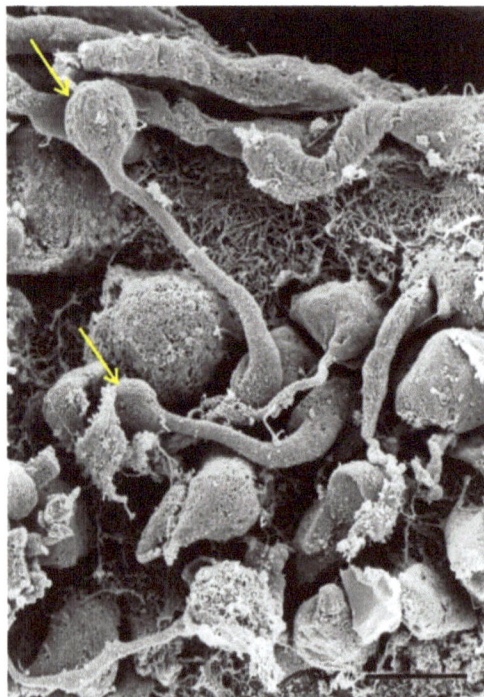

Figure 1.25ac.

The monkey retina reveals the formation of phagosome (yellow arrows) at the tip of some outer segments of the visual cells. Bar = 5 μm.

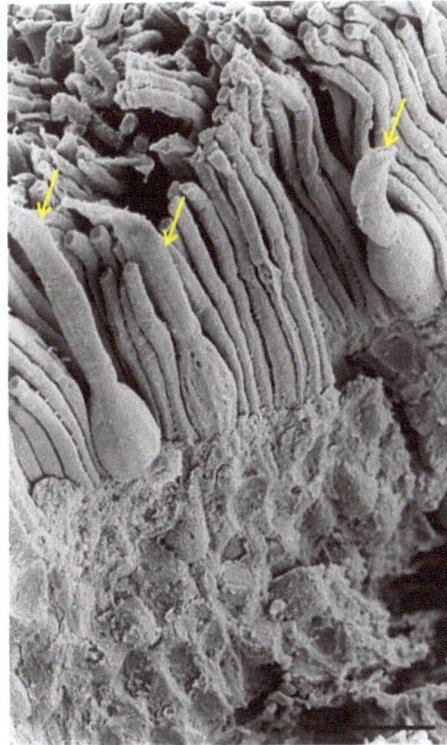

Figure 1.25ad.

Note that some single cones in the monkey retina have blade-like outer segments (arrows). Bar = 10 µm.

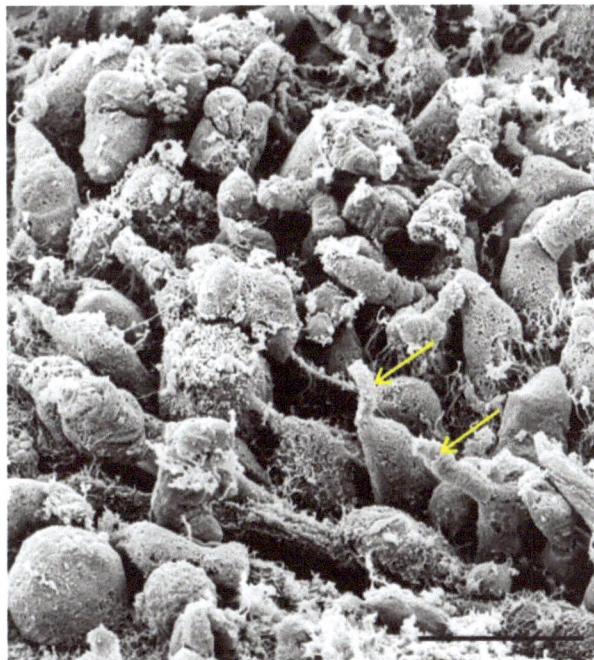

Figure 1.25ae.

Higher magnification showing many smaller visual cells which are probably still in their growing stage. The yellow arrows indicate the tiny outer segments noted in some cells. Bar = 10 µm.

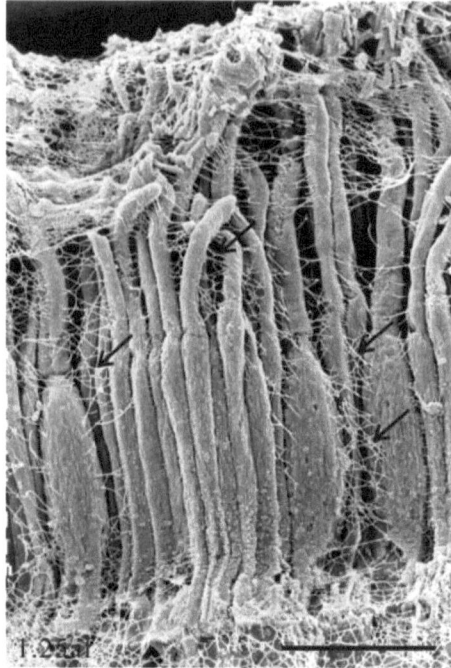

Figure 1.25af.

This scanning electron microscopy of the monkey visual cells shows many interconnections between cells (arrows). Bar = 10 μm.

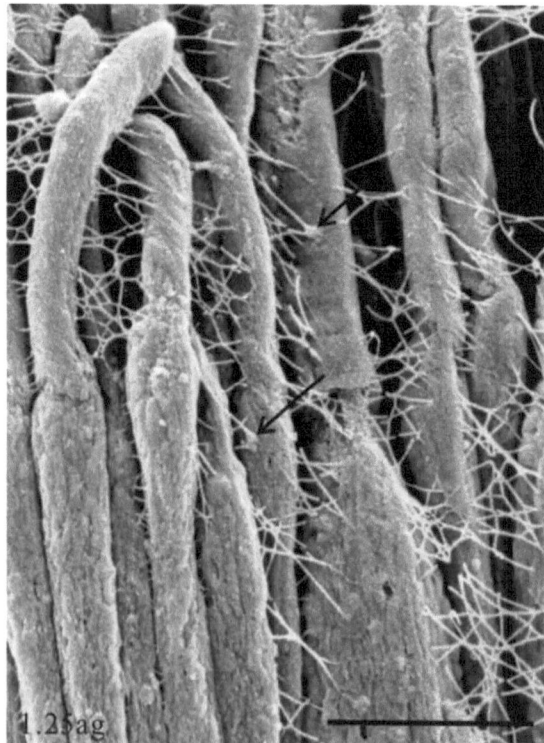

Figure 1.25ag.

Some of the fibers have dilated endings (arrows). Bar = 5 μm.

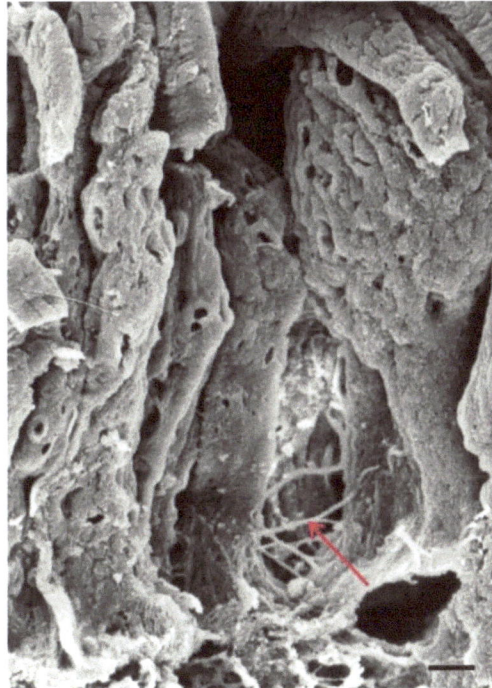

Figure 1.25ah.

Communication is enhanced via connections between visual cells (red arrow). Bar = 1 μm.

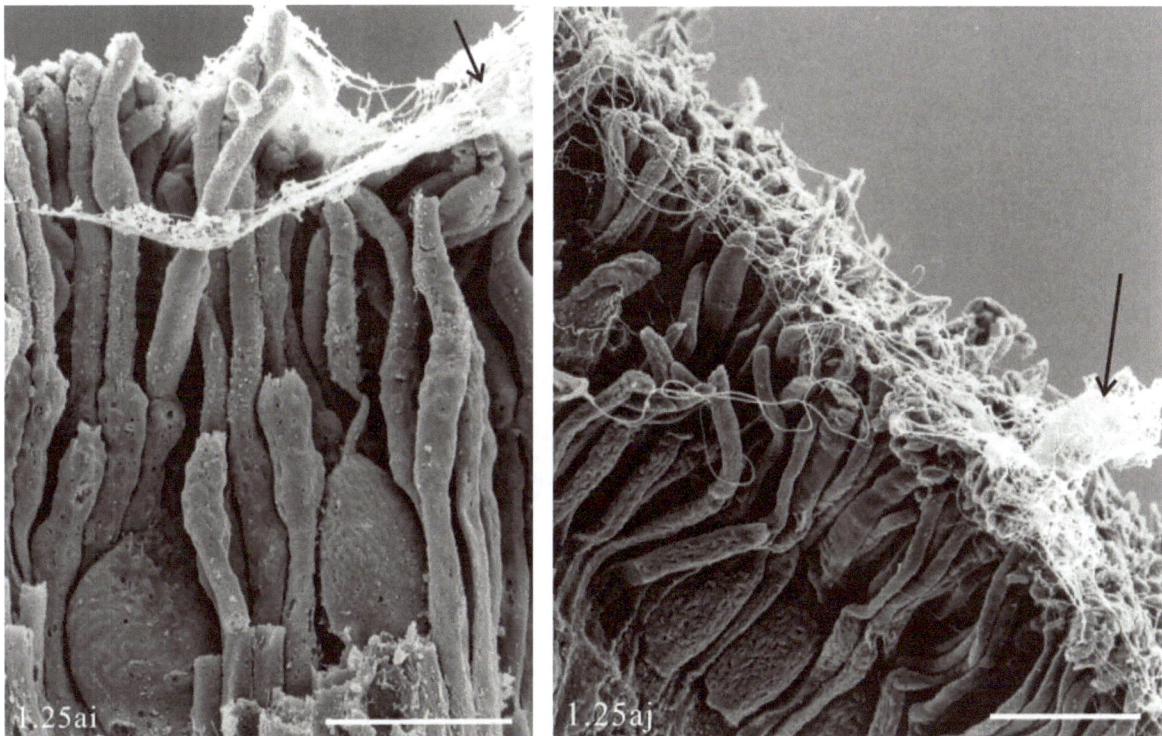

Figures 1.25ai and 1.25aj.

Monkey retina showing fibrils in the interreceptor matrix (arrows). Bar = 10 μm.

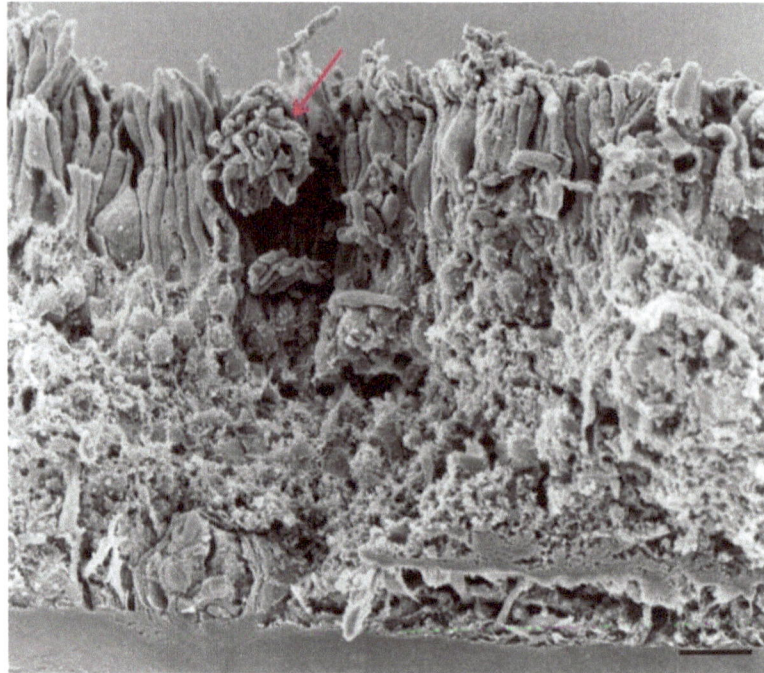

Figure 1.25ak.

A spherical ball of pigment cells (red arrow) invading the space between visual cells is seen. This is a pathological situation of the monkey retina. Bar =10 μm.

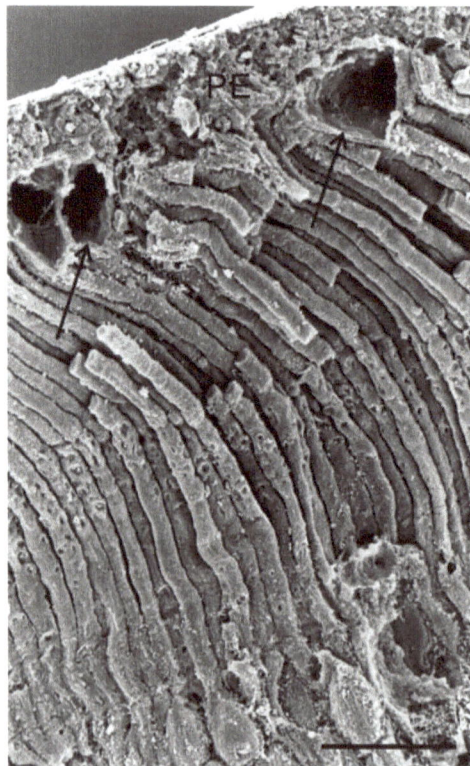

Figure 1.25al.

Arrows show large spaces for phagosomes in the ventricular surface of the pigment epithelium (PE). Bar = 10 μm.

26 MOUSE.

Mouse has retina with thick outer nuclear layer, of as much as 10 layers of cell bodies. The inner nuclear layer is relatively thinner with 7 to 8 layers of cell bodies. The ganglion cell layer is one layer thick as the typical vertebrate retina, having a continuous row of ganglion cells.

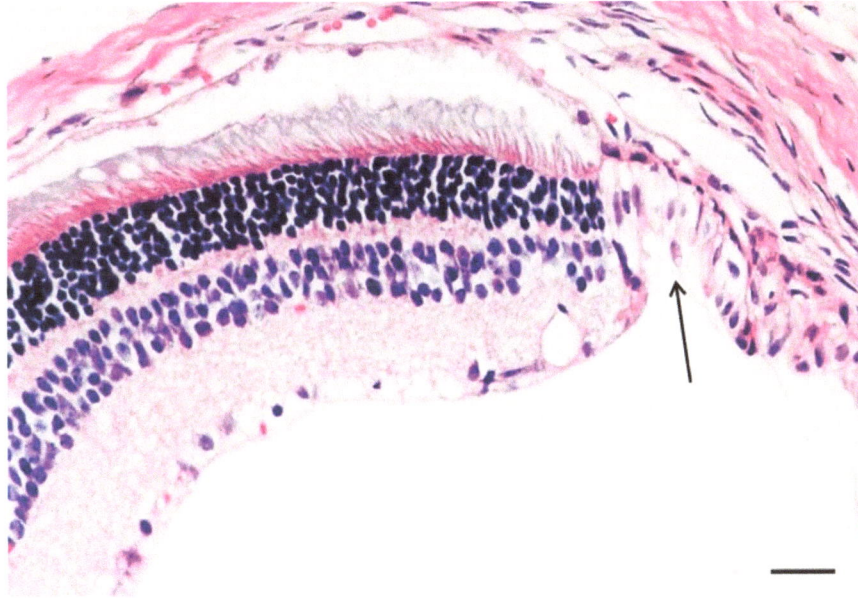

Figure 1.26a *Anterior retina near ora serrata.*

An abrupt transition (arrow) of the anterior retina of the mouse into the ora serrata is shown. Bar = 50 μm.

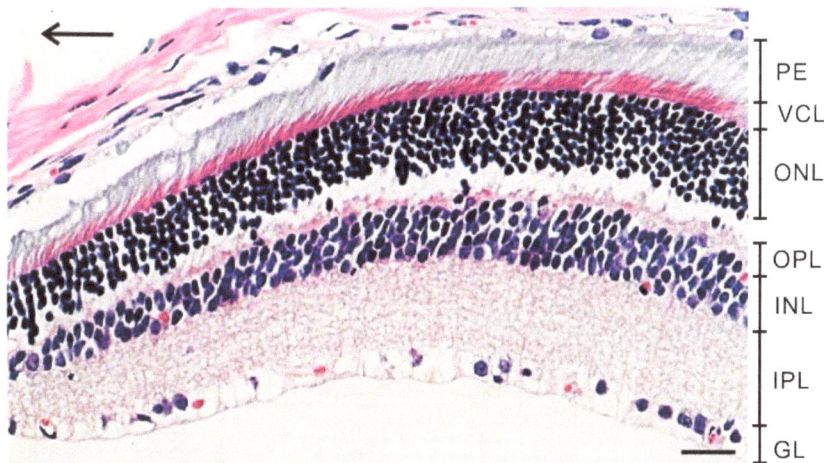

Figure 1.26b *Anterior retina.*

Different retinal layers of the mouse are identified. There is a gradual decrease of retinal thickness towards the ora serrata. The arrow denotes the location of the ora serrata. The pigment epithelium (PE) in mouse appears lighter in color than other animals, suggesting the presence of little pigment inside. Bar = 50 μm.

(GL - Ganglion cell layer; INL - Inner nuclear layer; IPL - Inner plexiform layer; ONL - Outer nuclear layer; OPL - Outer plexiform layer; PE - Pigment epithelium; VCL - Visual cell layer).

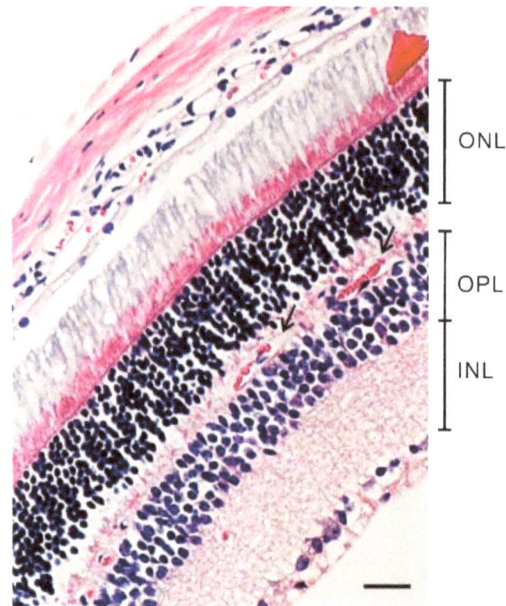

Figure 1.26c *Peripheral retina.*

The retina of the mouse consists of predominately rods and has a relatively thick outer nuclear layer (ONL), which is at times even thicker than the inner nuclear layer (INL). Some blood capillaries (arrows) are seen in the outer plexiform layer (OPL). Bar = 50 μm.

(INL - Inner nuclear layer; ONL - Outer nuclear layer; OPL – Outer plexiform layer).

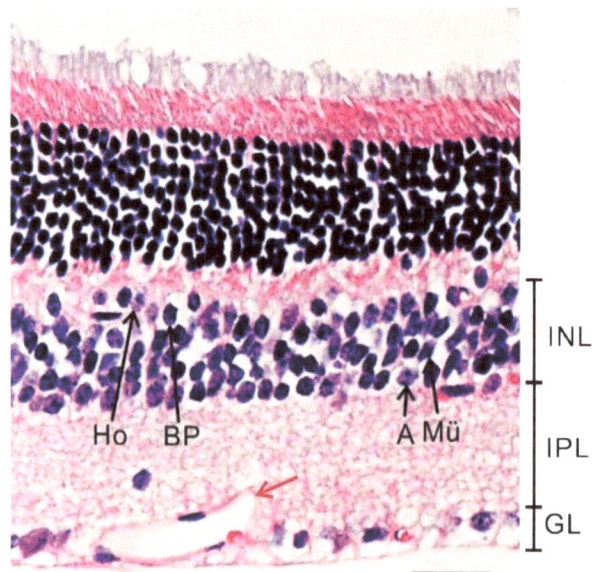

Figure 1.26d *Peripheral retina.*

An amacrine cell (A), bipolar cell (BP), horizontal cell (Ho), and Müller cell (Mü) are shown in the inner nuclear layer (INL). A blood capillary (red arrow) is also noted near the ganglion cell layer (GL). Bar = 50 μm.

(GL - Ganglion cell layer; INL - Inner nuclear layer; IPL - Inner plexiform layer).

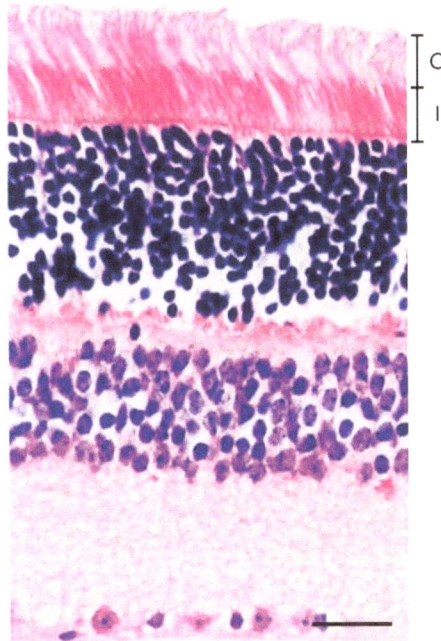

Figure 1.26e *Central retina.*

The central retina consists of many long and slender rods. Their inner (I) and outer (O) segments are distinguishable. Bar = 50 μm.

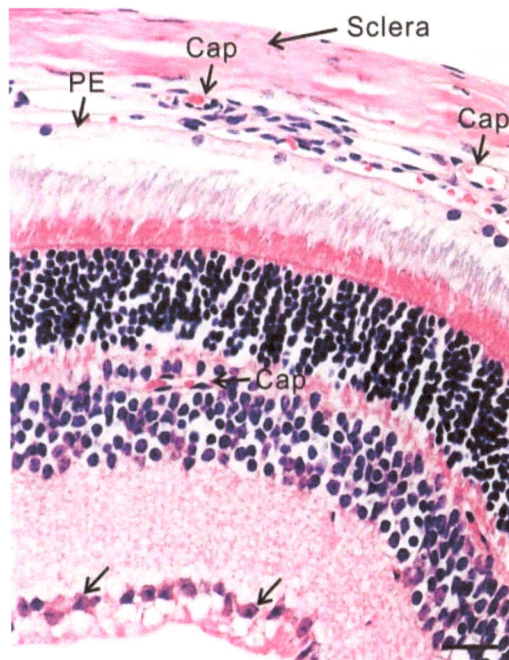

Figure 1.26f *Central retina.*

In this figure, the layer of sclera, choroid and pigment epithelium (PE) still exist external to the neural retina. Blood capillaries (Cap) are noted in the choroid layer as well as in the outer plexiform layer. Ganglion cells (arrows) appear as a row of cells in its own layer. Bar = 50 μm.

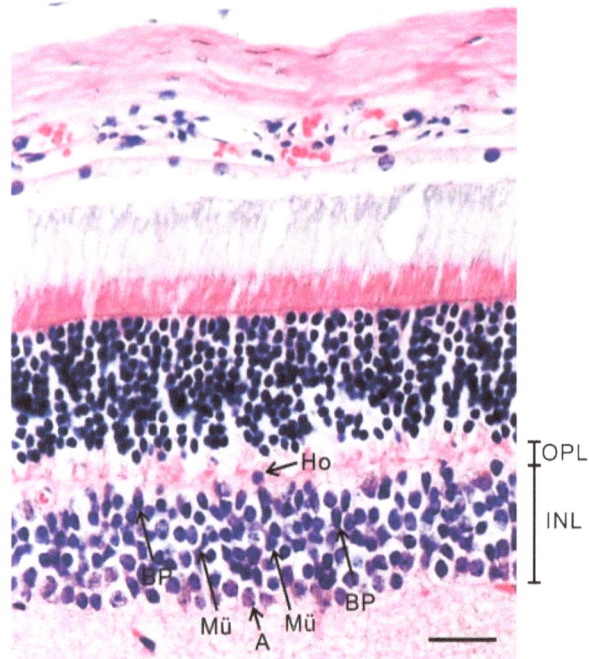

Figure 1.26g *Central retina.*

Near the outer plexiform layer (OPL), a horizontal cell (Ho) is noted. Besides, some other retinal cells such as amacrine cells (A), bipolar cells (BP), and Müller cells (Mü) are also identified. Bar = 50 µm.

(INL - Inner nuclear layer; OPL - Outer Plexiform layer).

27 PIG.

The pig has a retina which is comparative thinner than many other mammals. The outer nuclear layer is at least more than double the thickness of the inner nuclear layer. However, there are many types of visual cells. The ganglion cell layer features sparsely distributed ganglion cells.

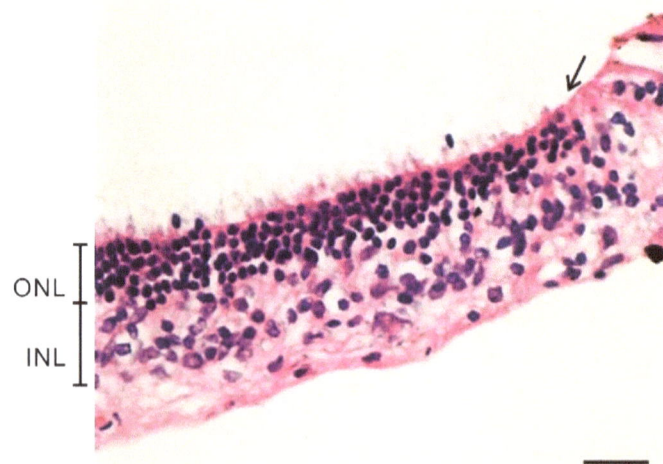

Figure 1.27a *Anterior retina near ora serrata.*

Retina of the pig near the ora serrata. Note 1) the decreasing number of visual cells (arrow); and 2) merging of the outer nuclear layer (ONL) with the inner nuclear layer (INL). Bar = 50 µm.

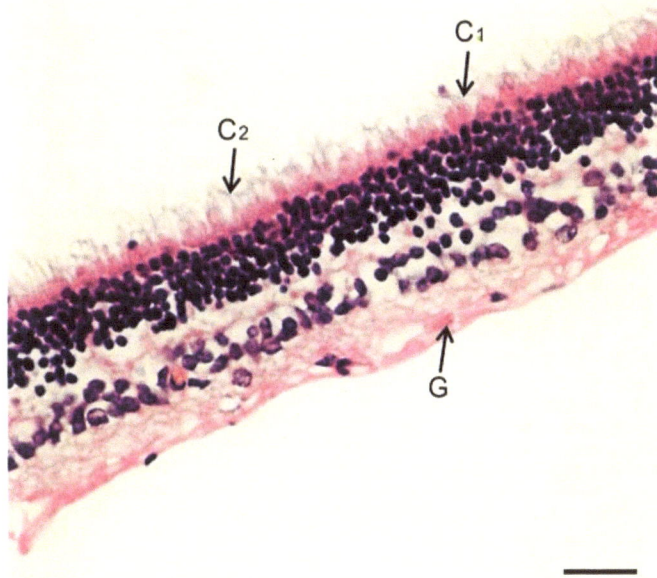

Figure 1.27b *Peripheral retina.*

Peripheral retina of the pig. Note cone-like cells C1 and C2 of different morphology. Also note the very few ganglion cells (G) present. Bar = 50 μm.

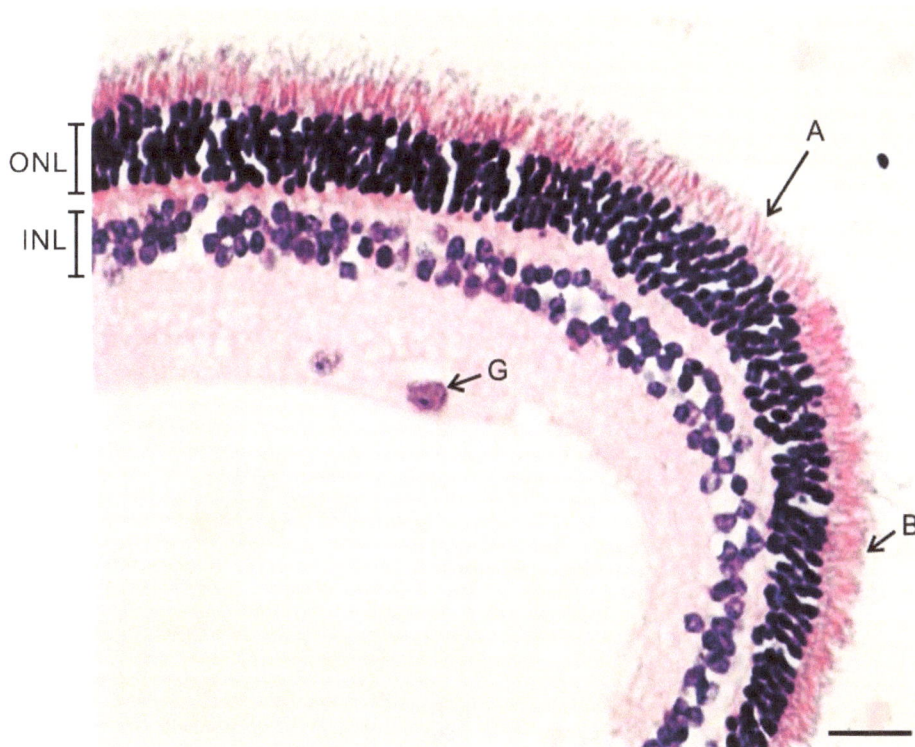

Figure 1.27c *Junction between peripheral and central retina.*

Note the rod-like cells present at region A and the increase in visual cell density at region B. The outer nuclear layer (ONL) is thicker than the inner nuclear layer (INL), and having more elongated cell nuclei. Ganglion cells (G) in this animal are not numerous in number. Bar = 50 μm.

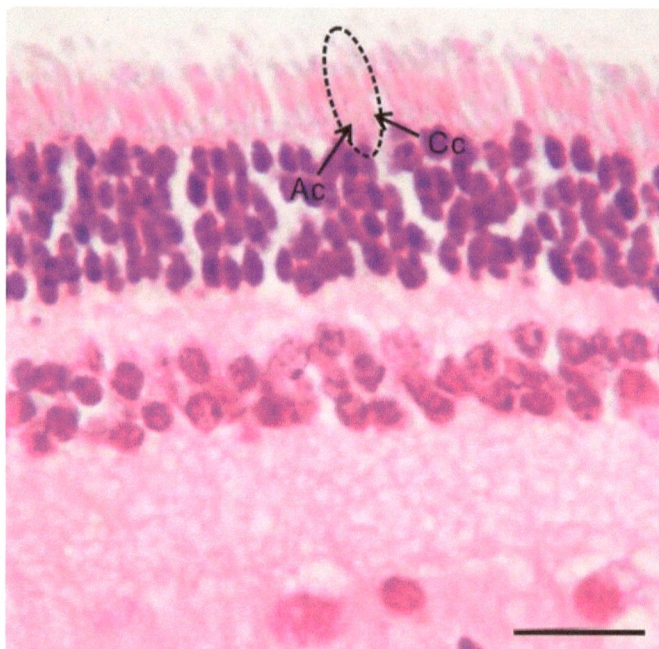

Figure 1.27d *Central retina.*

In the central retina, a double cone with shorter accessory (Ac) and taller chief cones (Cc) are noted (circle). Bar = 50 μm.

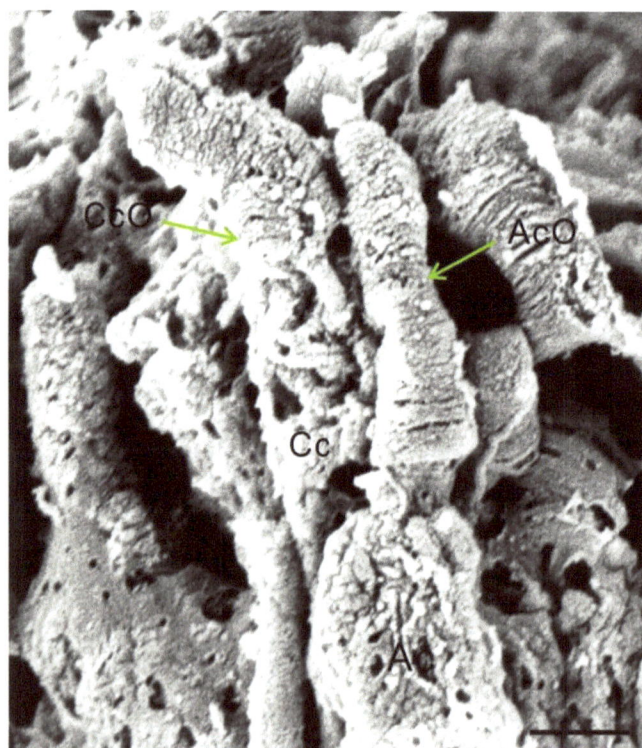

Figure 1.27e.

The double cone of the pig from an oblique view showing the broader inner segment of the accessory cone (Ac) and the slender inner segment of the chief cone (Cc). Chief cone outer segments (CcO) are always at a higher level than accessory cone outer segments (AcO). Bar = 1 μm.

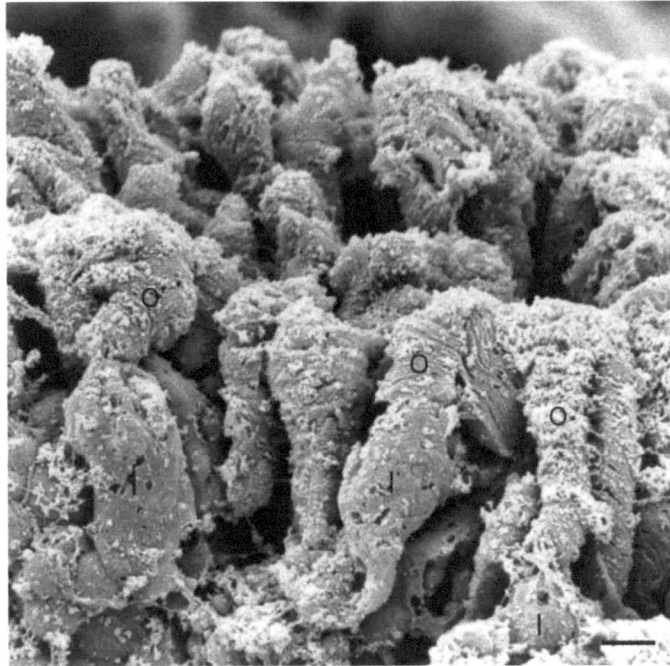

Figure 1.27f.

Note that the outer segments (O) and the inner segments (I) are both generally short in comparison with those of other vertebrates. Bar = 1 μm.

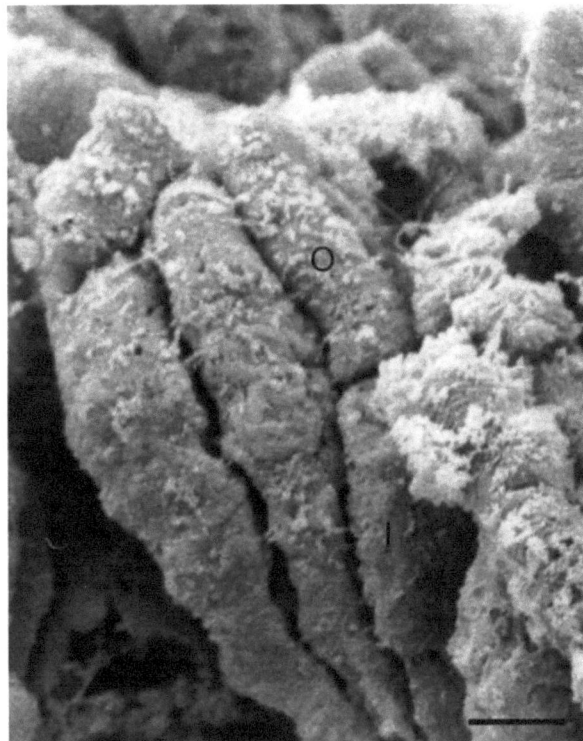

Figure 1.27g.

These visual cells with tall inner segments may be rods. "O" denotes the outer segment and "I" indicates the inner segment. Bar = 1 μm.

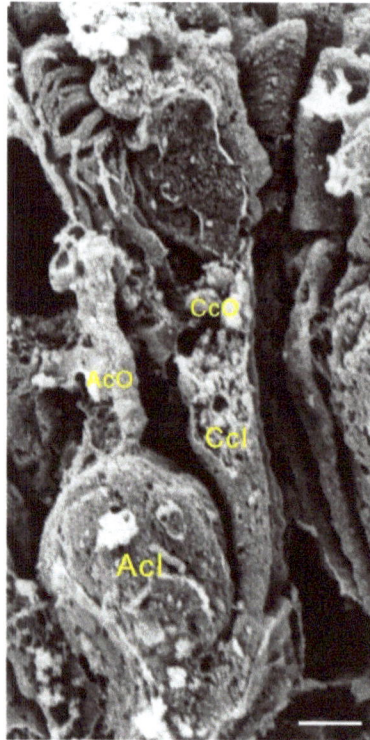

Figure 1.27h.

A frontal view of a double cone of the pig. The broader inner segment of the accessory cone (AcI) and the taller inner segment of the chief cone (CcI) are shown. The accessory cone outer segment (AcO) is better preserved than the ruptured outer segment of the chief cone (CcO). Bar = 1 μm.

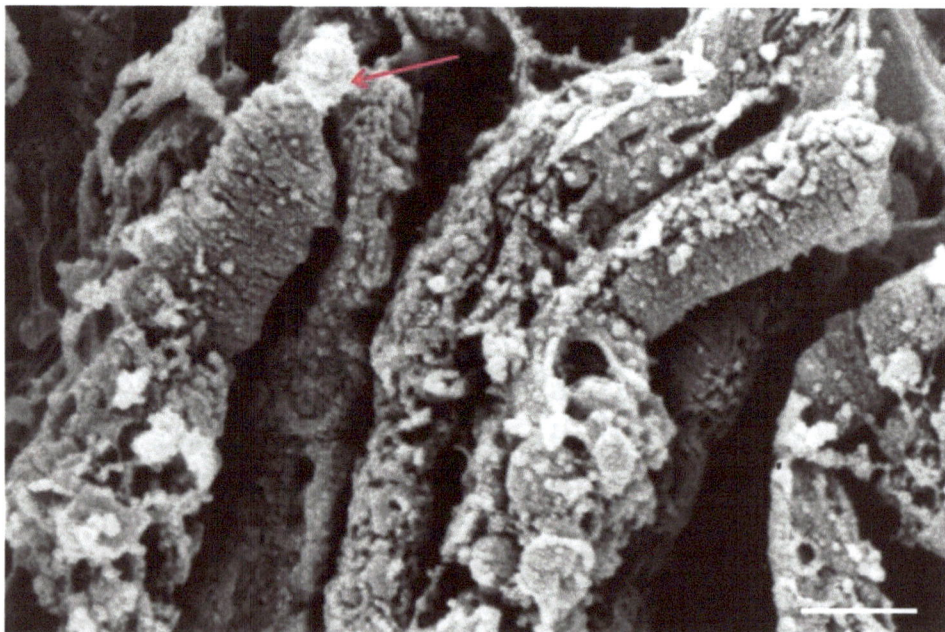

Figure 1.27i.

The red arrow indicates the shredding tip of the outer segment of a cone. Bar = 1 μm.

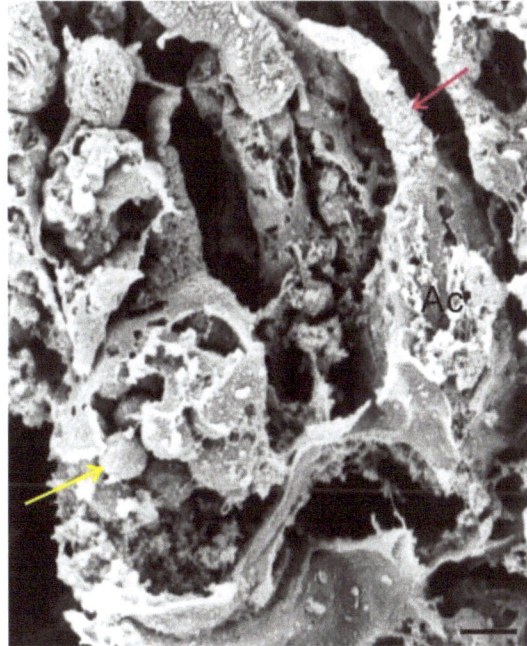

Figure 1.27j.

The outer segment (red arrow) of the accessory cone (Ac) has a very thin distal tip. Another inner segment of the accessory cone is cracked, reviewing round mitochondria (yellow arrow) within. Bar = 1 μm.

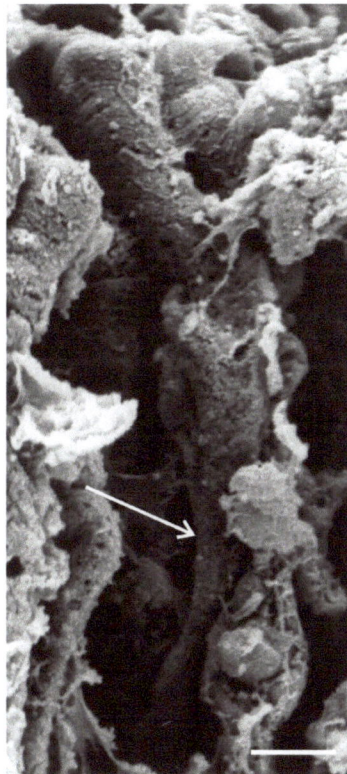

Figure 1.27k.

A chief cone (white arrow) with the diameter of the inner segment increasing distally is shown. Bar = 1 μm.

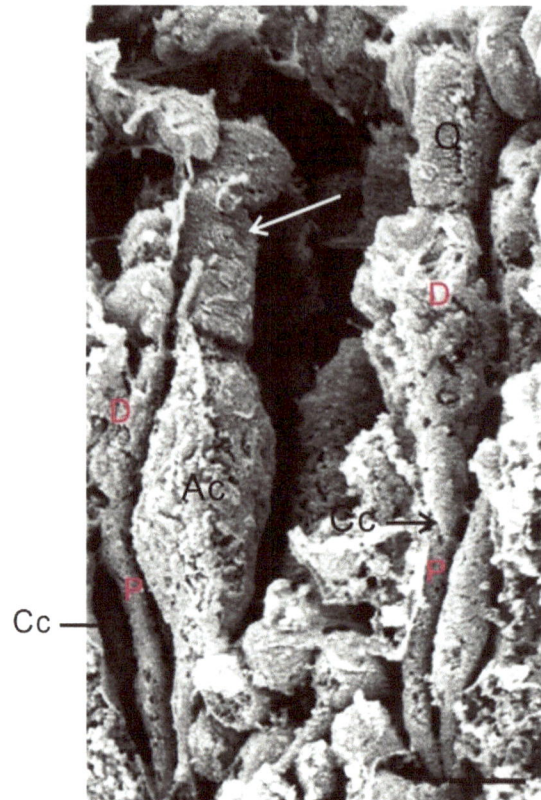

Figure 1.27l.

Sometimes accessory cones (Ac) can also have thicker outer segments (white arrow) but chief cone (Cc) in the pig always have inner segments with a dilated distal region (D) and a thin proximal region (P). "O" denotes the outer segment of the chief cone. Bar = 1 μm.

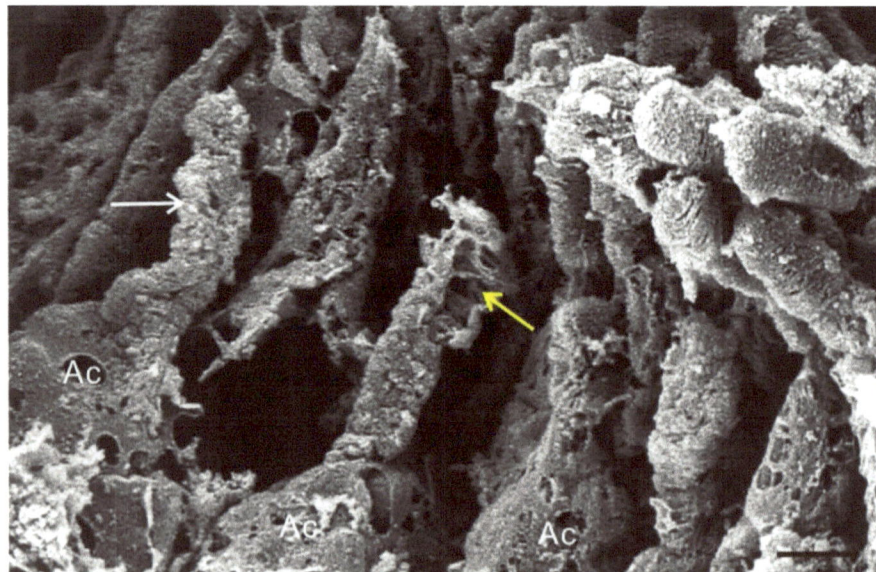

Figure 1.27m.

Distal accessory cones (Ac) with their outer segments (white arrow) are shown. Some membranes inside the outer segment are exposed (yellow arrow). Bar = 1 μm.

REFERENCES.

[1]   Collin SP, Collin HB. The foveal photoreceptor mosaic in the pipefish, Corythoichthyes paxtoni (Syngnathidae, Teleostei). Histol Histopathol 1999; 14(2): 369-82.

[2]   Azuma N. Molecular cell biology on morphogenesis of the fovea and evolution of the central vision. Nippon Ganka Gakkai Zasshi 2000; 104(12): 960-85.

[3]   Hess M. Triple cones in the retinae of three anchovy species: Engraulis encrasicolus, Cetengraulis mysticetus and Anchovia macrolepidota (Engraulididae, Teleostei). Vision Res. 2009; 49(12): 1569-82.

[4]   Collin SP, Lloyd DJ, Wagner HJ. Foveate vision in deep-sea teleosts: a comparison of primary visual and olfactory inputs. Philos Trans R Soc Lond B Biol Sci 2000; 355(1401): 1315-20.

[5]   Tucker VA. The deep fovea, sideways vision and spiral flight paths in raptors. J Exp Biol 2000; 203(Pt 24): 3745-54.

[6]   Tucker VA, Tucker AE, Akers K, Enderson JH. Curved flight paths and sideways vision in peregrine falcons (Falco peregrinus). J Exp Biol 2000; 203(Pt 24): 3755-63.

[7]   Packer O, Hendrickson AE, Curcio CA. Photoreceptor topography of the retina in the adult pigtail macaque (Macaca nemestrina). J Comp Neurol 1989; 288(1): 165-83.

[8]   Szél A, Röhlich P, Caffé AR, van Veen T. Distribution of cone photoreceptors in the mammalian retina. Microsc Res Tech 1996; 35(6): 445-62.

[9]   Ahnelt PK. The photoreceptor mosaic. Eye (Lond) 1998; 12 (Pt 3b): 531-40.

[10]   Collin SP, Davies WL, Hart NS, Hunt DM. The evolution of early vertebrate photoreceptors. Philos Trans R Soc Lond B Biol Sci 2009; 364(1531): 2925-40.

[11]   Kryger Z, Galli-Resta L, Jacobs GH, Reese BE. The topography of rod and cone photoreceptors in the retina of the ground squirrel. Vis Neurosci 1998; 15(4): 685-91.

[12]   Temple S, Hart NS, Marshall NJ, Collin SP. A spitting image: specializations in archerfish eyes for vision at the interface between air and water. Proc Biol Sci 2010 (E. Pub.).

[13]   Wagner HJ, Fröhlich E, Negishi K, Collin SP. The eyes of deep-sea fish. II. Functional morphology of the retina. Prog Retin Eye Res 1998; 17(4): 637-85.

[14]   Walls GL. The vertebrate eye and its adaptive radiation. Hafner, N.Y. 1942.

[15]   Wai SM, Kung LS, Yew DT. Novel identification of the different types of cones in the retina of the chicken. Cell Mol Neurobiol 2002; 22(2): 177-84.

[16]   Hart NS. The visual ecology of avian photoreceptors. Prog Retinal Eye Res 2001; 20(5): 675-03.

[17]   Cameron DA. Pugh Jr EN. Double cones as a basis for a new type of polarization vision in vertebrates. Nature 1991; 353: 161-4.

[18]   Wolf G. The visual cycle of the cone photoreceptors of the retina. Nutr Rev. 2004; 62(7 Pt 1): 283-6.

[19]   Shand J, Archer MA, Collin SP. Ontogenetic changes in the retinal photoreceptor mosaic in a fish, the black bream, Acanthopagrus butcheri. J Comp Neurol 1999; 412(2): 203-17.

[20]   Mizuno TA, Ohtsuka T. Quantitative study of apoptotic cells in the goldfish retina. Zoolog Sci 2009; 26(2): 157-62.

[21]   Sherry DM, Bui DD, Degrip WJ. Identification and distribution of photoreceptor subtypes in the neotenic tiger salamander retina. Vis Neurosci. 1998; 15(6): 1175-87.

[22]   Zhang J, Wu SM. Immunocytochemical analysis of photoreceptors in the tiger salamander retina. Vision Res 2009; 49(1): 64-73.

[23]   Davies WL, Cowing JA, Bowmaker JK, Carvalho LS, Gower DJ, Hunt DM. Shedding light on serpent sight: the visual pigments of henophidian snakes. J Neurosci 2009; 29(23): 7519-25.

[24]   Cottrill PB, Davies WL, Semo M, Bowmaker JK, Hunt DM, Jeffery G. Developmental dynamics of cone photoreceptors in the eel. BMC Dev Biol 2009; 9: 71.

[25]   Bowmaker JK, Loew ER, Ott M. The cone photoreceptors and visual pigments of chameleons. J Comp Physiol A Neuroethol Sens Neural Behav Physiol 2005; 191(10): 925-32.

[26]   Röhlich P, Szél A. Photoreceptor cells in the Xenopus retina. Microsc Res Tech. 2000 ; 50(5): 327-37.

[27]   Meyer-Rochow VB, Wohlfahrt S, Ahnelt PK. Photoreceptor cell types in the retina of the tuatara (Sphenodon punctatus) have cone characteristics. Micron 2005; 36(5): 423-8.

[28]   Sillman AJ, Carver JK, Loew ER. The photoreceptors and visual pigments in the retina of a boid snake, the ball python (Python regius). J Exp Biol 1999; 202 (Pt 14): 1931-8.

[29]   Sillman AJ, Johnson JL, Loew ER. Retinal photoreceptors and visual pigments in Boa constrictor imperator. J Exp Zool 2001; 290(4): 359-65.

[30]   Dieterich CE, Dieterich HJ. Electron microscopy of retinal tapetum (Caiman crocodilus). Albrecht Von Graefes Arch Klin

Exp Ophthalmol 1978; 208(1-3): 159-68.

[31] Cohen AI The fine structure of the visual receptors of the pigeon. Exp Eye Res 1963; 2: 88-97.

[32] Ladman AJ, Soper EM. Preliminary observations on the fine structure of Müller cells of the avian retina. 5 Int Congress E.M. 2: R6 1962.

[33] Shiragami M. Electron microscopic study on synapses of visual cells. 3. Morphologic classification of visual cell synapses and a peculiar type of synapses in chicken retina. Nippon Ganka Kiyo 1969a; 20(4): 430-438.

[34] Shiragami M. Electron microscopic study on synapses of visual cells. IV. [The ultrastructure of synapses in the midperipheral area of chicken retina. Nippon Ganka Kiyo 1969b; 20(4): 439-446.

[35] Hogan MJ, Alvarado JA, Weddell JE. The histology of the human eye. Philadelphia, W. B. Saunders, 1971.

[36] Dowling JE, Cowan WM. An electron microscope study of normal and degenerating centrifugal fiber terminals in the pigeon retina. Z Zellforsch Mikrosk Anat 1966; 71(1): 14-28.

[37] Cowan WM. Centrifugal fibres to the avian retina. Br Med Bull 1970; 26: 112-118.

[38] Yamada E, Ishikawa T. The fine structure of the horizontal cells in some vertebrate retinae. Cold Spring Harb Symp Quant Biol. 1965a; 30: 383-392.

[39] Ramón y Cajal S. The structure of the retina: A complete work. Translated by Thorpe SA, Glickstein M, Thomas CC. Springfield. 1972.

[40] Missotten L. The synapses in the human retina. In: Rochen JW, Ed. Structure of the eye. II. Symposium, The 8th International Congress of Anatomy, Stuttgart, Schattauer-Verlag, 1965.

[41] Cowan WM, Powell TP. Centrifugal fibres in the avian visual system. Proc R Soc Lond B Biol Sci. 1963; 158: 232-52.

[42] Dowling JE, Boycott BB. Neural connections of the retina: fine structure of the inner plexiform layer. Cold Spring Harb Symp Quant Biol 1965; 30: 393-402.

[43] Fine BS, Zimmerman LE. Muller's cells and the "middle limiting membrane" of the human retina. An electron microscopic study. Invest Ophthalmol 1962; 1: 304-326.

[44] Villegas GM. Ultrastructure of the human retina. J Anat 1964; 98: 501-513.

[45] Uga S, Smelser GK. Electron microscopic study of the development of retinal Müllerian cells. Invest Ophthalmol 1973b; 12(4): 295-307.

[46] Missotten L. A study of the rods of the human retina by means of the electron microscope. Ophthalmologica 1960; 140: 200-214.

[47] Dowling JE, Boycott BB. Organization of the primate retina: electron microscopy. Proc R Soc Lond B Biol Sci 1966; 166(2): 80-111.

[48] Allen RA. The retinal bipolar cells and their synapses in the inner plexiform layer. In: Straatsma, BR, Hall MO, Allen RA, Crescitelli F, Eds. The retina: Morphology, function and clinical characteristics. Los Angeles, University of California Press, 1969.

[49] Fine BS. Ganglion cells in the human retina, with particular reference to the macula lutea: An electron microscopic study. Arch Ophthal 1963; 69: 83-96.

[50] Villegas GM. Electron microscopic study of the vertebrate retina. J Gen Physiol 1960; 43(6) Suppl: 15-43.

[51] Cowan WM, Powell TP. Centrifugal fibres in the avian visual system. Proc R Soc Lond B Biol Sci 1963; 158: 232-252.

[52] Hogan MJ. The vitreous, its structure, and relation to the ciliary body and retina. Invest Ophthalmol 1963; 2: 418-445.

[53] Matsusaka T. The fine structure of the inner limiting membrane of the rat retina as revealed by ruthenium red staining. J Ultrastruct Res 1971; 36(3): 312-317.

[54] Salzmann M. The anatomy and histology of the human eyeball. Denticke, Chicago. 1912.

[55] Polyak SL. The retina. Chicago, University of Chicago Press, 1941.

[56] Wolff E. The anatomy of the eye and orbit. 6th Edition, WB Saunders, Philadelphia, 1968.

CHAPTER 2

Other Retinal Layers – From Development to Maturation (A Chicken Model)

Abstract: This chapter uses a chicken model to introduce different inner retinal layers from development to maturation. These retinal layers include outer nuclear layer, outer plexiform layer, inner nuclear layer, inner plexiform layer, ganglion cell layer and the nerve fibre layer. Horizontal cells, bipolar cells, Müller cells, amacrine cells and ganglion cells, which serve different functions in the eye, are also discussed in this chapter. The neuronal and Müller morphologies, forms of synaptic contacts and connections between neurons, and how they eventually develop are clearly depicted in sequences. Synaptic terminals in the outer nuclear layer, the cone pedicles and the rod spherules are laden with synaptic vesicles and synaptic ribbons. The presence of these organelles and their morphogenesis are clearly portrayed. Further, the 'dyad' and the conventional synapses in the inner plexiform layers are carefully presented.

Key Words: maturation, horizontal cell, bipolar cell, müller cell, amacrine cell, ganglion cell, cell process, dense body, astrocyte, nerve fiber >layer, internal limiting membrane, astrocyte

INTRODUCTION

The other retinal layers include the outer nuclear layer (photoreceptor cell bodies), the outer plexiform layer, the inner nuclear layer containing horizontal, bipolar, amacrine and Müller cells, the inner plexiform layer, the ganglion cell layer and the nerve fiber layer. The processes of the Müller cells form the external and internal limiting membranes. In this chapter, we shall use the chicken as a model to illustrate these layers.

OUTER NUCLEAR LAYER

The outer nuclear layer is composed of the nuclei of the photoreceptors. This layer is first distinguishable when the outer plexiform layer in the chicken initially appears at stage 36 (approximately 10 days of incubation), separating the inner nuclear layer from the outer nuclear layers. At later stages of chicken development (e.g. from stage 42 onward), the nuclei of the accessory cones may protrude above the level of the external limiting membrane.

OUTER PLEXIFORM LAYER

Light and electron microscopic data on the outer plexiform layer in the chicken and human retina [1-3] indicate its appearance subsequent to the formation of the inner plexiform layer. In the chick, this layer arises initially at stage 36, which agrees with Coulombre4 who first recorded it on the 9th to 10th day. Shiragami [5], on the other hand, notes the separation of the outer and inner nuclear layers to form the outer plexiform layer at a slightly earlier time (8th day).

Cellular maturation in the outer plexiform layer depends mainly on the development of the synaptic relationships between the terminals of photoreceptor cells and the processes of horizontal and bipolar cells. The significant morphological components of these terminals, e.g. synaptic ribbons and synaptic vesicles, and the relative frequency of these structures has been sequentially examined in the present work based on an approach adopted by Kim and Wenger [6] in their study on the formation of synapses in cultures of chick neural tube. Our study has revealed the appearance of dense junctions, for example, at stage 40 of chicken incubation when branches of bipolar and horizontal cells are already evident. Most dense junctions which are characterized by pre- and postsynaptic thickenings belong to horizontal cells and have synaptic vehicles. Such thickenings have been described in the adult turtle by Lasansky [7].

Synaptic ribbons and synaptic vesicles in the photoreceptor synaptic terminals, however, appear at a later date. Synaptic ribbons which are initially present at stage 42 were first reported in the eye of the rabbit and guinea pig by DeRobertis and Francis [8] and Sjöstrand [9]. Similar structures are also observed to be present in the cochlea [10] and the lateral line system [11]. In the chicken, these ribbons are found to arise by elongation of dense accumulations in the photoreceptors terminals. Similar suggestions have been made by Glees and Sheppard [12] in the chick. Cohen [13], on the other hand, believed that synaptic ribbons develop from invaginations of the synaptic membrane which breaks off and forms this structure. We have not been able to gather enough morphological support for this hypothesis.

David T. Yew, Maria S. M. Wai and Winnie W. Y. Li

Synaptic vesicles of the photoreceptor terminals also appear at stage 42 of chicken incubation. They are of various densities (some are dark-cored) and appear to surround the synaptic ribbons. Both the ribbons and vesicles are believed to be associated with the transmitting mechanism.

Early reports by Shiragami [14-16] indicated that synaptic ribbons and synaptic vesicles in photoreceptor synapses appear either at an earlier or a later time than that reported in this study. In one report, Shiragami [14] observed both synaptic ribbons and synaptic vesicles on the 11th day, and in another report [5], the 15th day. He also classified the synaptic terminals (or bodies) of the photoreceptors into three types. Type 1 closely resembles the pedicles of the single cones. Type 2 and 2' represent two closely applied pedicles (undoubtedly a double cone), and type 3 appears to represent a rod spherule. On the basis of this classification, he reported type 1 (single cone) and type 2 (double cone) synaptic terminals to be present on the 11th day, and type 3 (rod) terminals, the 19th day of chick development. According to our data, rod terminals are distinguishable several days earlier (stage 42). Perhaps, the methods employed for determining embryonic age may account for this discrepancy.

The nature of the transmitting material in any of the terminals of the outer plexiform layer is not known. No report has indicated the presence of either acetylcholine, aspartic acid, GABA, glutamic acid, glycine or histamine in this layer. In the frog, Wislocki and Sidman [17] have suggested the possible presence of adrenergic fibers. Dark-cored vesicles have been associated with adrenergic endings [18, 19]. On occasions, we have observed them in the photoreceptor terminals, but unfortunately, they are not very abundant. We have never observed dark-cored vesicles in the perikarya of the horizontal cells.

Our data indicate that the outer plexiform layer is morphologically equipped to transmit impulses as early as stage 42 (approximately 16 days of incubation in the chicken), a time when the outer segments also begin to form (stage 42). These morphological findings seem to coincide with the initial appearance of visual pigments (16th to 17th day) [20,21] and the first recorded electroretinogram (ERG) (16th to 19th day) [21-27], and together they all appear to point in the direction of the functional maturation of the external retinal layers around 16 – 17 days of development in the chicken.

Histochemical data on the outer plexiform layer of the chicken are scarce. Kojima et al. [28] reported the presence of succinic dehydrogenase in this layer. In mammals, however, additional enzymes and chemicals have been found, e.g. acid phosphatase [29, 30], GIP polysaccharide [31], glycogen [32, 33], phosphorylase [34]. Thus, in the mammal, it seems that this layer is responsible for some storage activity as well as involvement in the energy pathway (as in the chicken).

HORIZONTAL CELLS

The exact function of horizontal cells is a matter of much dispute. In 1958, MacNichol and Svaetichin [35] reported the presence of an S potential in the horizontal cells of fish. The S potential is usually a hyperpolarizing or depolarizing response to illumination, showing a spatial summation within a uniform receptive field. This potential generally covers a large area of the retina [36, 37] and suggests lateral transmission or lateral spread [38]. Lateral transmission involves a spread of polarization from one horizontal cell to another, a phenomenon called coupling [39]. Two main factors support this phenomenon: (1) the presence of tight junctions between adjacent horizontal cells, as in the fish [40-43], and (2) diffusion of procion yellow dye from one horizontal cell to its neighbor, as when injected into goldfish and dogfish retinas [39,44]. Recently, Naka and Nye [45] noted that there are more than one lateral transmission system.

Nilsson and Crescitelli [46] studied the relationship between retinal development and embryonic components of the electroretinogram (ERG) in the frog, and indicated that the first ERG to appear is the "a wave" which has a negative (hyperpolarizing) main component. This wave is usually regarded as being characteristic of photoreceptor function, provided the outer segments reach a certain length [47]. Nevertheless, intracellular recordings from horizontal cells also show a negative wave response [37] which may contribute to this embryonic "a wave".

The horizontal cells using the chick embryo in this atlas has revealed that in early stages, they are oval in shape with short processes resembling human horizontal cells [40]. Prominent Golgi bodies, mitochondria, rough endoplasmic reticulum and free ribosomes complemented by neurotubules are also present; the rough endoplasmic reticulum increases in amount with further development. All of these organelles are found in other species as well, e.g. tortoise, carp, shark, ray [40], although human horizontal cells are devoid of neurotubules [40] and are characterized by the presence of Kolmer's crystalloids which consist of longitudinal bodies with ribosomes surrounded by unit membranes [40, 48]. Such crystalloids have not been observed in the chicken.

In some species, e.g. carp, shark, ray [40], goldfish and dogfish [39,44], the horizontal cells are arranged into two distinct layers. In the chicken, however, the internal layer is neither continuous nor distinct.

The existence of a neurotransmitter in horizontal cells is still a speculation. The presence of dense bodies observed in our study may indicate that these cells are adrenergic as reported by Ehinger and Falck [49] in the monkey. Yet, in the chicken, only light-cored vesicles are observed in the horizontal cell terminals of horizontal- horizontal junctions. It is thus possible that these cells may be cholinergic as reported by Koelle [50] in the chick and Nichols and Koelle [51] in mammals and birds.

Histochemical studies of mammalian horizontal cells have revealed the presence of acid phosphatase30 and glycogen35,52. In the chicken, however, glycogen is not observed, although positive reactions for disulfide and sulfhydryl (enzyme active sites) groups are obtained.

DIFFERENTIATION OF HORIZONTAL CELLS

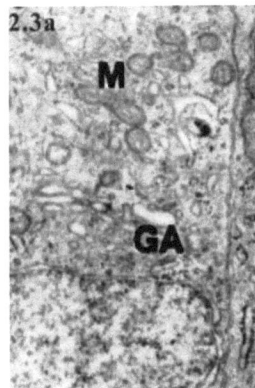

Figure 2.3a. *(stage 38).*

The cell ends bluntly with no projections. Note presence of mitochondria (M) and Golgi apparatus (GA). X14,400.

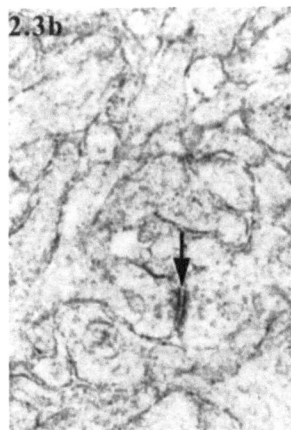

Figure 2.3b. *(stage 40).*

Horizontal-horizontal synapse (arrow). Dark-cored vesicles are not observed. X22,500.

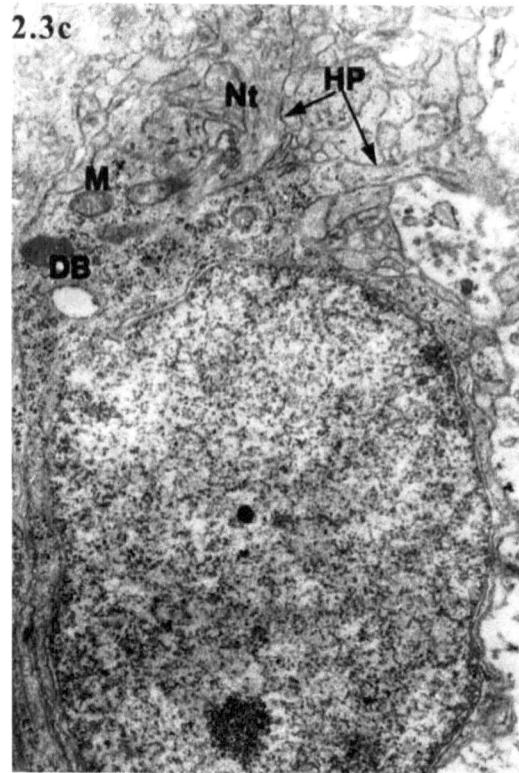

Figure 2.3c. *(stage 40).*

Projections (HP) from horizontal cells enter outer plexiform layer. Neurotubules (Nt), mitochondria (M), dense body (DB) and rough endoplasmic reticulum are present in horizontal cell cytoplasm. X14,400.

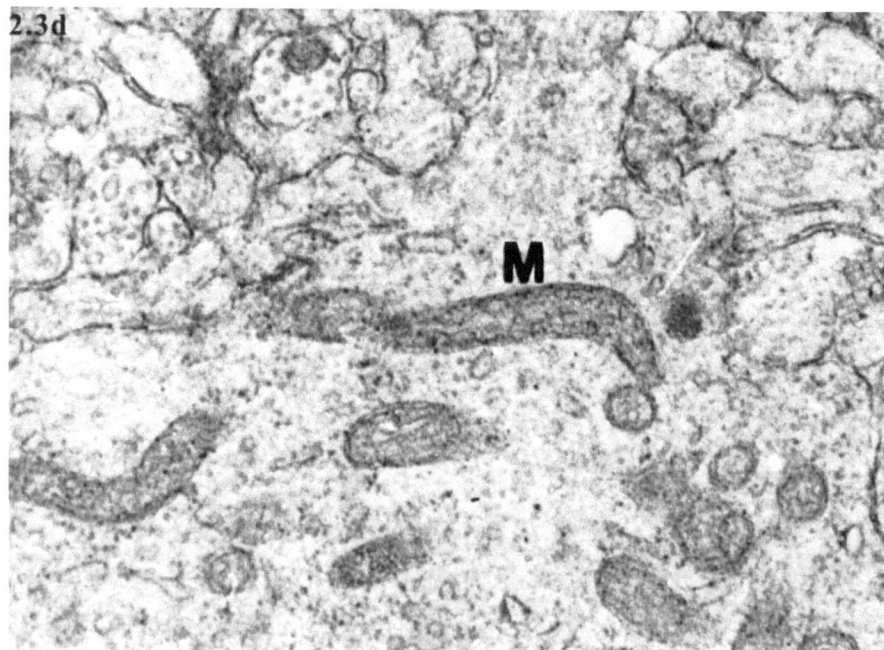

Figure 2.3d. *(stage 42).*

Dark-staining mitochondria (M) in horizontal cell cytoplasm. X22,500.

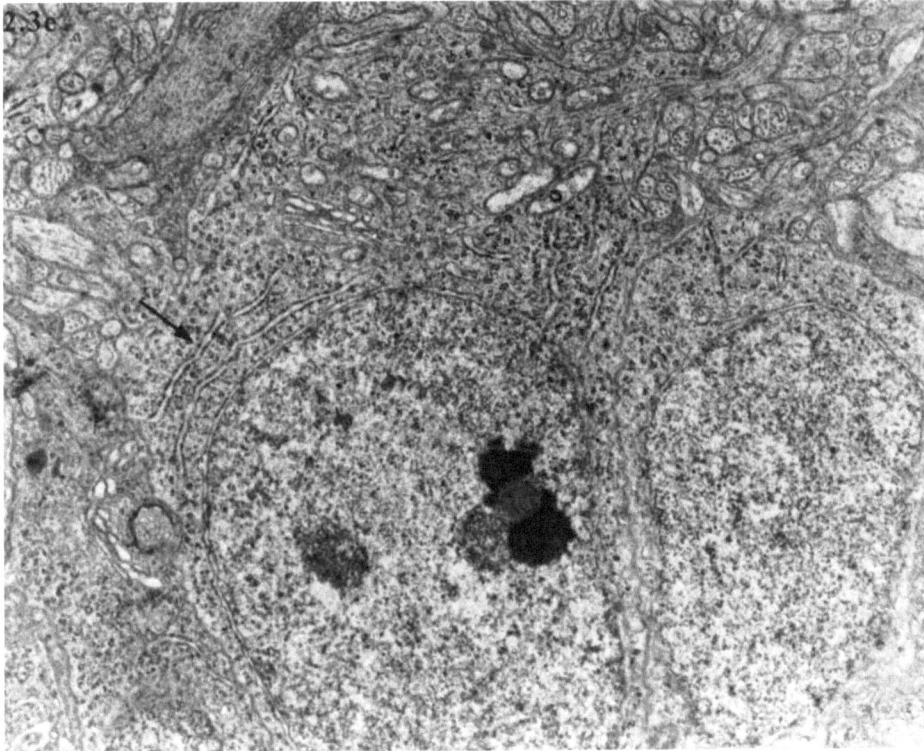

Figure 2.3e. *(stage 45).*

Piliing up of rough endoplasmic reticulum (arrows). X14,400.

BIPOLAR CELLS

Bipolar cells are derivatives of the outer neuroblastic layer [1, 3]. In the early 2/3 of retinal development when the outer plexiform layer appears, the bipolar cells occupy eight to ten layers and still retain their spindle shape, whereas the horizontal cells are confined to about one single layer and are rounder in appearance.

Bipolar cells have dendrites projecting to the outer plexiform and axon forming dyads with ganglion and amacrine cells. Inside the dyad, there are synaptic ribbon [20, 21].

Many types of bipolar cells have been described. Ramón y Cajal [53], utilizing the Golgi technique, found two types (outer and inner) of bipolar cells in the chicken retina on the basis of nuclear size and the pattern of dendritic branching. Type I bipolar cells (outer bipolars) had large nuclei and short dendritic branches while inner bipolars cells has smaller nucleus and long main dendritic trunk. This is similar in fish to chicken [53].

In higher vertebrates, Ramón y Cajal [53] described three types of bipolar cells: (1) rod bipolar with dendritic clusters – which leave the cell body at an acute angle, (2) cone bipolars with horizontal clusters, and (3) giant bipolars. Polyak [54], in "The Vertebrate Visual System", further clarified and confirmed this bipolar classification as mop, brush and midget bipolars.

The mop bipolars were described by Tartuferi [55] in 1887 (cited by Ramón y Cajal [25]) and equal as rod bipolar by Ramón y Cajal [53].

Midget bipolar have short fibers which divide at the external part of the outer plexiform layer. They make no synapses with rods and are monosynaptic. They had been described by Merkel [56], then Ramón y Cajal [53], Kolmer [57], Dowling and Boycott [58], Boycott and Dowling [59] and Hogan *et al.* [60].

Mop bipolars are rod bipolars, brush and midget bipolars are cone bipolars.

All bipolars have neurotubules, endoplasmic reticulum and mitochondria. Some have a long prominent Golgi apparatus and is structurally different from the others [61, 62].

Bipolar cells are cholinergic [63,64] and Shen [65] confirmed that acetylcholinesterase is present in the axons of these cells.

Histochemically, the bipolar cell layer is relatively unreactive. Succinic dehydrogenase in the chick [28], acid phosphatase and phosphorylase in mammals [30, 34] are also documented.

Rebollo [66] and Coulombre [67] noted the existence of Nissl bodies in bipolar cells while glycogen is reported in the bipolar cell layer of the guinea pig [32] and in the carp [68] but is absent in the chick.

Landolt's Clubs

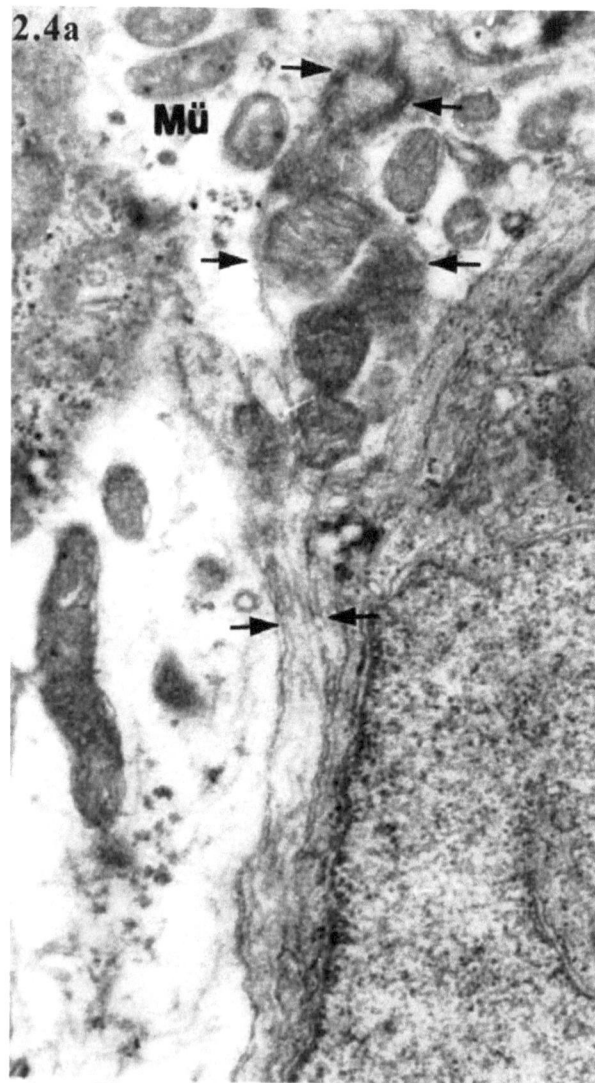

Figure 2.4a. *(stage 38).*

Protrusion of Landolt's club (arrows). Mü – Müller fiber (cell). X22,500.

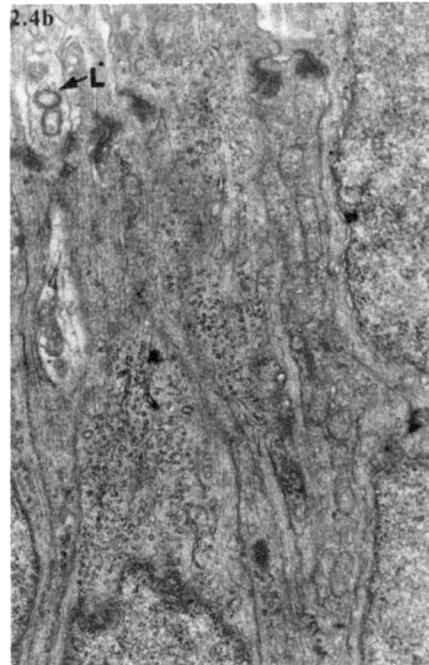

Figure 2.4b. *(stage 45).*

Protruded Landolt's club (L) with a pair of centrioles. X14,400.

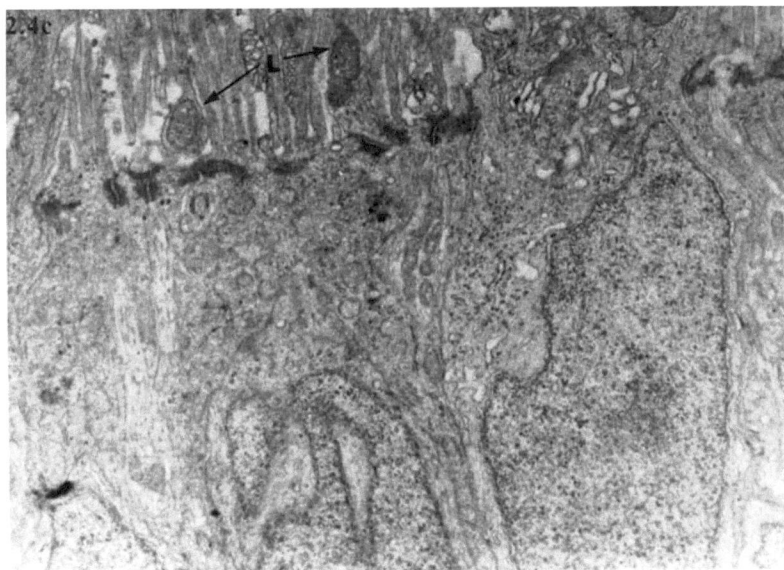

Figure 2.4c. *(stage 45).*

Landolt's clubs (L) with mitochondria inside. X14,400.

MÜLLER CELLS

At the beginning of retinal differentiation, Müller fibers usually have their cell bodies located close to the presumptive ganglion cells, but as development progresses, and as their main trunks elongate, the cell bodies become displaced further externally until they are finally lodged at the level between the bipolar and amacrine cells.

We have classified the gross development of Müller cells into two phases. Phases I is characterized by the formation of the two main trunks (external and internal) from the cell body. Duke-Elder and Cook [69] have reported this initial phase in human embryos of the third month. In the chick, the internal trunk reaches the internal limiting membrane at around stage 30, whereas the external trunk does not arrive at the primitive external limiting membrane until stage 38. The inner segments appear one day earlier (stage 37) and may be responsible for the delayed arrival of the external trunk at the external limiting membrane, although one could speculate that the greater distance the external trunk must travel before reaching the primitive external limiting membrane may also account for this display. The terminal portion of the external trunk interdigitate between the receptor cells (formerly joined by desmosomes). New desmosomes develop immediately between the Müller and receptor cells (except double cones) and the definitive external limiting membrane is now established. In the second phase of development, horizontal branches project out from both external and internal trunks and microvilli are formed at the terminal portion of the external trunk. A similar sequence in the development of Müller cells has been observed in the rat by Weidman and Kuwabara [70].

Concomitant with the above morphogenetic changes, Müller cells undergo cytological maturation which likewise appears to take place in two phases. Initially, there is a relatively large number of rough endoplasmic reticulum and mitochondria, contrary to the study of Uga and Smelser [71], which reports smooth instead of rough endoplasmic reticulum in the rabbit. This is followed by a phase of less rough endoplasmic reticulum and mitochondria but more microtubules. Meller and Glees [72] also mentioned the presence of Golgi complex in chicken Müller cells, which we failed to observe. The exact function of Müller fibers is unknown although there are many speculations. The presence of microtubules in Müller cells seems to make these cells chiefly responsible for impulse transport and/or nutrient transport. However, they may also act as insulators by wrapping themselves around different circuits.

Histochemically, the presence of glycogen in Müller cells is reported in many instances (Shimizu and Maeda [32] in the guinea pig; Nakayama [73] in human embryos; Raviola and Raviola [48] in the rabbit; Kuwabara and Cogan [74] mainly in rabbit and guinea pig; Agarwal *et al.* [33] and Magalhàes and Coimbra [75] in the rabbit). However, the presence of these particles is not detected in chick embryos under the light or electron microscope. Other materials observed in Müller cells include succinic dehydrogenase in the chick [28], nucleoside phosphatase in the rabbit [76] and cholinesterase activity in various mammals [63].

Development of Müller Cells

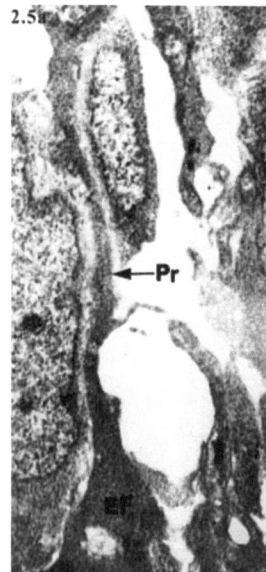

Figure 2.5a. *(stage 30).*

Müller cells showing main trunk projections (Pr). The internal projection forms the end foot (EF), a part of the internal limiting membrane. X8,640.

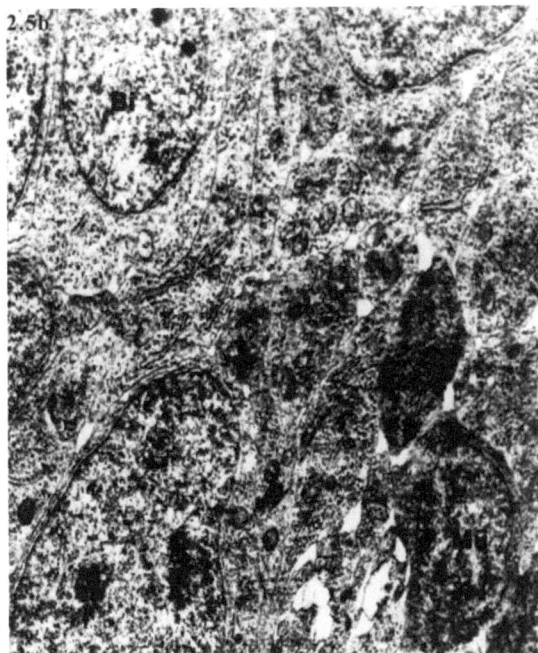

Figure 2.5b. *(stage 36).*

Inner nuclear layer showing bipolar cells (Bi) in telophase and a Müller cell (Mü). X14,400.

DEVELOPMENT OF MÜLLER CELLS

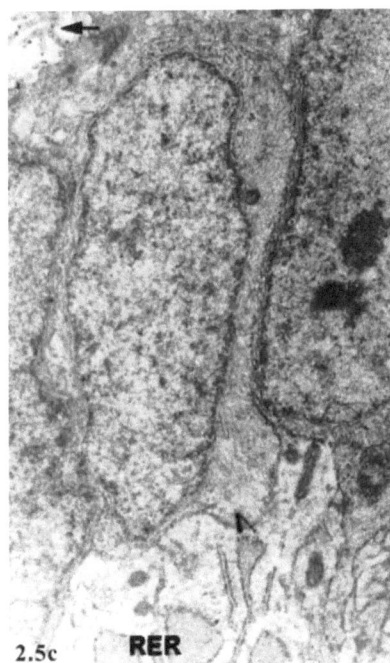

Figure 2.5c. *(stage 42).*

Projection of Müller microvilli (arrow). Note dilated rough endoplasmic reticulum (RER) in region of outer plexiform layer. X14,400.

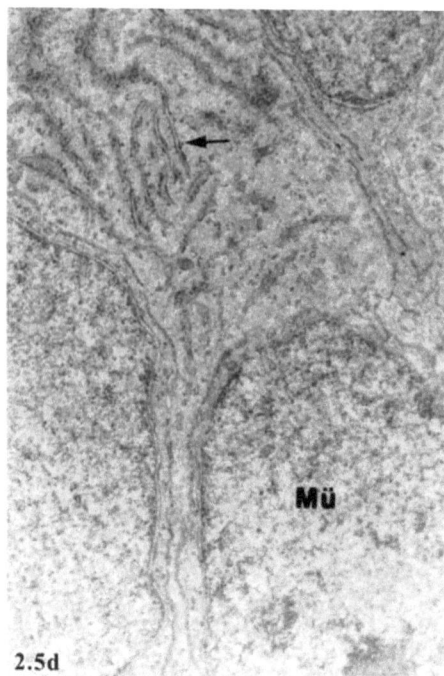

Figure 2.5d. *(stage 42).*

Inner nuclear layer showing rough endoplasmic reticulum (arrow) in Müller cells (Mü). Such alignment first appears at stage 40.

FURTHER DEVELOPMENT OF MÜLLER CELLS

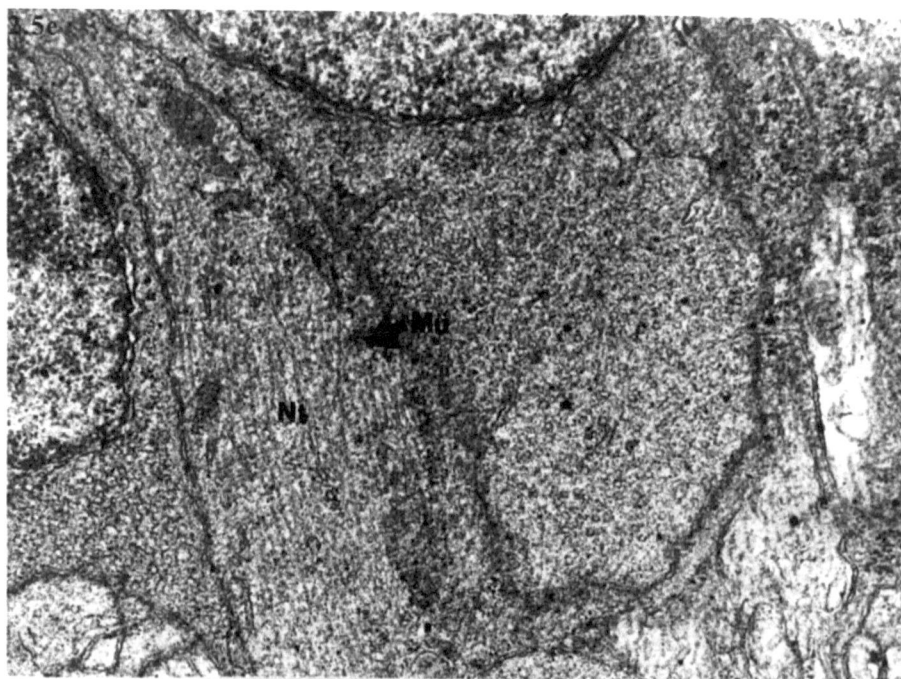

Figure 2.5e. *(newly hatched).*

Müller cells (Mü) near the outer plexiform layer. Note the tremendous amount of neurotubules (Nt), few endoplasmic reticulum and mitochondria in this region. X30,400.

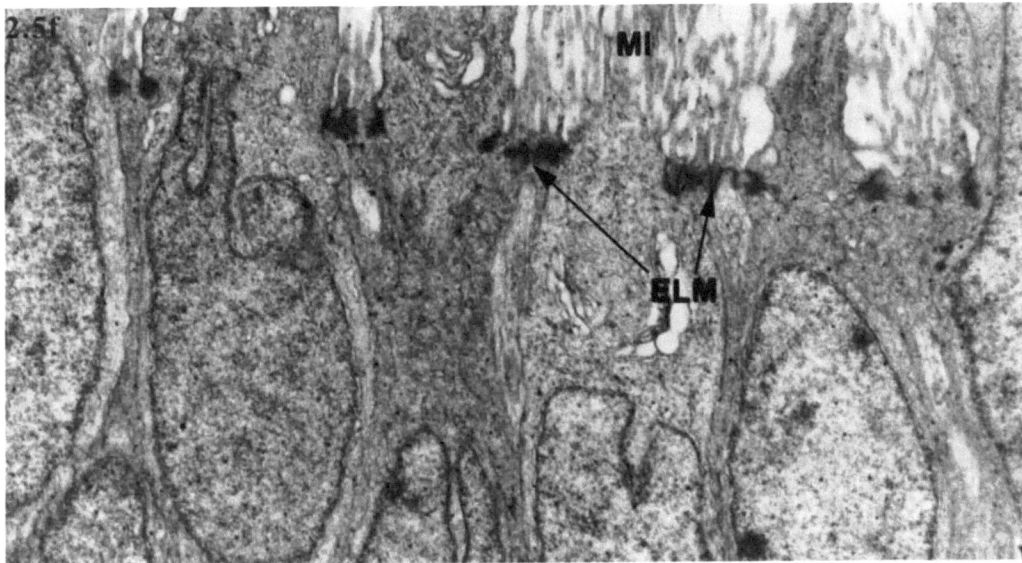

Figure 2.5f. *(newly hatched).*

Projections of microvilli (Mi) above the level of external limiting membrane (ELM). X10,560.

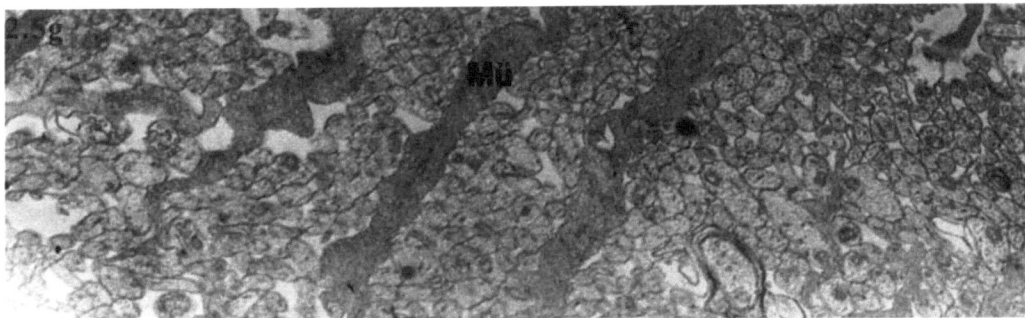

Figure 2.5g. *(stage 45).*

Projection of secondary Müller (Mü) branches into the nerve fiber layer. X14,400.

AMACRINE CELLS

Amacrine cells are important cells in the inner nuclear layer of the retina. Together with bipolar and ganglion cells, they participate in the formation of "dyads" in the inner plexiform layer.

The amacrine cell probably aids in the transmission of impulses through two routes, both of which are indirect when compared to the main pathway, namely, that which goes directly from bipolar to ganglion cells at the "dyads". The pathways in which amacrine cells participate involve amacrine-amacrine contacts observed in the study of Dowling [47] as well as in the present study. First, an amacrine cell receives an impulse through contact with the bipolar cell in the "dyad". Next, the impulse is communicated to neighboring amacrine cells which in turn either relay the impulse to the ganglion cell of a neighboring "dyad", or to a lesser extent, to a ganglion cell that is in contact with the latter amacrine cell but not in a "dyad" (*i.e.* no bipolar cell contacts). In these respects, amacrine cells serve as a secondary mechanism in impulses transmission by amplifying the principal pathway.

Dowling and Werblin [77] and Dowling [47] discovered in rabbit, ground squirrel and mudpuppy an equal number of a second kind of "dyads" involving bipolar plus amacrine-amacrine pairings co-existing with those involving bipolar plus amacrine-ganglion pairings. However, on the chick, no such amacrine-amacrine paired "dyads" are detected. Furthermore, Dowling [47] reported that the intracellular electrical activity of amacrine cells is mainly in an on-and-off fashion which seems particularly suitable for mediating motion-sensing responses. On this basis, the author speculated that since the former three species of animals are natural preys in their wild state, motion-sensing activities are important to their survival. Perhaps, because the chick is less prone to predators, this second type of "dyads" is not developed in this species.

Morphologically, the many types of amacrine cells can only be identified by silver impregnation [53] and thus, are indistinguishable on an ultrastructural basis [60]. Under the electron microscope, all types of amacrine cells possess rough endoplasmic reticulum, free ribosomes, Golgi apparatus, centrioles and dense bodies. The nuclei may or may not be indented, and thus unlike those of the higher species (Hogan *et al.* [60] in the human).

Embryologically, amacrine cells are a product of the inner neuroblastic layer [3]. This layer is composed of three types of cells: Müller, amacrine and ganglion cells. For example, in the chicken, at stage 35, the amacrine cells, followed by the Müller cells, migrate externally (toward the bipolar and horizontal cells) to form the inner nuclear layer and the gap remaining between the ganglion and amacrine cells becomes the inner plexiform layer. Apparently, amacrine and ganglion cells are among the first cells to develop in the retina, a proposition suggested by Coulombre [53] in the chick and Morest [54] in the neonatal rat.

In the chicken, the amacrine cells become morphologically discernible at stage 36, as pointed out by Coulombre [4]. They are not the very first retinal cells to differentiate; they follow the ganglion cells by several days. Development of the amacrine cells proceeds in two phase: (1) the prolongation of processes and the appearance of intracytoplasmic dense bodies (both at stage 37) (Olney [79] in albino mice), and (2) the increase in ribosomes (stage 42). The ribosomes are initially free and subsequently become aligned around the nuclei as rough endoplasmic reticulum (stage 45). Concomitant with these changes, the size of the amacrine cells also gradually increases.

Synaptic vesicles are seen in the amacrine cells in the inner plexiform layer by stage 40, when "dyad" formation takes place between bipolar and ganglion cells. Synaptic contacts between amacrine and ganglion cells without the involvement of "dyads" are not seen until around hatching in the chicken (stage 45), which leads one to assume that maturation of this kind of amacrine-ganglion pathway does not occur until this time.

Several different types of neurotransmitter material have been suggested to reside in the amacrine cells (table XIX). Nichols *et al.* [80] (in nonprimate mammals), Ehinger and Falck [81] (in amphibians, reptiles, birds and primates), Kramer [82] (in mammals), and Kramer *et al.* [83] (in mammals) believe it to be adrenergic in nature. Boycott *et al.* [84]. (cited by Kramer *et al.* [83]) suggest a special amacrine cell type, equivalent to the large amacrine cells described by us in the light microscope, secretes an adrenergic material – dopamine. Hebb [63], however, detected acetylcholinesterase in the adult amacrine cells of various vertebrates. Shen [65] also reported acetylcholinesterase activity in the amacrine cells in the chick around the 6th day, although our study has shown that synaptic vesicles are not present at this time and that the amacrine cells themselves cannot be recognized as separate entities even with the electron microscope. Moreover, ultrastructural indications of adrenergic material, e.g. dark- cored vesicles are not, for instance, in amacrine-amacrine contacts (Coupland [18,19] hypothesized that dark-cored vesicles are adrenergic). Ehinger and Falck [81] found GABA in the rabbit's amacrine cells. Neal and Inversen [85] suggested that GABA may also be present in rat amacrine cells. Other neurotransmitter substances such as glycine have also been implicated in the rabbit [86].

The presence of enzymatic active sites has been suggested by the sulfhydryl positivity we obtained in the histochemical studies of the amacrine cells. These enzymes include succinic dehydrogenase [28], ATPase [87], acid phosphatise [30] and alkaline phosphatise [66]. An increase of RNA was seen also in these cells around hatching in the chicken [66].

AMACRINE CELL DEVELOPMENT

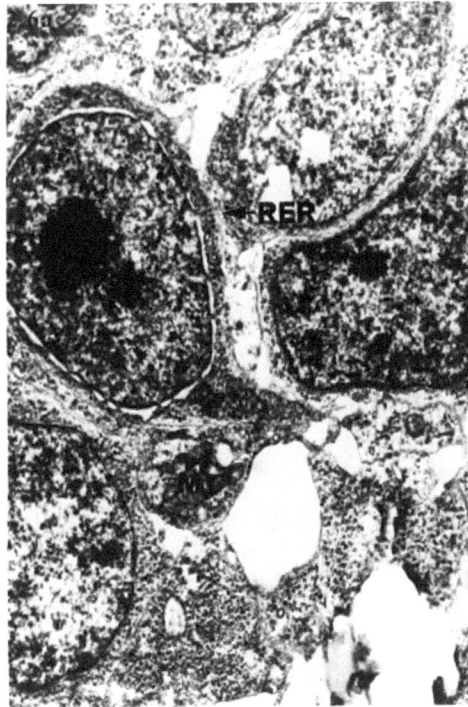

Figure 2.6a. *(stage 36).*

Mitochondria (M) and rough endoplasmic reticulum (RER) are the only organelles present. X14,400.

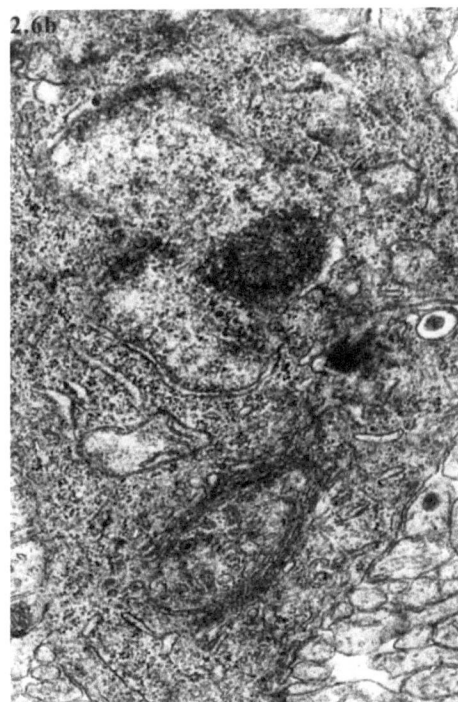

Figure 2.6b. *(stage 37).*

Unusual indented nucleus. X22,500.

AMACRINE CELL DEVELOPMENT

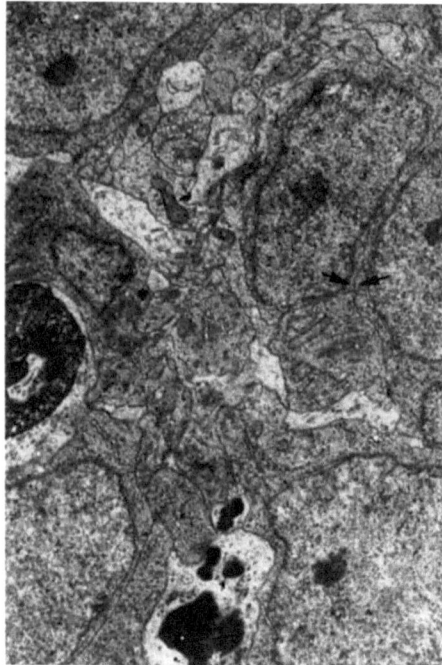

Figure 2.6c. *(stage 37).*

Note close contact between cells (arrows). X8,960.

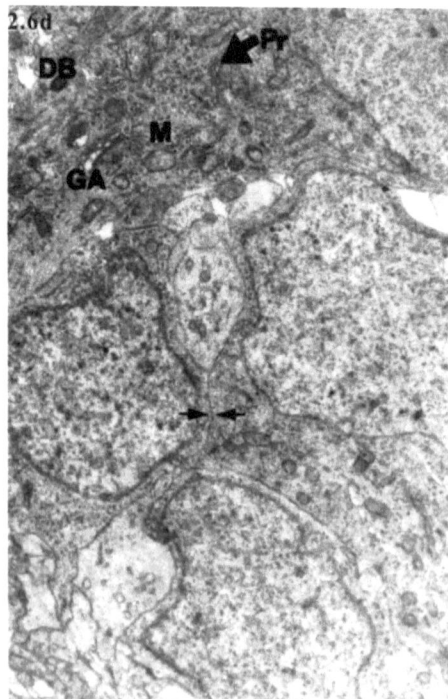

Figure 2.6d. *(stage 37).*

Amacrine cell projection (Pr). Note presence of rough endoplasmic reticulum, mitochondria (M), Golgi apparatus (GA) and dense bodies (DB). Amacrine-amacrine contact is indicated by arrows. X8,960.

FURTHER DEVELOPMENT OF AMACRINE CELLS

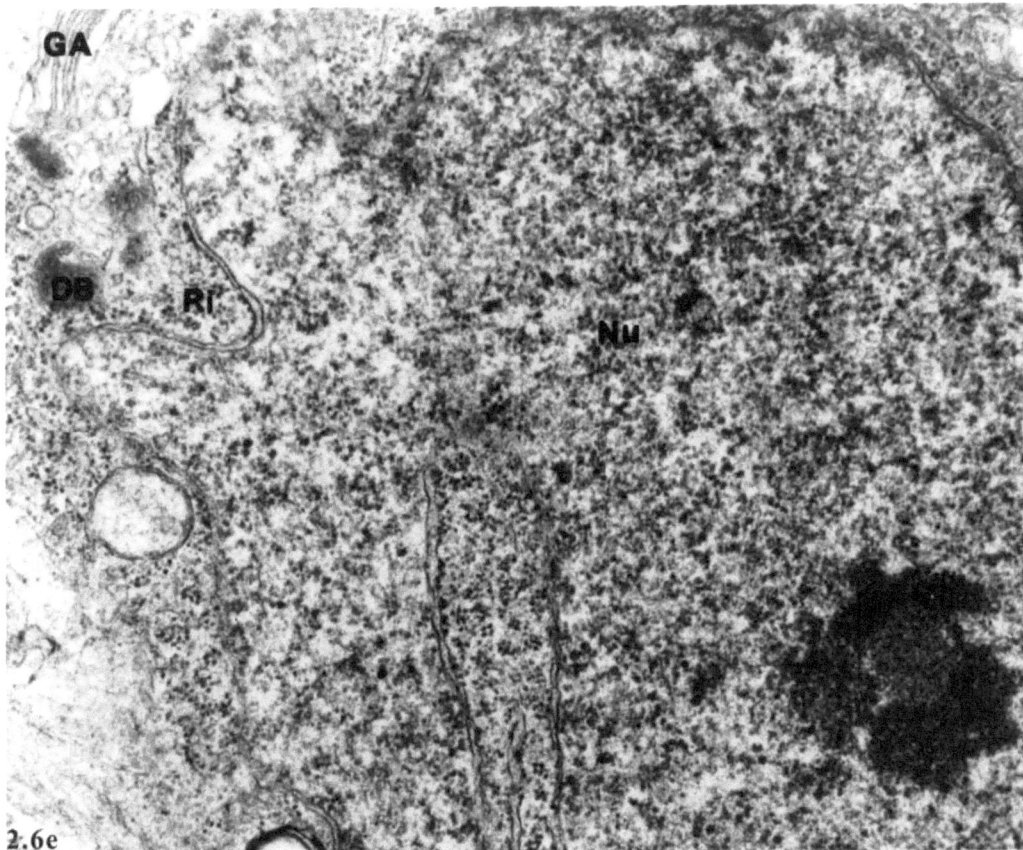

Figure 2.6e. *(stage 42).*

Ribosomes (Ri) are numerous around the nucleus (Nu). Note presence of Golgi apparatus (GA) and dense bodies (DB). X30,400.

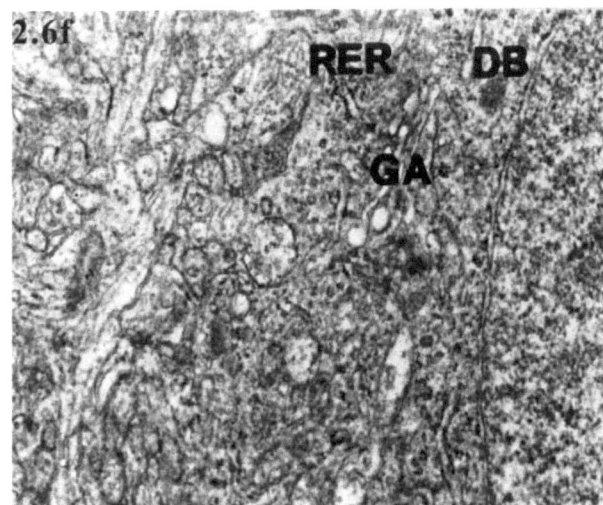

Figure 2.6f. *(stage 45).*

Golgi apparatus (GA), rough endoplasmic reticulum (RER) and dense bodies (DB). X14,400.

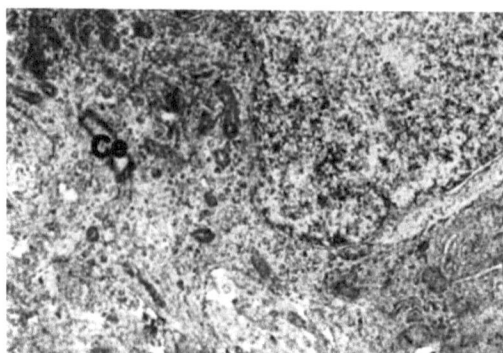

Figure 2.6g. *(stage 45).*

Centriole (Ce). X14,400.

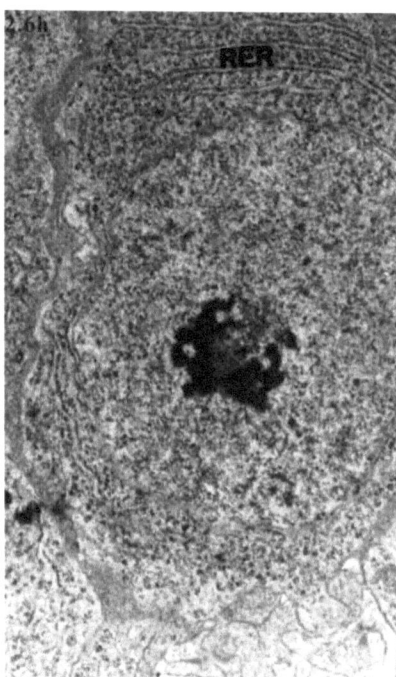

Figure 2.6h. *(stage 45).*

Stacking up of rough endoplasmic reticulum (RER). X14,400.

INNER PLEXIFORM LAYER

There have been relatively few studies on the specific morphogenesis of the inner plexiform layer. Light microscopically, this layer in the chick embryo has been investigated by Weysse and Burgess [88], Mann [1], Coulombre [4] and Shen [65]. Electron microscopic data are lacking for chicken although Olney [79] and Weidman and Kuwabara [89] have studied the genesis if this layer in mice and rat respectively, and found, for example, that the maturation of this layer occurs in an orderly fashion with the appearance of dense junction followed by the appearance of synaptic vesicles and synaptic ribbons. These studies, although failing to establish the specific cellular components involved in this layer, have made admirable attempts to initiate embryological studies of this complex layer.

Extensive ultrastructural data on the inner plexiform layer in the adult chicken [90], adult primates [58], frogs [91] and the human [60] have helped us to identify the three basic cell types in the developing chicken inner plexiform layer and to determine their synaptic relationships.

In this atlas, we show that the differentiation of bipolar axons occurs in two phases. In the first phase (stage 37), the axons are projected into the further inner plexiform layer. And, in the second phase (stage 40), contacts are made with processes from ganglion and amacrine cells forming "dyads." Synaptic ribbons and synaptic vesicles make their appearance at this time (stage 40), and thus, all structural components are present for normal functioning.

In the meantime (stage 40), processes from amacrine cells have acquired dense bodies in their cytoplasm and synapse with each other to form the so-called conventional synapses (or dense junctions) characterized by the presence of pre- and postsynaptic thickenings with vesicles on the presynaptic side. The initial appearance of these junctions at this stage (approximately 14 days of incubation) is also reported by Sheffield and Fischman [70]. In later stages (45 to hatching), two more advances are seen: (1) the initial appearance of amacrine-ganglion cell junctions, and (2) the formation of a second type of amacrine-amacrine cell junctions, which has vesicles on both pre- and postsynaptic sides, *i.e.* reciprocal control. Dowling [13] postulated that there are two types of amacrine-amacrine contacts in the plexiform layer, one type with excitatory synapses and the other with inhibitory synapses. Perhaps, the reciprocal type is inhibitory (feedback), whereas the conventional type mentioned before is excitatory, thus making amacrine cells directionally selective (personal speculation).

Like the bipolar cells, the ganglion cell processes also develop in two phases. In the first phase (stage 40), dense bodies and a few neurotubules appear in the cytoplasm of these processes. During the second phase (stages 45 to hatching), the formation of amacrine-ganglion cell synapses take place.

Thus, our findings indicate that the transmitting pathway form bipolar to ganglion cells (and thus the optic nerve) becomes established by stage 40, although the synaptic relationships between amacrine and ganglion cells are not completed until several days later (stage 45).

Electron microscopic observations present here further indicate the presence of certain particles in the inner plexiform layer, which are suspected to be glycogen, although we could not detect it in the light microscope by the PAS reaction. Agarwal *et al.* [33] reported the presence of granular glycogen in this layer in the rabbit and the enzyme, phosphorylase, responsible for the breakdown of glycogen has been reported by Shanthaveerappa and Bourne [30] in the rabbit and squirrel monkey. Amemiya [31] localized glucose-1-phosphatase, which synthesizes polysaccharide, in the rat. The above results hint at a possible presence of glycogen in this layer.

DEVELOPMENT OF INNER PLEXIFORM LAYER (STAGES 37-40)

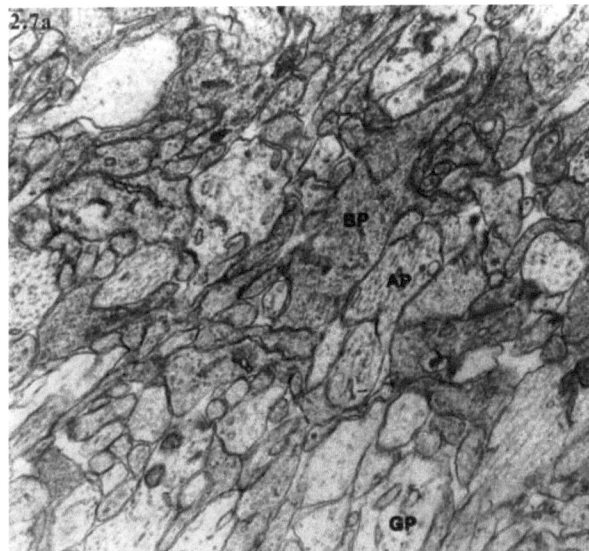

Figure 2.7a. (stage 37).

Presumptive processes of bipolar (BP), amacrine (AP) and ganglion (GP) cells in the inner plexiform layer. X30,400.

DEVELOPMENT OF INNER PLEXIFORM LAYER (STAGES 37-40)

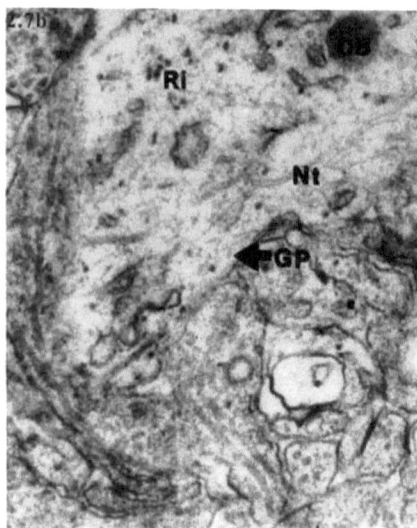

Figure 2.7b. *(stage 37).*

Ganglion cell process (GP) with a few neurotubules (Nt), dense bodies (DB) and groups of ribosomes (Ri). X47,500.

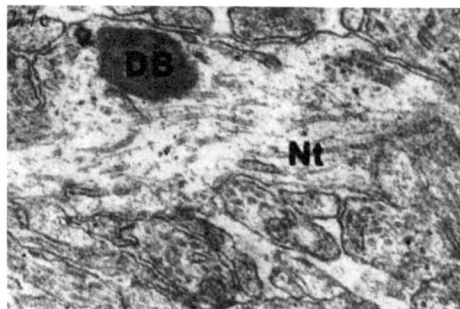

Figure 2.7c. *(stage 40).*

Ganglion cell process showing a large dense body and a few neurotubules (Nt). X30,400.

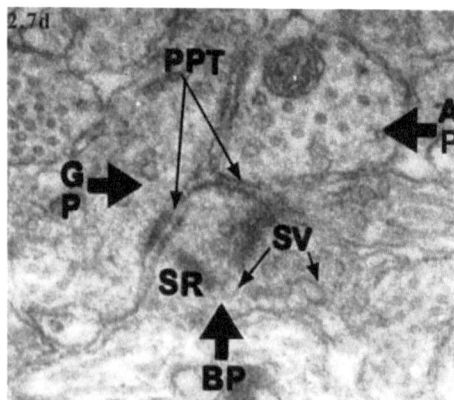

Figure 2.7d. *(stage 40).*

"Dyad" formation between processes of bipolar (BP), ganglion (GP) and amacrine (AP) cells. Note synaptic vesicles (SV), pre- and postsynaptic thickenings (PPT). X47,500.

INNER PLEXIFORM LAYER, STAGE 40

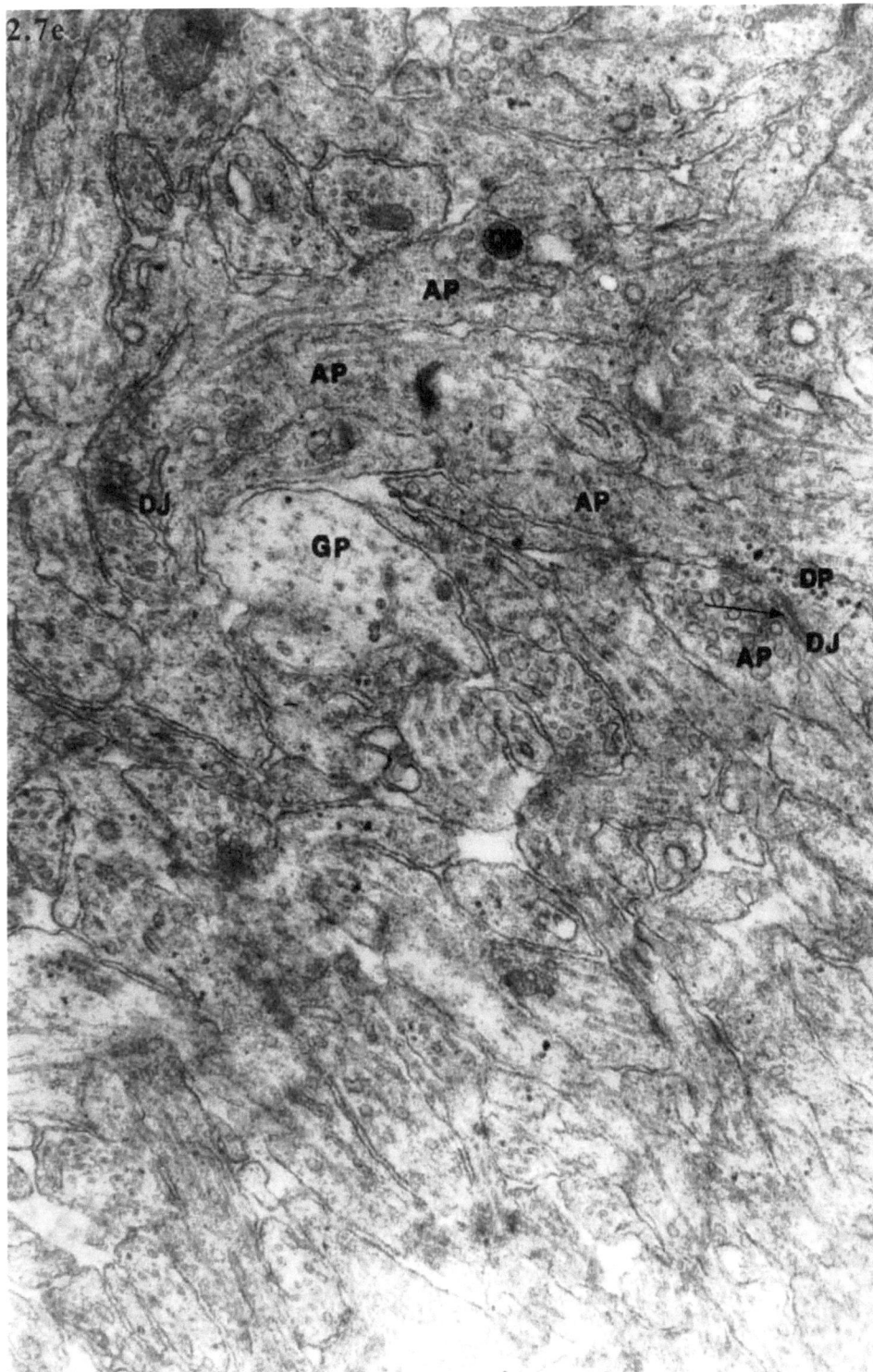

Figure 2.7e.

Amacrine cell processes (AP) containing dense bodies (DB), dense junctions (DJ) and dense particles (DP). Note that one amacrine cell process synapses on another at one point (light arrow). A ganglion cell process (GP) is also indicated. X30,400.

INNER PLEXIFORM LAYER, STAGE 42

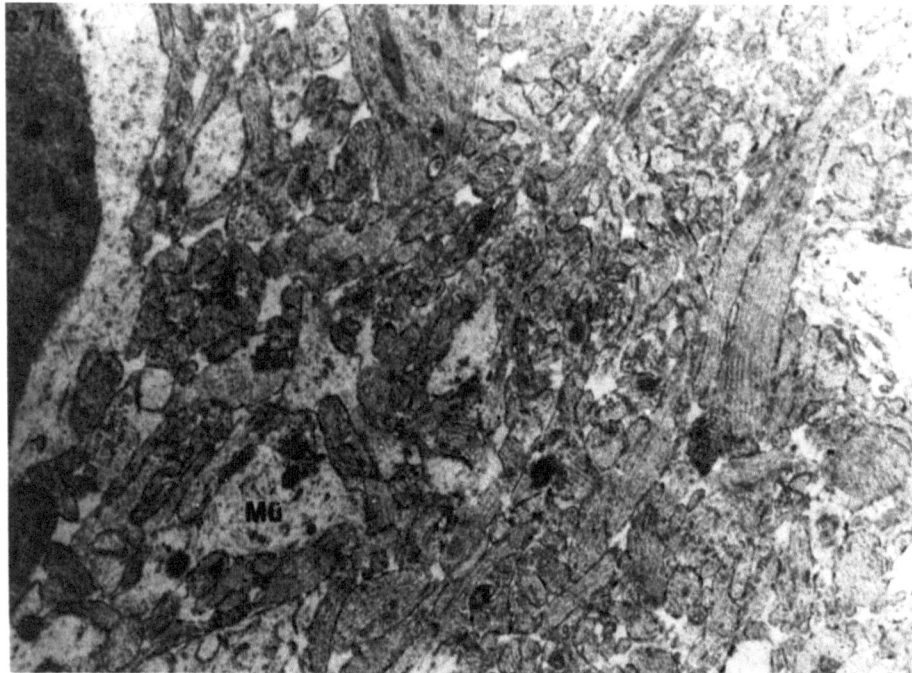

Figure 2.7f.

Electron lucent Müller fiber (Mü) branches project into the spaces between the other cell processes. X14,400.

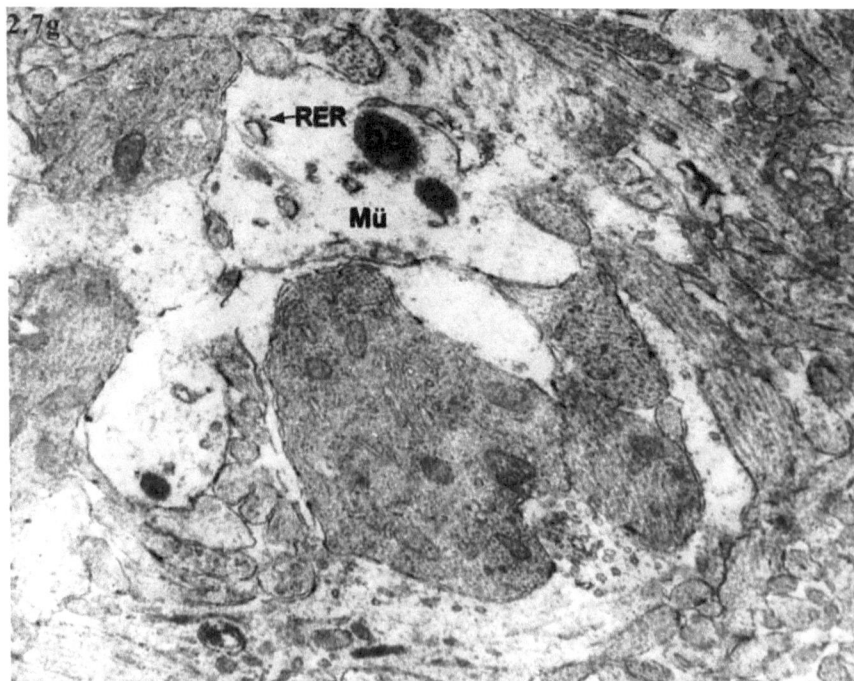

Figure 2.7g.

Higher magnification of Müller fiber (Mü) branches which have short rough endoplasmic reticulum (RER) and dense bodies (DB). X30,400.

INNER PLEXIFORM LAYER, STAGE 45 – NEWLY HATCHED

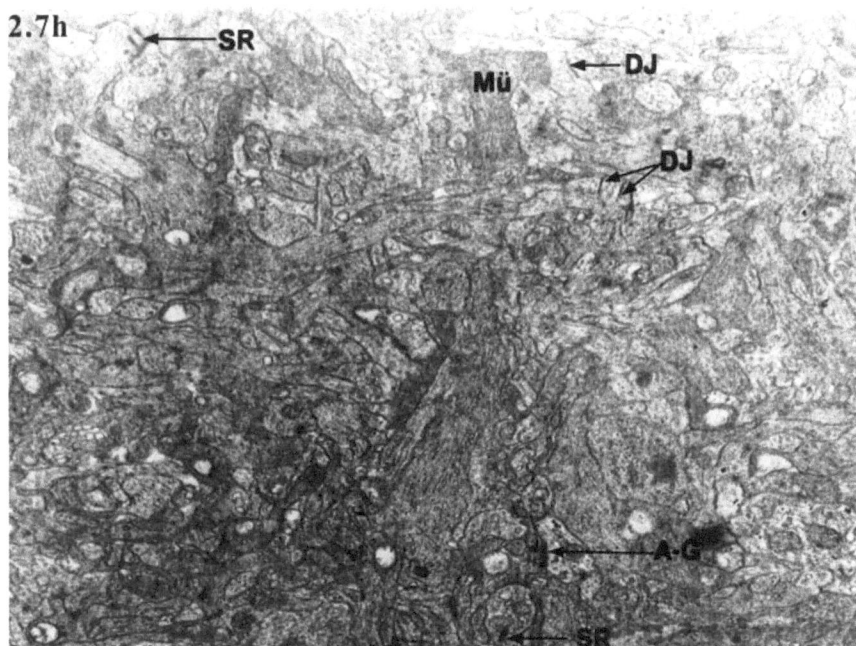

Figure 2.7h. *(stage 45).*

Note increase in amount of synaptic ribbons (SR) and dense junctions (DJ). Also note presence of amacrine-ganglion (A-G) synapse. Müller fibers (Mü) are more electron dense at this stage. X14,400.

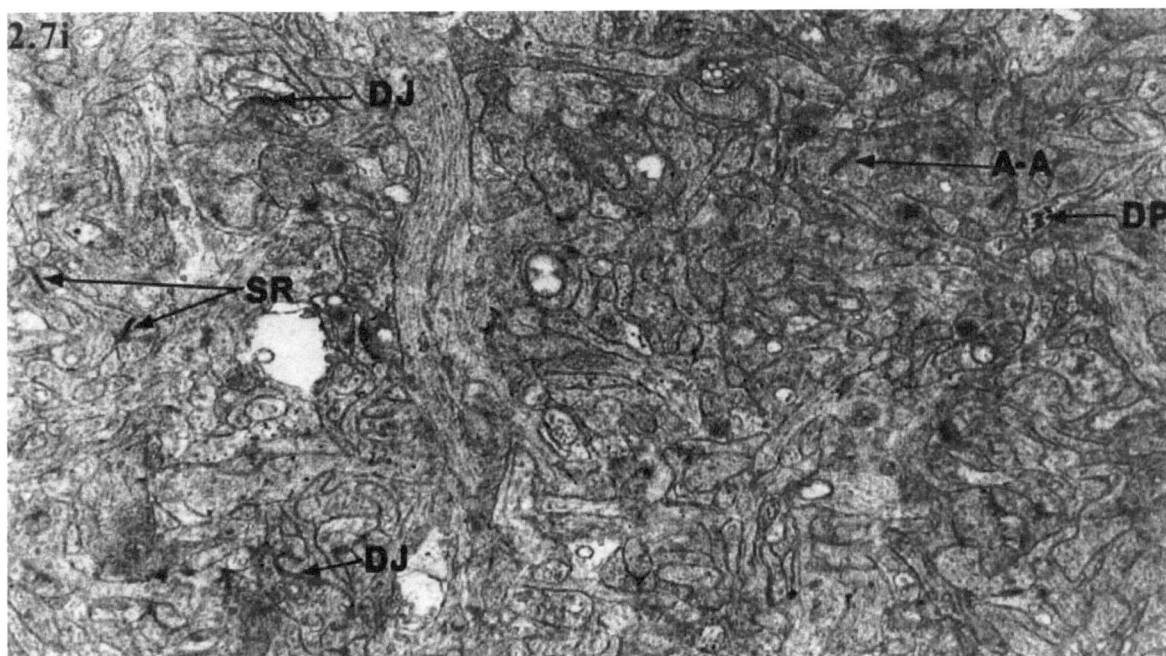

Figure 2.7i. *(stage 45).*

Again note increase in amount of synaptic ribbons (SR) and dense junctions (DJ). Also note amacrine-amacrine (A-A) contact with reciprocal control (synaptic vesicles on both opposing sides). DP – dense particles. X14,400.

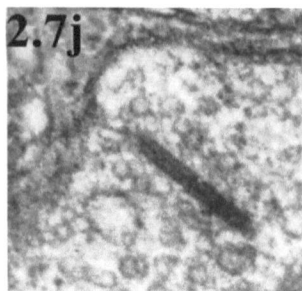

Figure 2.7j. *(newly hatched).*

Bipolar cell process in inner plexiform layer showing synaptic ribbon (five layers) and vesicles of two sizes. X30,400.

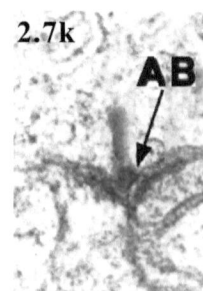

Figure 2.7k. *(newly hatched).*

Bipolar cell process in inner plexiform layer showing synaptic ribbon and arciform body (AB). X30,400.

GANGLION CELL LAYER

Ganglion cells accept impulse information from bipolar and amacrine cells and transmit such impulses to the central nervous system through the nerve fiber layer and optic nerve. The various synaptic relationships of the ganglion cells occur in the inner plexiform layer and have been discussed in that section.

Ramón y Cajal [53] distinguished different types of ganglion cells on the basis of their cytological appearance and the stratification of their processes by using the silver technique. However, the same cytological organelles and arrangement present in these variations of the ganglion cell make them indistinguishable either by routine staining in light microscope or under the electron microscope.

It has been repeatedly demonstrated that during vertebrate development, ganglion cells are the first neuronal cells to separate from the non-differentiable neuroepithelial mass and form a discrete layer [93, 94]. In the chicken, O'Rahilly and Meyer [95] initially detected ganglion cells at stage 18 (3.5 days of incubation), whereas in the English sparrow, Slonaker [96] recorded their appearance on the fourth day of incubation. In the human, Magitot [97] observed ganglion cell presence in the central retina in six to eight week old embryos. Mann [3] later found that ganglion cells begin to migrate at 10 mm. C.R. and by 18 mm. C.R., a distinct ganglion cell layer is formed. And, according to O'Rahilly [98], this process occurs between horizon XII and XVII which starts at around 4 weeks of age. In the rat, on the other hand, ganglion cells do not begin to differentiate until after birth [78].

The stratification of the ganglion cell layer has been studied in the amphibian by Cameron [93] who noted that ganglion cells are initially organized into two layers which later become one. In the chick embryo, Weysse and Burgess [88] found three rows at first, and Coulombre [4] observed a single layer at 8 to 10 days of incubation, which agrees with the present study (stage 37). Under the electron microscope, a "pseudo' layering can be observed up to stage 36. The cells form two layers in some areas but not in other regions in the same section. It seems possible that ganglion cell stratification may be different in different regions of the retina. Extensive studies of retinal development have established that the central and upper parts of the retina differentiate earlier than the peripheral and lower parts, as expressed in Mann's [2] classical lecture, "The regional differentiation of the vertebrate retina", delivered to the Royal College of Surgeons. Since then, this information has appeared in practically all textbooks of visual development.

Ganglion Cell Nucleus in Development

In the course of ganglion cell development, constrictions of nuclei are often observed. These constrictions may indicate a process of amitosis as suggested by Cameron [93] in his studies on amphibian retina.

Ganglion Cell Cytoplasm in Development

With respect to ganglion cell fine structure, Fisher and Jacobson [99], in their study of Xenopus embryos, reported three progressive stages of development: (1) the appearance of endoplasmic reticulum and Golgi apparatus, (2) the appearance of mitochondria and macrofilaments, and (3) the presence of Nissl bodies. Our data on the chick vary slightly with these observations. Initially, we detected endoplasmic and mitochondria (stage 30) followed by Golgi apparatus and dense bodies (stage 37). The endoplasmic reticulum begins to stack up in the choroidal side of the cell at stage 37 to form Nissl bodies which subsequently (stage 42) exhibit strong RNA positivity as previously shown by Eichner [100] and Rebollo [66]. Finally, Nissl body formation occurs throughout the cell by stage 45. In other light microscopic studies, Coulombre [67] described the initial appearance of Nissl bodies at a much later time (17 days of incubation) which may be due to his use of incubation days, an often inaccurate estimation of developmental age. As mentioned previously, the staging of embryos from external morphological criteria is far more superior and useful because this method permits accurate comparison of the developmental state by different investigators.

Nissl Bodies

The development of retinal ganglion cell Nissl bodies has been reported in other animals, e.g. the puppy [101], human [73]. In the rabbit, Radnot and Lovas [102] referred to them as subsurface cristae. The functional significance of Nissl bodies is primarily in the synthesis of protein material, and may be closely related to the maturation of the ganglion cells, and thus, the maturation of the retina itself. It is noteworthy, for example, that the adult electroretinogram (ERG) is first obtained at stage 45 (19 to 20 days of incubation) [21, 24, 27] when Nissl body formation is completed (personal observation).

Neurotransmitter in Ganglion Cells

It is also possible that the functional maturation of ganglion cells depends on the production of transmitter material. Shen [65] reported acetylcholinesterase in ganglion cells (in the 4th day chick embryo), thus confirming previous results by Hebb [63] and Leplat and Gerebtzoff [64]. Other groups of researchers, De Iraldi and Etcheverry [103] and Ehinger [104], suggested catecholamine or GABA instead. Whatever the neurotransmitter is, the synthesis of this material is closely related to the Golgi apparatus. It is stored in dense bodies which initially appear in ganglion cell cytoplasm at stage 37, and later in the processes at stage 40 (see section on inner plexiform layer). These bodies become more electron dense at stage 45, probably due to an increase in materials in the package.

Other components of the chicken ganglion cells are essentially similar to those described in higher species, e.g. human [105]. Micro- and macrofilaments are rarely, if ever, observed in the ganglion cell bodies themselves. Their presence in the processes has been discussed in the section on the inner plexiform layer.

DEVELOPMENT OF GANGLION CELL LAYER

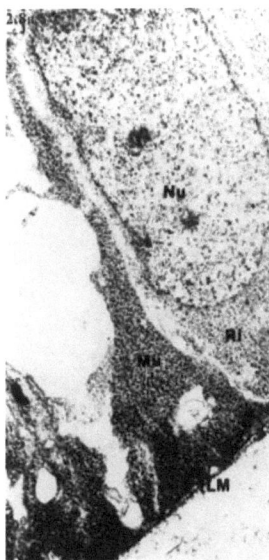

Figure 2.8a. *(stage 30).*

Ganglion cell layer. Nucleus (Nu) of ganglion cell is shown. The cell contains a lot of ribosomes (Ri). The main trunk of Müller fiber (Mü) is near the ganglion cell forming a part of the internal limiting membrane (ILM). X14,400.

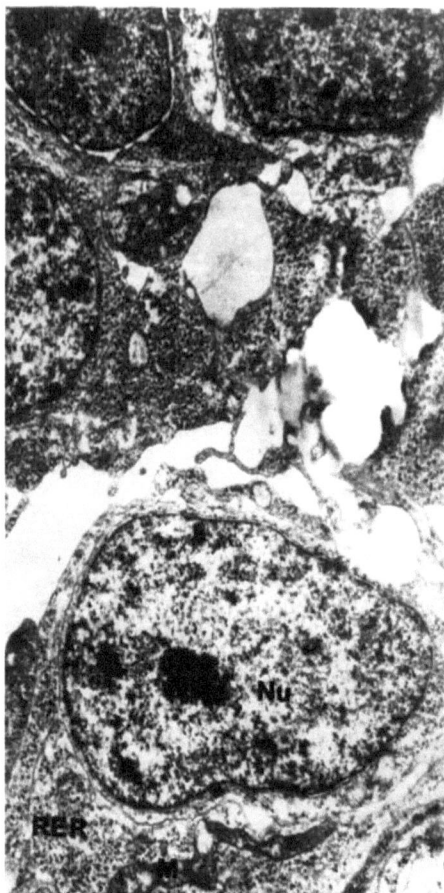

Figure 2.8b. *(stage 36).*

Ganglion cell with a nucleus (Nu), mitochondria (M) and rough endoplasmic reticulum (RER). X14,400.

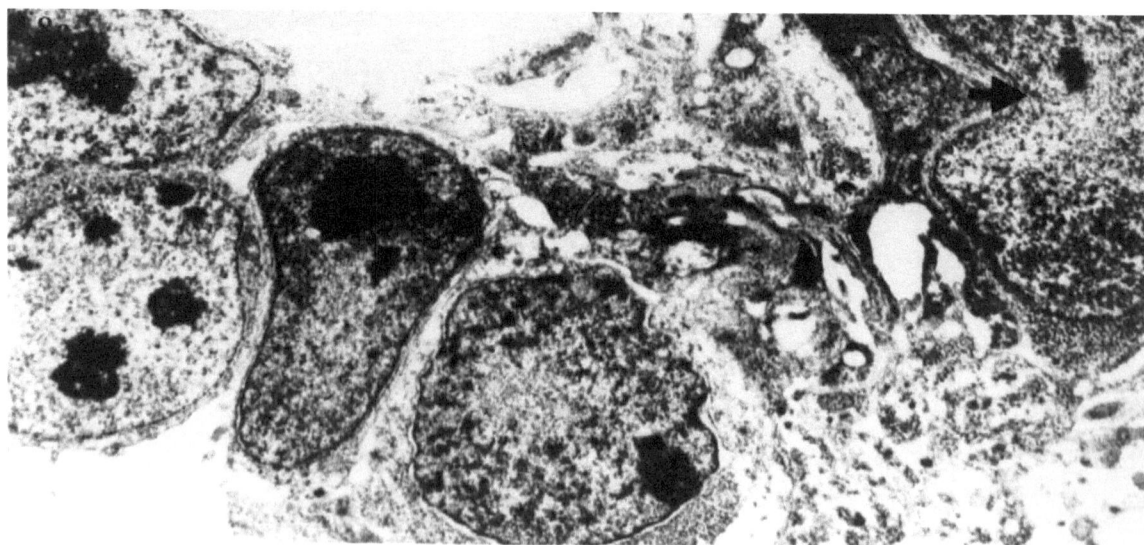

Figure 2.8c. *(stage 36).*

Note constriction of one ganglion cell body (arrow) and a tendency of pseudolayering. X10,500.

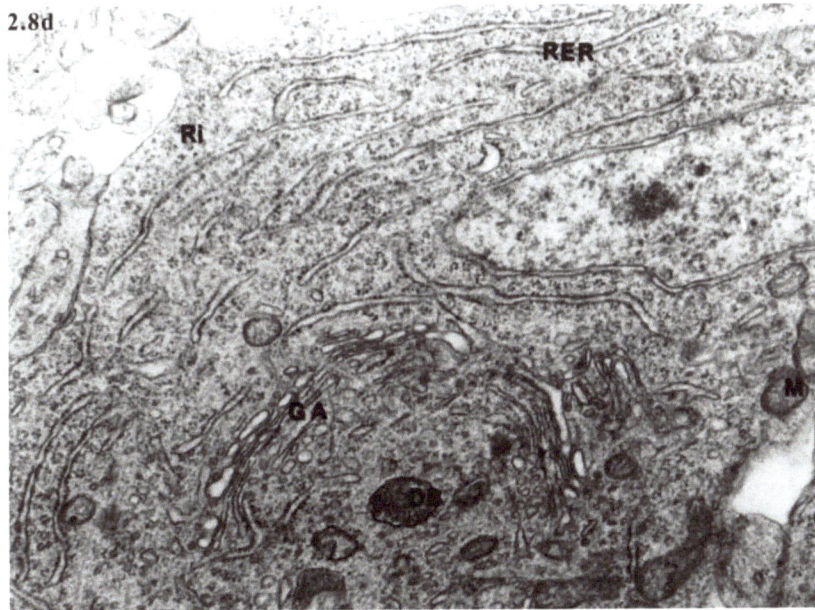

FURTHER DEVELOPMENT OF GANGLION CELL LAYER

Figure 2.8d. *(stage 37).*

Ganglion cell showing the beginning of the stacking of rough endoplasmic reticulum (RER), the presence of ribosomes (Ri), Golgi apparatus (GA), dense bodies (DB) and mitochondria (M). X30,400.

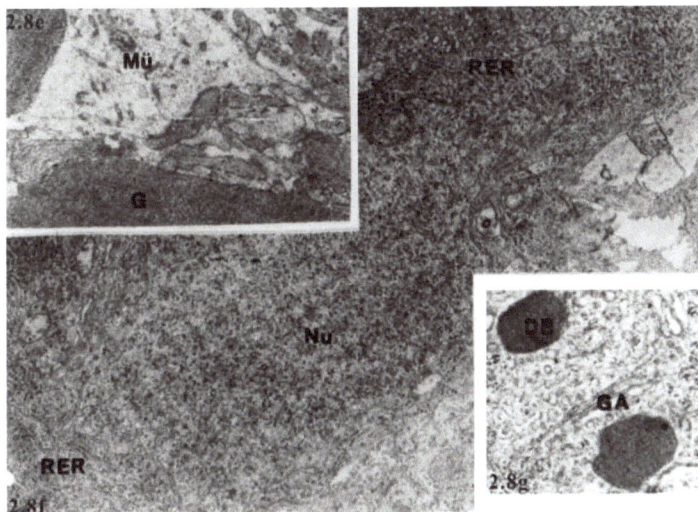

Figure 2.8e. *(stage 42).*

Ganglion cell (G) layer surrounded by new branches of Müller fiber (Mü) which have a light contrast.

Figure 2.8f. *(stage 45).*

Ganglion cell showing rough endoplasmic reticulum (RER) surrounding all sides of the nucleus (Nu). X30,400.

Figure 2.8g. *(newly hatched).*

Homogeneous dense body (DB) within a ganglion cell. Note its close association with the Golgi apparatus (GA). X30,400.

NERVE FIBER LAYER AND INTERNAL LIMITING MEMBRANE

The nerve fiber layer is comprised mainly of non-myelinated ganglion cell axons which arise very early in development. Coulombre [4] reported the presence of the nerve fiber layer in four to five day old chick embryos. Both O'Rahilly and Meyer [106] and Rogers [107], using silver technique, found nerve fibers to appear much earlier (stage 18; 65 hours). O'Rahilly and Meyer [95] further confirmed their observations in 1959, and reported that these nerve fibers reach the brain by stage 23 (3.5 days to 4 days of incubation). In the human, Magitot [76] observed the appearcance of the nerve fiber layer in the second month of human development (about 45 mm. C.R. [108]). O'Rahilly [98], using staged human embryos, reported its presence in horizon XIX (47.5 days).

The number of nerve fibers in the nerve fiber layer steadily increases with development. In the chicken, as example, by stage 37, when photoreceptors first begin to appear, these nerve fibers have already acquired the functional organelles: mitochondria, neurotubules and vesicles. At stage 42, there is an increase in Müller branching around the axons.

The myelinated fibers within the nerve fiber layer undoubtedly comprise centrifugal fibers which represent the efferent system to the retina from the central nervous system [109]. These fibers were first described in the avian retina by Ramón y Cajal [110] using the Golgi technique. Dogiel [111] confirmed the presence of these fibers by using methylene blue technique, and traced them to the optic nerve. These fibers originate from the isthmo-optic nucleus located midway between the nucleus of the fourth cranial nerve and the medial edge of the optic tectum. The isthmo-optic tract was discovered by Perlia [112] in 1889 (cited by Cowan [113]) and the route of the isthmo-optic tract was proposed by Wallenberg [114] in 1898 (cited by Cowan [113]). The transmission of these fibers in the retina has been studied by Maturana and Frenk [115] and Dowling and Cowan [116]. The former group even classified the fibers into convergent and divergent fibers with the convergent type penetrating farther into the inner nuclear layer, although most of them tended to adhere onto the soma and processes of amacrine cells. The electron microscopic appearance of the endings of these myelinated fibers is still unclear. Dowling and Cowan [116] observed that they are larger than ordinary synaptic endings in the inner plexiform layer (often up to 8 μm in diameter) and are packed with synaptic vesicles. Our study indicates that synaptic vesicles of large size are present in the nerve fiber layer (and very occasionally, around the amacrine cells in the inner plexiform layer) as early as stage 37, several days before myelinated fibers can be observed (stage 45) in the nerve fiber layer. Perhaps, these endings represent newly projected terminals of centrifugal fibers which become myelinated later.

Our observation also shows that myelinated fibers are larger than average non-myelinated fibers, and that contacts with Müller branches is an essential prerequisite for myelination. From these data, we may speculate that Müller fibers may take the place of Schwann cells or oligodendroglia in this type of myelination. Thus, our data appear to substantiate Ladman and Soper's [117] findings in the pigeon and gull. The embryogenesis of conspicuous amounts of myelinated fibers is observed at stage 45, around hatching in the chicken. At which time, they are present throughout the entire thickness of the nerve fiber layer.

The function of centrifugal fibers is still under study. Holden [118-121] suggested that they act to suppress sigals – such as to suppress lateral monocular fields. He also found that electrical stimulation of the optic nerve can excite the isthmo-optic nucleus. On the other hand, Ogden and Miller [122], using electroretinography, indicates that these fibers may serve as tonic inhibitors of "retinal oscillation".

The internal limiting membrane is first observed at stage 23 (3.5 to 4 days) in the chick [95]. In the human, Mann [3] first recognized this layer in embryos of 12 mm. C.R., and Nakayama [73], in fetuses of three months. The structure of the internal limiting membrane is found to be essentially the same as that described in mammals [123,124]. Our results suggest that the early (stage 30) internal limiting membrane contains all of the adult components: Müller end feet, a gap and an electron dense layer of acid mucopolysaccharide (also known as hyaloid membrane), despite a slight difference in the thickness of the acid mucopolysaccharide layer as development proceeds.

Histochemically, a trace of acid mucopolysaccharide is also confirmed in the internal limiting membrane.

Figure 2.9a.

Astrocytes (figure 2.9a) and microglia can be found internal to the ganglion cells and in between nerve fibers. The microglia is frequently located in disease retina [125,126]. Astrocytes, on the other hand, are usually observed in normal retina, but may increase in certain diseases [125,127].

REFERENCES

[1]   Mann IC. The process of differentiation of the retinal layers in vertebrates. Br J Ophthalmol 1928a; 12(9): 449-478.

[2]   Mann IC. The regional differentiation of the vertebrate retina. Am J Ophthalmol 1928b; 11: 515-526.

[3]   Mann IC. The development of the human eye. 2nd Ed. Grune & Stratton Inc., New York. 1950.

[4]   Coulombre AJ. Correlations of structural and biochemical changes in the developing retina of the chick. Am J Anat 1955; 96(1): 153-189.

[5]   Shiragami M. Electron microscopic study on synapses of visual cells in chick embryo. Nippon Ganka Gakkai Zasshi 1968; 72: 232-245.

[6]   Kim SU, Wenger EL. De novo formation of synapses in cultures of chick neural tube. Nat New Biol 1972; 236(66): 152-153.

[7]   Lasansky A. Basal junctions at synaptic endings of turtle visual cells. J Cell Biol. 1969; 40(2): 577-581.

[8]   DeRobertis E, Francis CM. Electron microscopic observations on synaptic vesicles in synapses of retinal rods and cones. J Biophys Biochem Cytol 1956; 2: 307-318.

[9]   Sjöstrand FS. Ultrastructure of retinal rod synapses of the guinea pig as revealed by three dimensional reconstruction from serial sections. J Ultrastruct Res 1958; 2: 122-170.

[10]   Smith CA, Sjöstrand FS. Structure of the nerve endings on the external hair cells of the guinea pig cochlea as studied by serial sections. J Ultrastruct Res 1961; 5: 523-556.

[11] Hama K. Some observations on the fine structure of the lateral line organ of the Japanese sea eel Lyncozymba nystromi. J Cell Biol 1965; 24: 193-210.

[12] Glees P, Sheppard BL. Electron microscopical studies of the synapses in the developing chick spinal cord. Z Zellforsch Mikrosk Anat 1964; 62: 356-362.

[13] Cohen AI. The fine structure of the visual receptors of the pigeon. Exp Eye Res 1963; 2: 88-97.

[14] Shiragami M. Electron microscopic study on synapses of visual cells. I. The ultrastracture on synapses of the visual cells in chick embryo Nippon Ganka Kiyo 1967; 18(1): 24-34.

[15] Shiragami M. Electron microscopic study on synapses of visual cells. 3. Morphologic classification of visual cell synapses and a peculiar type of synapses in chicken retina. Nippon Ganka Kiyo 1969a; 20(4): 430-438.

[16] Shiragami M. Electron microscopic study on synapses of visual cells. IV. [The ultrastructure of synapses in the midperipheral area of chicken retina. Nippon Ganka Kiyo 1969b; 20(4): 439-446.

[17] Wislocki GB, Sidman RL. The chemical morphology of the retina. J Comp Neurol 1954; 101(1): 53-99.

[18] Coupland RE. Electron microscopic observations on the structure of the rat adrenal medulla: I. The ultrastructure and organization of chromaffin cells in the normal adrenal medulla. J Anat 1965a; 99: 231-254.

[19] Coupland RE. Electron microscopic observations on the structure of the rat adrenal medulla: II. Normal innervation. J Anat. 1965b; 99 (Pt 2): 255-272.

[20] Bliss AF. The chemistry of daylight vision. J Gen Physiol 1946; 29(5): 277-297.

[21] Witkovsky P. An ontogenic study of retinal function in the chick. Vision Res 1963; 3: 341-355.

[22] Goto M. The ontogenetic study on electroretinogram of chick. Nippon Seirigaku Zasshi 12: 67-73.

[23] Peters JJ., Vonderahe A.R., Powers I.H. Electrical studies of functional development of the eye and optic lobes in the chick embryo. J Exp Zool 1958; 39: 459-468.

[24] Garcia-Austt E, Patetta-Queirolo MA. Electroretinogram of the chick embryo. I. Onset and development. Acta Neurol Latinoam 1961; 7: 178-189.

[25] Sedlácek J. Development of ocular evoked potentials in chicken fetuses. Cesk Fysiol 1967; 16: 240-241.

[26] Blozovski D, Blozovski M. Comparatie development of the electroretinogram and visual evoked potentials of the optic lobe, cerebellum and telencephalon, in the chick. J Physiol (Paris) 1968; 60(1): 33-50.

[27] Ookawa T. Further studies on the ontogenetic development of the chick electroretinogram. Poult Sci 1971; 50(4): 1185-1190.

[28] Kojima K, Okuda S, Tomita K, Majima Y. Succinic acid dehydrogenase in the visual cells of the human retina. Nippon Ganka Gakkai Zasshi 1957; 60: 1776-1779.

[29] Lessell S, Kuwabara T. Phosphatase histochemistry of the eye. Arch Ophthalmol 1964; 71: 851-860.

[30] Shanthaveerappa TR, Bourne GH. Histochemical demonstration of thiamine pyrophosphatase and acid phosphatases in the Golgi region of the cells of the eye. J Anat 1965; 99: 103-117.

[31] Amemiya T. Cytochemical and electron microscopic demonstration of polysaccharide synthesized by enzyme activities in synapses of the rat retina. Nippon Ganka Gakkai Zasshi 1970; 74(4): 286-294.

[32] Shimizu N, Maeda S. Histochemical studies on glycogen of the retina. Anat Rec 1953; 116(4): 427-437.

[33] Agarwal LP, Lamba PA, Mohan M, Batta RK. Histochemical study of retinal glycogen. I. Normal and starvation. Orient Arch Ophthal 1964; 2: 191-199.

[34] Shanthaveerappa TR, Weitzman MB, Bourne GH. Studies on the distribution of phosphorylase in the eyes of the rabbit and the squirrel monkey. Histochimie 1966; 7: 80-95.

[35] MacNichol EJ, Svaetichin G. Electric responses from the isolated retinas of fishes. Am J Ophthalmol 1958; 46(3 Part 2): 26-40.

[36] Tomita T, Tosaka T, Watanabe K, Sato Y. The fish EIRG in response to different types of illumination. Jpn J Physiol 1958; 8(1): 41-50.

[37] Norton AL, Spekreijse H, Wolbarsht ML, Wagner HG. Receptive field organization of the S-potential. Science 1968; 160(831): 1021-1022.

[38] Naka KI, Rushton WA. The generation and spread of S-potentials in fish (Cyprinidae). J Physiol 1967; 192(2): 437-461.

[39] Kaneko A. Physiological and morphological identification of horizontal, bipolar and amacrine cells in goldfish retina. J Physiol 1970; 207(3): 623-633.

[40] Yamada E, Ishikawa T. The fine structure of the horizontal cells in some vertebrate retinae. Cold Spring Harb Symp Quant Biol 1965a; 30: 383-392.

[41] O'Daly JA. ATPase activity at the functional contacts between retinal cells which produced S-potential. Nature 1967; 216(5122): 1329-1331.

[42] Stell WK. The structure and relationships of horizontal cells and photoreceptor-bipolar synaptic complexes in goldfish retina. Am J Anat 1967; 121(2): 401-423.

[43]   Witkovsky P, Dowling JE. Synaptic relationships in the plexiform layers of carp retina. Z Zellforsch Mikrosk Anat 1969; 100(1): 60-82.

[44]   Kaneko A. Electrical connexions between horizontal cells in the dogfish retina. J Physiol 1971; 213(1): 95-105.

[45]   Naka KI, Nye PW. Role of horizontal cells in organization of the catfish retinal receptive field. J Neurophysiol 1971; 34(5): 785-801.

[46]   Nilsson SE, Crescitelli F. A correlation of ultrastructure and function in the developing retina oof the frog tadpole. J Ultrastruct Res 1970; 30(1): 87-102.

[47]   Dowling JE. Organization of vertebrate retinas. Invest Ophthalmol. 1970; 9(9): 655-680.

[48]   Uga S, Nomura T, Ikui H. Observations on Kolmer's crystalloid in the human retina. Nippon Ganka Kiyo 1969; 20(10): 933-938.

[49]   Ehinger B, Falck B. Adrenergic retinal neurons of some new world monkeys. Z Zellforsch Mikrosk Anat. 1969; 100(3): 364-375.

[50]   Koelle GB, Friedenwald JS. The histochemical localization of cholinesterase in ocular tissues. Am J Ophthalmol 1950; 33(2): 253-256, illust.

[51]   Nichols CW, Koelle GB. Comparison of the localization of acetylcholinesterase and non-specific cholinesterase activities in mammalian and avian retinas. J Comp Neurol 1968; 133(1): 1-16.

[52]   Kuwabara T, Cogan DG. Ann Histochim. 1963; 8: 223-228.

[53]   Ramón y Cajal S. The structure of the retina: A complete work. Translated by Thorpe SA, Glickstein M, Thomas CC. Springfield. 1972.

[54]   Polyak SL. The vertebrate visual system. Chicago, University of Chicago Press, 1957.

[55]   Tartuferi F. Arch. per le sc med 1887; 11:335. (Cited by Ramón y Cajal, 1972)

[56]   Merkel F. Uber die macula des menschen und die ora serrata einiger wirbelthiere. W. Englemann, Leizig. 1869.

[57]   Kolmer W. Die netzhaut (retina). In: Handbuch der mikroskopischen Anatomie des menschen (V. Möllendorff) vol. 3 part 2, Haut und Binnesorgane Kolmer W, Lauber H, Eds. Springer, Berlin. 1936.

[58]   Dowling JE, Boycott BB. Organization of the primate retina: electron microscopy. Proc R Soc Lond B Biol Sci 1966; 166(2): 80-111.

[59]   Boycott BB, Dowling JE. Organization of the primate retina. Light microscopy. Philos Trans R Soc Lond B Biol Sci 1969; 255: 109-184.

[60]   Hogan MJ, Alvarado JA, Weddell JE. The histology of the human eye. Philadelphia, W. B. Saunders, 1971.

[61]   Yew DT, Meyer DB. Two types of bipolar cells in the chick retinal development. Experientia 1975; 31(9): 1077-1078.

[62]   Missotten L. The synapses in the human retina. In: Rochen JW, Ed. Structure of the eye. II. Symposium, The 8th International Congress of Anatomy, Stuttgart, Schattauer-Verlag, 1965.

[63]   Hebb CO. Acetylcholine metabolism of nervous tissue. Pharmacol Rev 1954; 6(1): 39-43.

[64]   Leplat G, Gerebtzoff MA. Localization of acetylcholinesterase and diphenolic mediators in the retina. Ann Ocul (Paris) 1956; 189(1): 121-128.

[65]   Shen SC. Changes in enzymatic patterns during development. In: A symposium on the chemical basis of development, McElroy WB, Glass B, Eds. Johns Hopkins Press, Baltimore 1958.

[66]   Rebollo MA. Some aspects of the histogenesis of retina. Acta Neurol Latinoam 1955; 1: 142-147.

[67]   Coulombre AJ. Cytology of the developing eye. Int Rev Cytol 1961; 11: 161-190.

[68]   Gourevitch A. Histological localization of glycogen in the retina of fish and its consumption by light. J Physiol (Paris). 1954; 46(2): 633-641.

[69]   Duke-Elder S, Cook C. Normal and abnormal development. Systems of Ophthalmology. Vol. 3, Mosby CV, St. Louis. 1963.

[70]   Weidman TA, Kuwabara T. Postnatal development of the rat retina. An electron microscopic study. Arch Ophthalmol 1968; 79(4): 470-484.

[71]   Uga S, Smelser GK. Electron microscopic study of the development of retinal Müllerian cells. Invest Ophthalmol. 1973 Apr; 12(4): 295-307.

[72]   Meller K, Glees P. The differentiation of neruoglia-Müller-cells in the retina of chick. Z Zellforsch Mikrosk Anat 1965; 66(3): 321-332.

[73]   Nakayama K. Histochemical study on the human fetal retina in the course of development. J Clin Ophthalmol (Tokyo) 1957; 11: 1024-1032.

[74]   Raviola E, Raviola G. Histochemical research on the retina of the rabbit during its postnatal development. Z Zellforsch Mikrosk Anat. 1962; 56: 552-572.

[75]   Magalhàes MM, Coimbra A. Electron microscope radioautographic study of glycogen synthesis in the rabbit retina. J Cell Biol. 1970; 47(1): 263-275.

[76] Ofuchi Y. Electron microscopic histochemistry of nucleoside phosphatases of the retina. I. Fine structural localization of "ATPase" in the pigment epithelium and the visual cell. Nippon Ganka Kiyo 1968; 19(4): 543-554.

[77] Dowling JE, Werblin FS. Organization of retina of the mudpuppy, Necturus maculosus. I. Synaptic structure. J Neurophysiol. 1969; 32(3): 315-338.

[78] Morest DK. The pattern of neurogenesis in the retina of the rat. Z Anat Entwicklungsgesch 1970; 131(1): 45-67.

[79] Olney JW. An electron microscopic study of synapse formation, receptor outer segment development, and other aspects of developing mouse retina. Invest Ophthalmol 1968; 7(3): 250-268.

[80] Nichols CW, Jacobowitz D, Hottenstein M. The influence of light and dark on the catecholamine content of the retina and choroid. Invest Ophthalmol 1967; 6(6): 642-646.

[81] Ehinger B, Falck B. Autoradiography of some suspected neurotransmitter substances: GABA glycine, glutamic acid, histamine, dopamine, and L-dopa. Brain Res 1971; 33(1): 157-172.

[82] Kramer SG. Dopamine: A retinal neurotransmitter. I. Retinal uptake, storage, and light-stimulated release of H3-dopamine *in vivo*. Invest Ophthalmol 1971; 10(6): 438-452.

[83] Kramer SG, Potts AM, Mangnall Y. Dopamine: a retinal neurotransmitter. II. Autoradiographic localization of H3-dopamine in the retina. Invest Ophthalmol 1971; 10(8): 617-624.

[84] Boycott B, Dowling J, Fisher S, Lolb H, Laties A. A new amacrine cell in the vertebrate retina. Presented at Spring National Meeting, Assoc. for Research in Vision and Ophthalmology, April 30, 1971. (cited by Kramer *et al.*, 1971).

[85] Neal MJ, Iversen LL. Autoradiographic localization of 3 H-GABA in rat retina. Nat New Biol 1972; 235(59): 217-218.

[86] Bruun A, Ehinger B. Uptake of the putative neurotransmitter, glycine, into the rabbit retina. Invest Ophthalmol 1972; 11(4): 191-198.

[87] Oishi T. Electron microscopic-histochemical studies of ATPase in the human retina. Nippon Ganka Gakkai Zasshi 1967; 71(8): 1323-1332.

[88] Weysse AW, Burgess WS. Histogenesis of the retina. Am Nat 1906; 40: 611-637.

[89] Weidman TA, Kuwabara T. Development of the rat retina. Invest Ophthalmol 1969; 8(1): 60-69.

[90] Dowling JE, Boycott BB. Neural connections of the retina: fine structure of the inner plexiform layer. Cold Spring Harb Symp Quant Biol 1965; 30: 393-402.

[91] Dowling JE. Synaptic organization of the frog retina: an electron microscopic analysis comparing the retinas of frogs and primates. Proc R Soc Lond B Biol Sci 1968; 170(19): 205-228.

[92] Sheffield JB, Fischman DA. Intercellular junctions in the developing neural retina of the chick embryo. Z Zellforsch Mikrosk Anat 1970; 104(3): 405-418.

[93] Cameron J. The Development of the Retina in Amphibia: an Embryological and Cytological Study: Part II. J Anat Physiol 1905; 39(Pt 3): 332-348.5.

[94] Hollyfield JG. Histogenesis of the retina in the killifish, Fundulus heteroclitus. J Comp Neurol. 1972; 144(3): 373-380.

[95] O'Rahilly R, Meyer DB. The early development of the eye in the chick Gallus domesticus (stages 8 to 25). Acta Anat (Basel) 1959; 36(1-2): 20-58.

[96] Slonaker JR. The development of the eye and its accessory parts in the English sparrow. J Morphol 1921; 35: 263-357.

[97] Magitot A. Etude sur le dévelopment de la rétine humaine. Ann Ocul (Paris) 1910; 143: 241-282

[98] O'Rahilly R. The early development of the eye in staged human embryos. Contrib Embryol 1966; 259: 1-59.

[99] Fisher S, Jacobson M. Ultrastructural changes during early development of retinal ganglion cells in Xenopus. Z Zellforsch Mikrosk Anat 1970; 104(2): 165-177.

[100] Eichner D. Topochemistry of the retina. Buch Augenarzt 1955; (23): 29-35.

[101] Perry HB. Degenerations of the dog retina. L. Structure and development of the retina of the normal dog. Am J Ophthalmol 1953; 37: 385-404.

[102] Radnot M, Lovas B. The subsurface cisternae of the ganglion cells of the retina. Ann Ocul (Paris) 1968; 201(3): 279-284.

[103] De Iraldi AP, Etcheverry GJ. Granulated vesicles in retinal synapses and neurons. Z Zellforsch Mikrosk Anat 1967; 81(2): 283-296.

[104] Ehinger B. Autoradiographic identification of rabbit retinal neurons that take up GABA. Experientia 1970; 26(10): 1063-1064.

[105] Yamada E, Tokuyasu K, Iwaki S. The fine structure of the retina studied with electron microscope. III. Human retina. J Kurume Med Assoc 1958b; 21: 1979-2027.

[106] O'Rahilly R, Meyer DB. Correlations between the development of the eye and embryonic staging in the chick. Anat Rec 1955; 121: 346.

[107] Rogers KT. Early development of the optic nerve in the chick. Anat Rec. 1957; 127(1): 97-107.

[108] Staflova J. Relation of the size of the eye to the age and length in human ontogenesis. Am J Obstet Gynecol 1971; 110(1): 126-128.

[109] Cowan WM, Powell TP. Centrifugal fibres in the avian visual system. Proc R Soc Lond B Biol Sci 1963; 158: 232-252.

[110] Ramón y Cajal S. Sur la morphologie et les connexions des éléments de la rétine des oiseaux Anat Anz 1889 4: 111-121.

[111] Dogiel AS. Zür frage über den bau der nervenzellen und über das verhaltnis ihnes achsencylinder-(nerven)-fortsatzes zu den protoplasmefortsätzen (dendriten). Arch f Mikr Anat 1893 41: 67-87.

[112] Perlia R. Albrecht v. Graefes Arch Ophthal 1889; 35: 20. (Cited by Cowan, 1970)

[113] Cowan WM. Centrifugal fibres to the avian retina. Br Med Bull 1970; 26: 112-118.

[114] Wallenberg A. Neurol Zentbl 1898; 17: 532. (Cited by Cowan, 1970)

[115] Maturana HR, Frenk S. Synaptic connections of the centrifugal fibers in the pigeon retina. Science 1965; 150(694): 359-361.

[116] Dowling JE, Cowan WM. An electron microscope study of normal and degenerating centrifugal fiber terminals in the pigeon retina. Z Zellforsch Mikrosk Anat 1966; 71(1): 14-28.

[117] Ladman AJ, Soper EM. Preliminary observations on the fine structure of Müller cells of the avian retina. 5 Int Congress E.M. 2: R6 1962

[118] Holden AL. Two possible visual functions for centrifugal fibres to the retina. Nature 1966; 212(5064): 837-838.

[119] Holden AL. Types of unitary response and correlation with the field potential profile during activation of the avian optic tectum. J Physiol. 1968a; 194(1): 91-104.

[120] Holden AL. Antidromic activation of the isthmo-optic nucleus. J Physiol 1968b; 197(1): 183-198.

[121] Holden AL. The centrifugal system running to the pigeon retina. J Physiol 1968c; 197(1): 199-219.

[122] Ogden TE, Miller RF. Studies of the optic nerve of the rhesus monkey: nerve fiber spectrum and physiological properties. Vision Res 1966; 6(9): 485-506.

[123] Tsuboi T. Study on the internal limiting membrane of the retina (preliminary report). Nippon Ganka Kiyo 1968; 19(1): 20-26.

[124] Matsusaka T. The fine structure of the inner limiting membrane of the rat retina as revealed by ruthenium red staining. J Ultrastruct Res 1971; 36(3): 312-317.

[125] Tang J, Tang I, Ling EA, Wu Y, Liang F. Juxtanodin in the rat olfactory epithelium: specific expression in sustentacular cells and preferential subcellular positioning at the apical junction belt. Neuroscience 2009; 161(1): 249-58.

[126] Zou YY, Lu J, Poon DJ, Kaur C, Cao Q, Teo AL, Ling EA. Combustion smoke indices up-regulated expression of vascular endothelial growth factor, aquaporin 4, nitric oxide synthases and vascular permeability in the retina of adult rats. Neuroscience 2009; 160(3): 698-709.

[127] Lam TK, Chan WY, Kuang GB, Wei H, Shum As, Yew DT. Differential expression of glial fibrillary acidic protein (GFAP) in the retinae and visual cortices of rats with experimental renal hypertension. Neurosci Lett 1995; 198(3): 165-8.

CHAPTER 3

Developing Retinae of Different Species

Abstract: Development of the retina is a highly correlated event and the morphogenesis for different retinal layers, which arise from the outer and inner neuroblastic layers, are different. Some of the animals have neonatal retinal developments, like the mouse and rat, while the humans at term have a well developed eye. In this chapter, 4 species of mammals (European rabbit, ICR mice, SD rat and humans) are used to clearly illustrate the progressive variations in the structures of the retinae during development, and specifically the dates of the events are listed for easy reference of readers to use these species in future research. The former three animals are used by many as experimental subjects and the readers need an introductory knowledge on them. The introduction in the chapter brings forth relationship between higher CNS targets and the retina in development. It includes de novo views which need to be evaluated by the readers.

Key Words: development, human, chicken, rodent, stages, clila, outer segments, higher CNS centers, light influence, scanning electron microscopy, light microscopy

INTRODUCTION

In human development at 10-11 weeks of gestation, the retina is divided into outer and inner neuroblastic layers by the layer of Chevitz. The presumptive inner segments emerge from the retina at 16 weeks of gestation. By the 19th week of gestation, the inner segments elongate; the outer segments appear by 24-25 weeks of gestation [1,2]. Apart from the human data, many studies have been published on the development of chicken and rodents. It is generally accepted that the retina begins with the formation of the presumptive inner plexiform layer, resulting in the separation of the ganglion cell layer from the mass of cell bodies that subsequently form the outer and inner nuclear layers with an outer plexiform layer between [3,4]. Finally, from the outer nuclear layer, the inner segments begin to appear. These inner segments have cilia and are round or oval initially. Subsequently, stacks of discs appear from the dilated cilia which then form the outer segments. At the same time, there is an elongation of the inner segments [5]. This is the general pattern of retinal development. In the chicken, all these are accomplished by about 14 days of incubation while specialized organs inside the inner segments such as the glycogen bodies are visible by 17 days of incubation [3]. Both the human and the chicken retina develop prenatally while the rodent develops neonatally.

The development of the retina correlates well with the sequential development of the higher visual centers. For example, in the quail, optic fibers reach the optic tectum by 10 days of incubation, a time when the retina acquires inner segments [6]. During development, as in any species, there are more cells generated than necessary and hence there is degeneration of the extra cells. This is particularly evident in the late stages of development and in the ganglion cell layer [7]. Normally, the development of the retina begins in the center and spreads peripherally, and is usually completed at birth (but not for rodents that develop neonatally). Also, there are exceptions in certain deep sea fish and the lamprey [8]. Development of the retina is also subject to light influences. For instance, intense light (laser) would damage the visual cells and inner nuclear layer in development [9]. Different wavelengths of light can affect retinal development differently. Far red light decreases growth of the outer segment while red light increases growth of the retina [10]. Once the development of the retina starts, it will proceed as genetically determined; further development does not rely on the linkage with the brain, as in anencephalic babies [11].

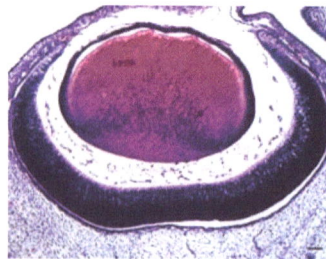

Figure 3.1a. *4 weeks prenatal.*

This figure shows an eye of a 4 weeks prenatal rabbit. Note the presence of a lens in the center and the developing retina. There are still many cell nuclei in the lens. Bar = 50 µm.

David T. Yew, Maria S. M. Wai and Winnie W. Y. Li

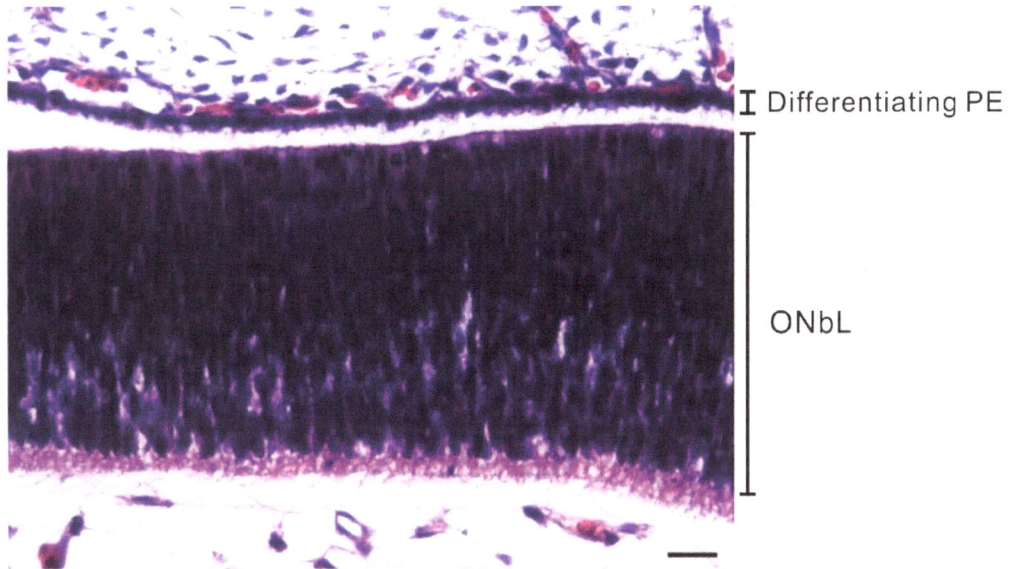

Figure 3.1b. *4 weeks prenatal.*

A high magnification of the retina. At this developmental stage, the retina only appears as a thick layer of differentiating neuroblastic layer (ONbL), visual cells are not yet developed. Bar = 20 μm.

(PE - Pigment epithelium).

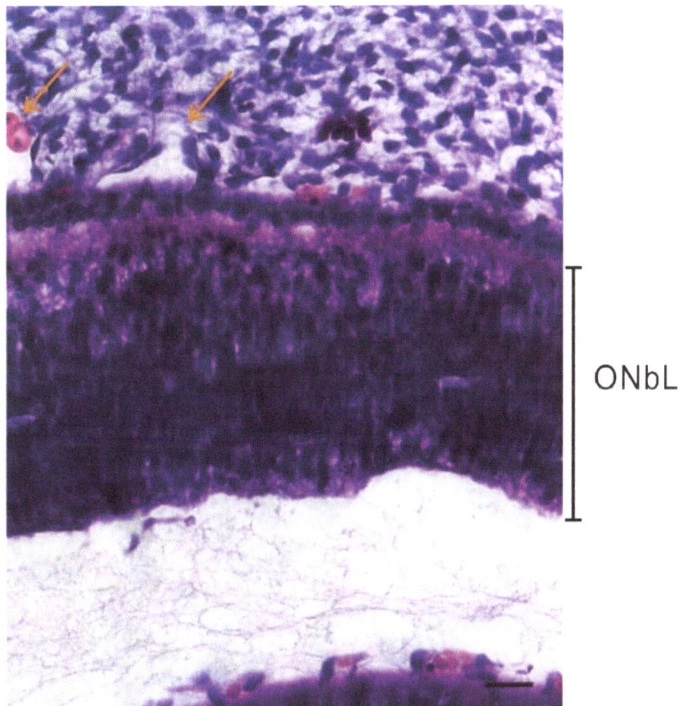

Figure 3.1c. *4 weeks prenatal.*

A retina from another rabbit at prenatal 4 weeks of age. Again, a single layer of differentiating neuroblastic cells is noted. Arrows are indicating the blood vessels. Bar = 20 μm.

(ONbL – Differentiating neuroblastic layer).

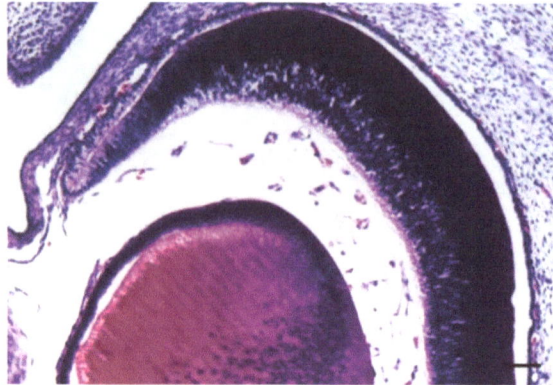

Figure 3.1d. *4 weeks prenatal.*

The cells in the most regions of the retina align into a compact layer with some migrating cells going towards the vitreous surface of the retina. However, near the ora serrata, only compact cells can be found. Bar = 50 μm.

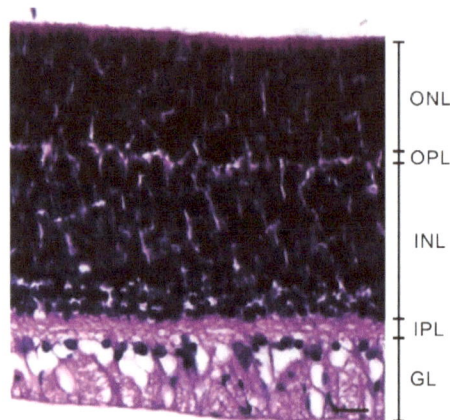

Figure 3.1e. *2 weeks prenatal.*

The retina of rabbit at prenatal 2 weeks of age has begun to differentiate into an outer nuclear layer (ONL) and an inner nuclear layer (INL). In between the two layers is a thin outer plexiform layer (OPL). Moreover, a thicker fiber layer which is the inner plexiform layer (IPL) together with the ganglion cell layer (GL) are also observed at this stage. Bar = 20 μm.

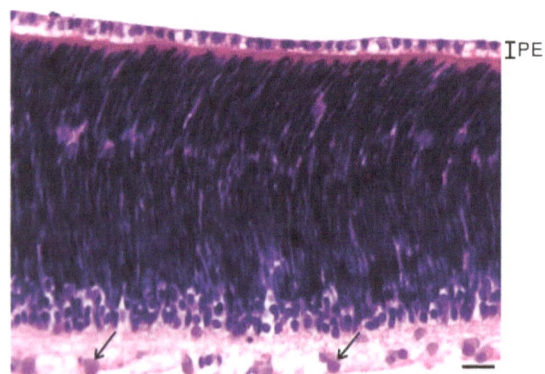

Figure 3.1f. *2 weeks prenatal.*

Another retina of a 2 weeks prenatal rabbit. Similar stage of differentiation is noted as in figure 3.1e. However, this figure displays a layer of early pigment epithelial layer (PE), in which a line of single epithelial cells is clearly shown. Arrows are indicating the large ganglion cells in this retina. Bar = 20 μm.

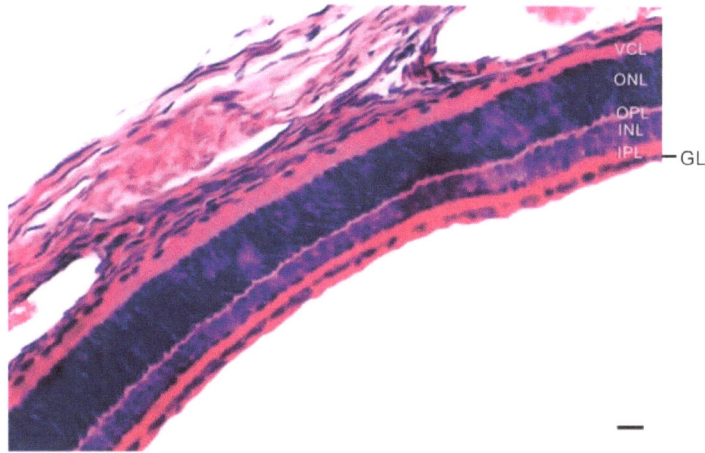

Figure 3.1g. *2 weeks postnatal.*

By 2 weeks postnatal, the retina is fully differentiated into in the visual cell layer (VCL), outer nuclear layer (ONL), outer plexiform layer (OPL), inner nuclear layer (INL), inner plexiform layer (IPL) and ganglion cell layer (GL). Bar = 50 μm.

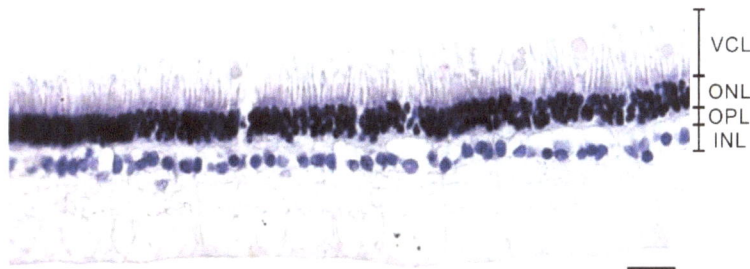

Figure 3.1h. *Adult.*

This figure shows the retina of an adult rabbit with distinctive layers of cells and fibers. The outer nuclear layer (ONL) is composed of about 2 to 3 rows of visual cell bodies with sizes smaller than those forming the inner nuclear layer (INL). Bar = 20 μm.

(OPL - Outer plexiform layer; VCL - Visual cell layer).

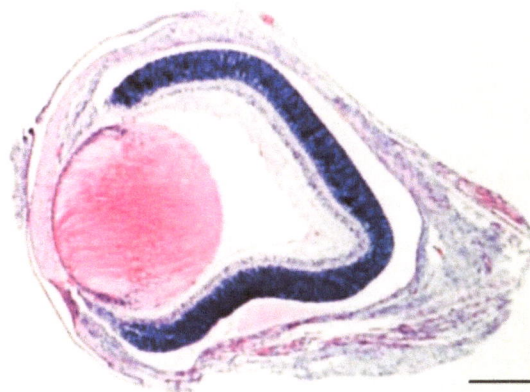

Figure 3.2a. *Postnatal day 7.*

A section of the mouse retina shows the lens and retina. Bar = 400 μm.

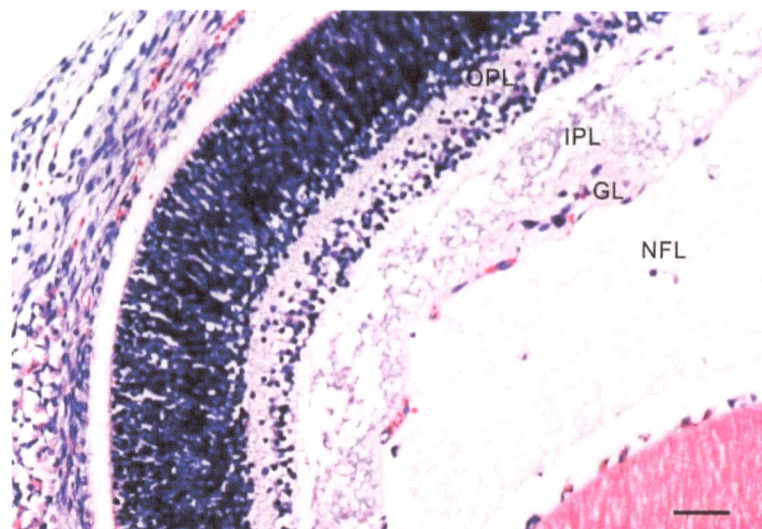

Figure 3.2b. *Postnatal day 7.*

A higher power view of figure 3.2a. Visual cells are not identifiable at this stage of development by light miscroscope, but the ganglion cell layer (GL), nerve fiber layer (NFL) layer, inner plexiform layer (IPL) and outer plexiform layer (OPL) are observed. Bar = 50 mm.

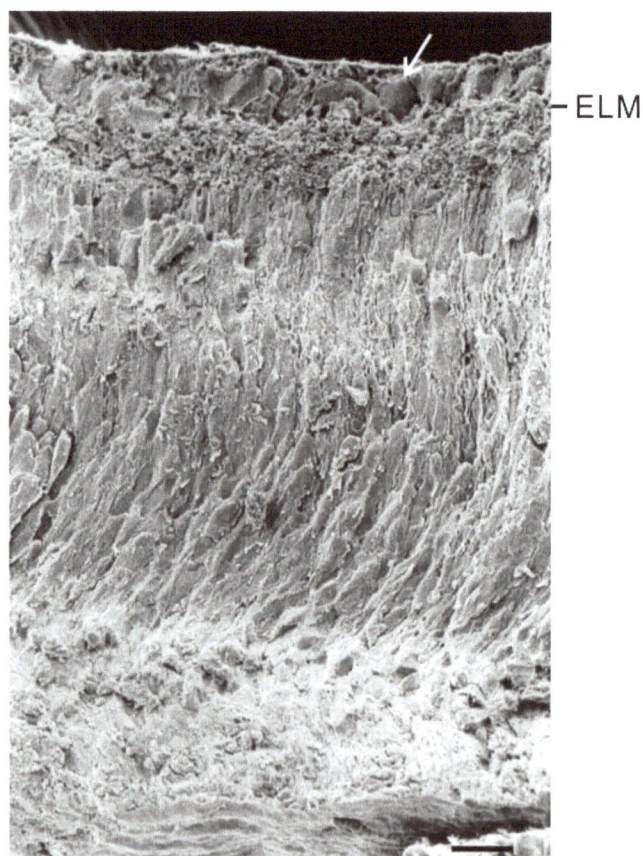

Figure 3.3a. *Postnatal day 3.*

Retina of a rat at day 3 postnatally. Note the protrusion of presumptive inner segments (arrow) beyond the external limiting membrane (ELM). Bar = 10 μm.

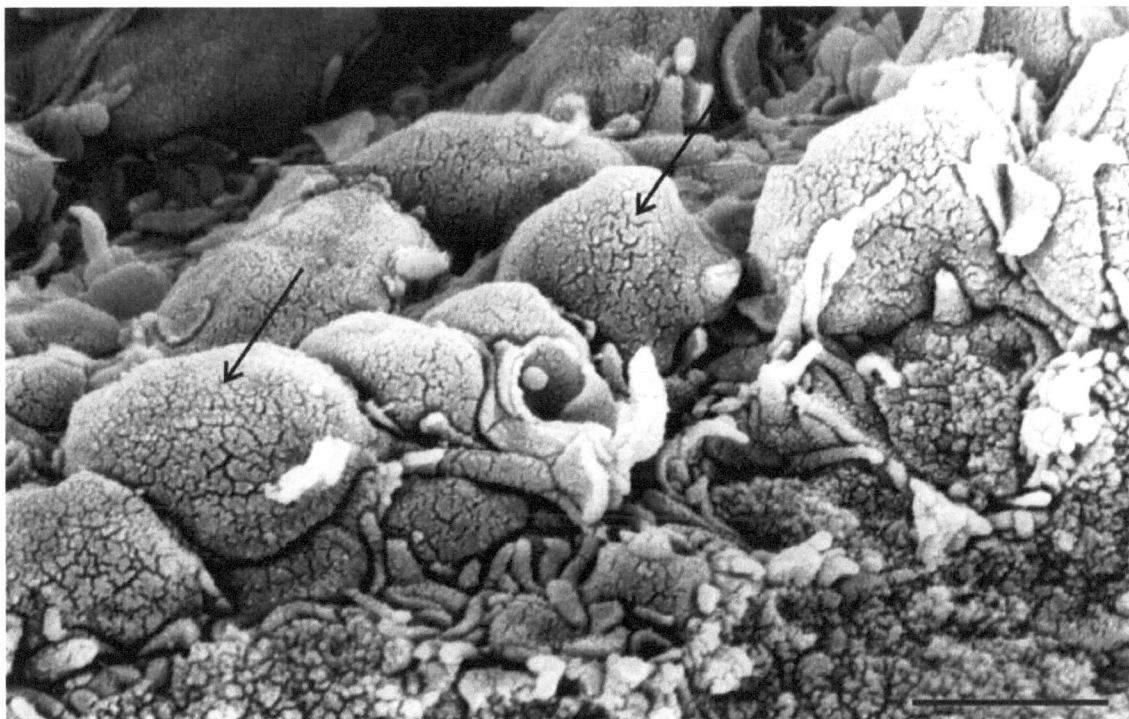

Figure 3.3b. *Postnatal day 3.*

On day 3 postnatally, the rat retina shows many bulges of inner segments (arrows). Bar = 1 μm.

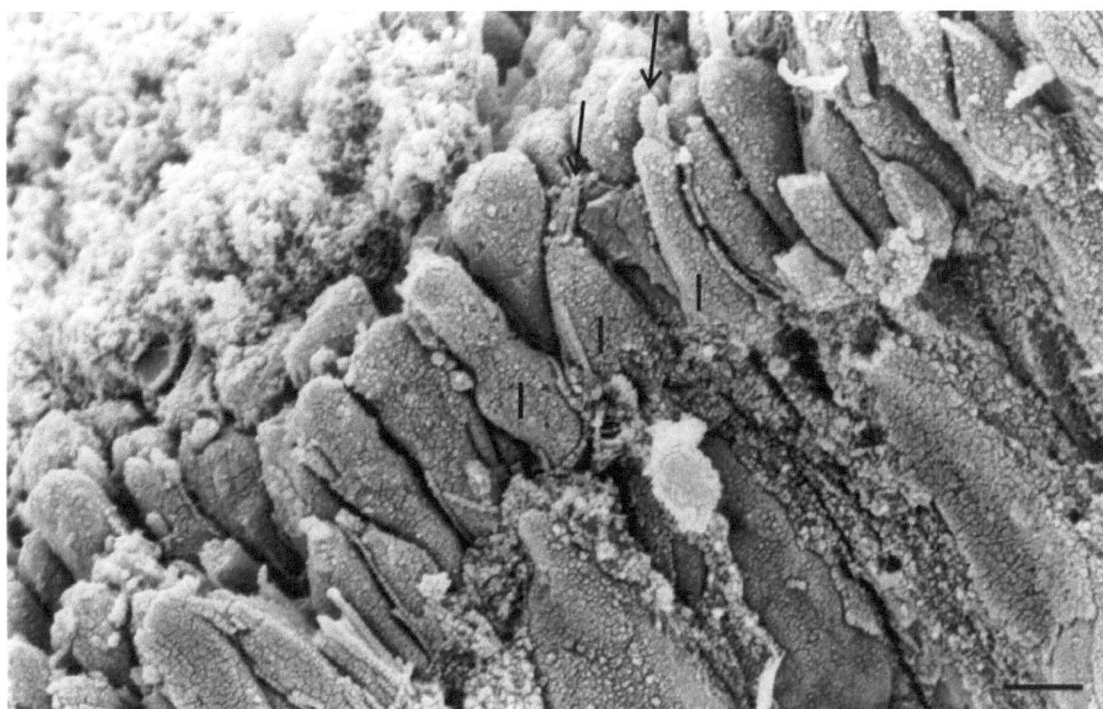

Figure 3.3c. *Postnatal day 7.*

The 1 week old rat retina shows elongated inner segments (I) of various shapes and sizes. Some even form a cilium (arrows) on top of the inner segment. Bar = 1 μm.

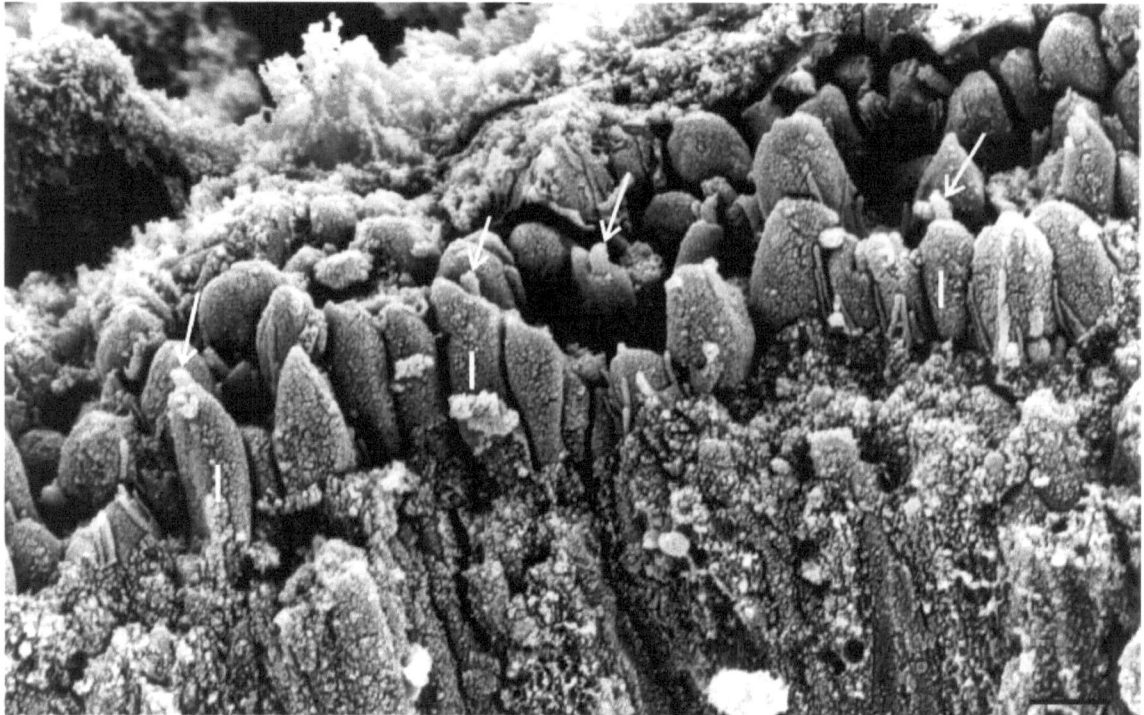

Figure 3.3d. *Postnatal day 7.*

Another region of a rat retina harvested on day 7 postnatally. As in figure 3.3c, visual cells appear as various shapes and sizes which may be of different developmental stages or different cell types. The protruded cilia in this region are short (yellow arrows). Bar = 1 mm.

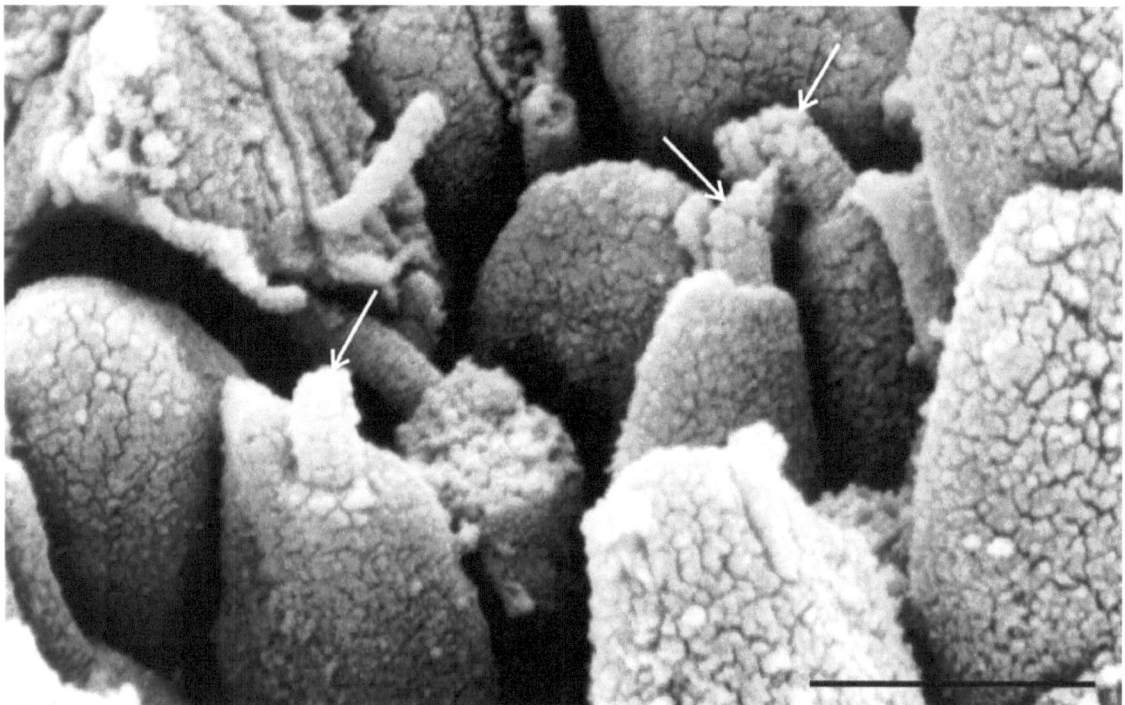

Figure 3.3e. *Postnatal day 7.*

Highly magnified visual cells with short cilia (arrows) growing out of the inner segments. Bar = 1 μm.

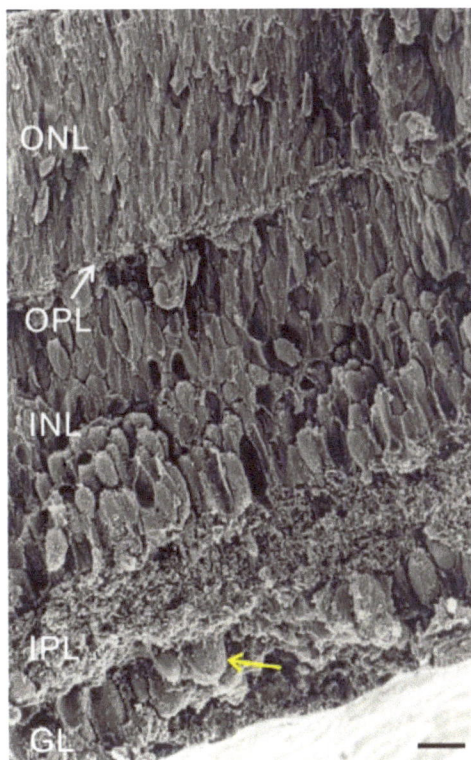

Figure 3.3f. *Postnatal day 7.*

At 1 week of age, the rat retina has differentiated into several layers, including the outer nuclear (ONL), outer plexiform (OP), inner nuclear (IN), inner plexiform (IP) and ganglion cell layers (GL). Large ganglion cells are clearly noted (yellow arrow). Bar = 10 μm.

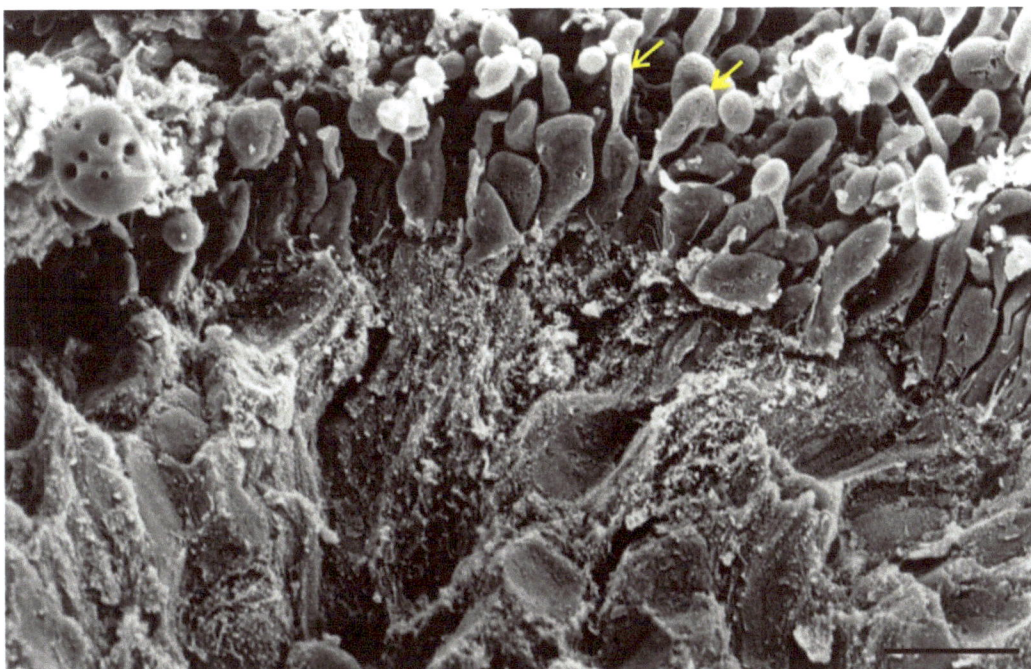

Figure 3.3g. *Postnatal day 10.*

Rat retina at postnatal day 10 appear to have longer outer segments (yellow arrows). Bar = 10 μm.

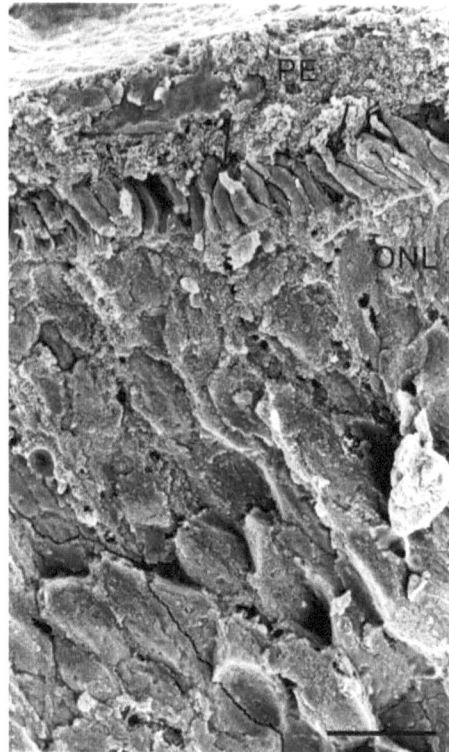

Figure 3.3h. *Postnatal day 11.*

The central retina normally develops faster than the peripheral retina in animals (e.g. SD rat). At this stage of development, most outer segments of the visual cells are already seen (arrows). The outer nuclear layer (ONL) is shown in the figure. Bar = 10 μm.

(PE - Pigment epithelium).

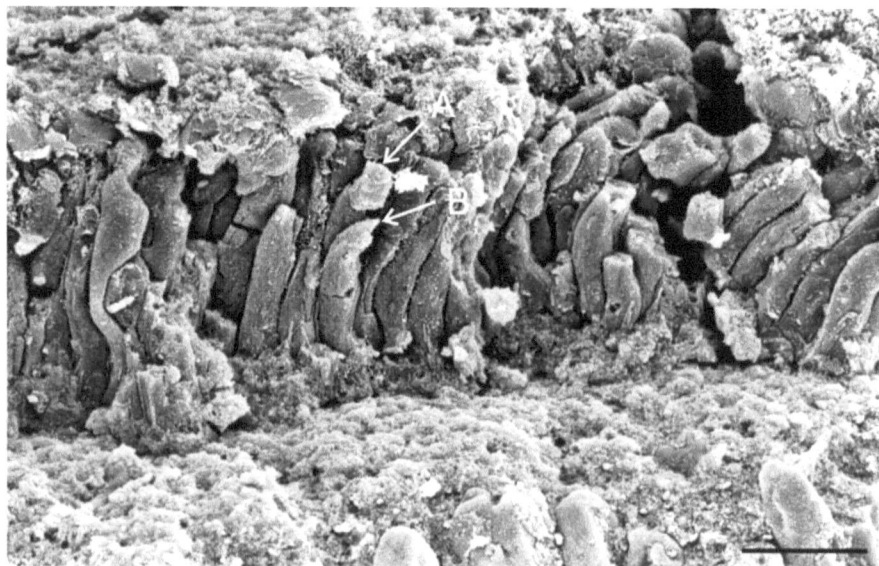

Figure 3.3i. *Postnatal day 11.*

The central retina of the rat at 11 days postnatal shows round (A) and pointed (B) outer segments, indicating different types of visual cells. Bar = 1 μm.

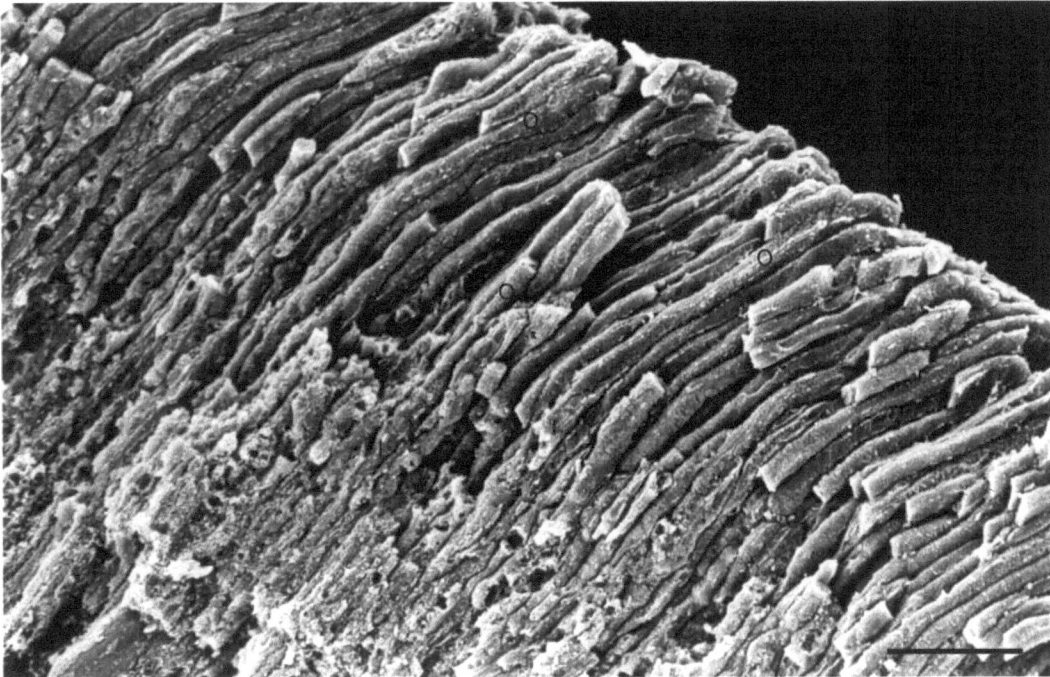

Figure 3.3j. *Postnatal day 14.*

14 days old retina of the rat showing visual cells with adult-like outer (O) and inner segments (I). Bar = 10 μm.

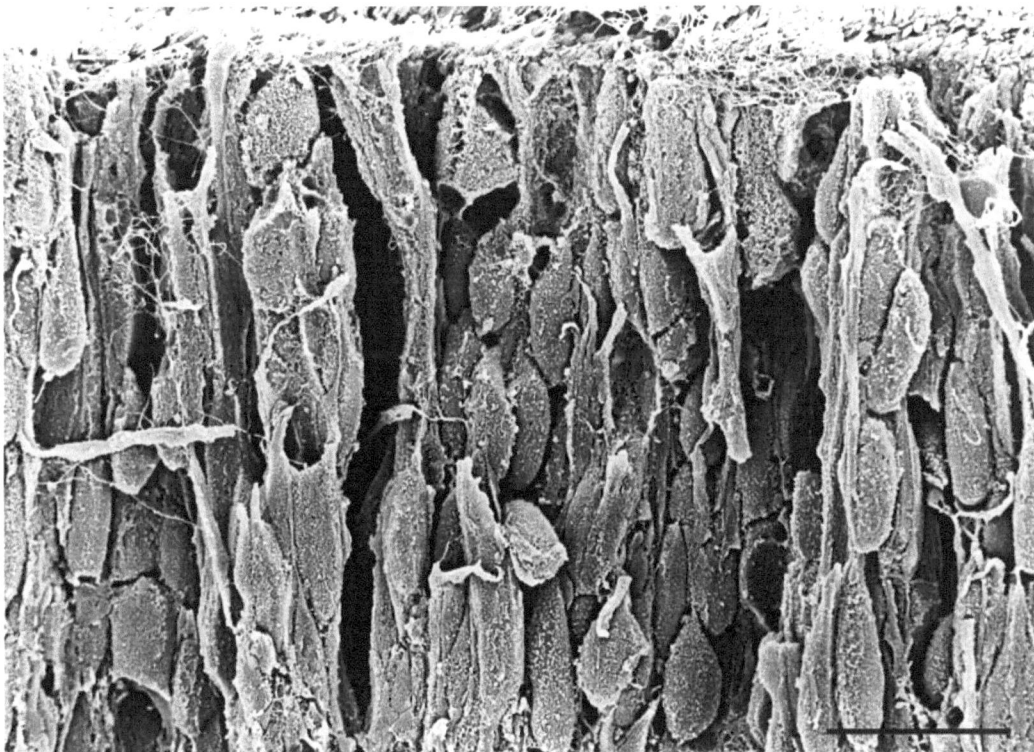

Figure 3.4a. *5 weeks of gestation.*

Scanning electron micrograph of a human retina at 5 weeks of gestation. Note that the retina at this stage of development is undifferentiated, with only a single layer. Bar = 10 μm.

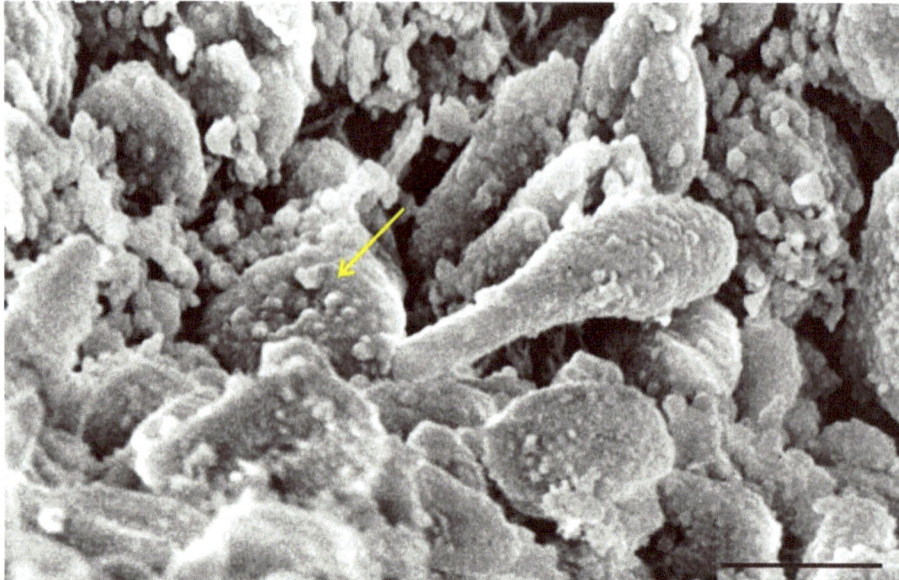

Figure 3.4b. *16 weeks of gestation.*

Human retina at 16 weeks of gestation. Note the projection of presumptive inner segment cells from the surface (arrow) of retina. Bar = 1 μm.

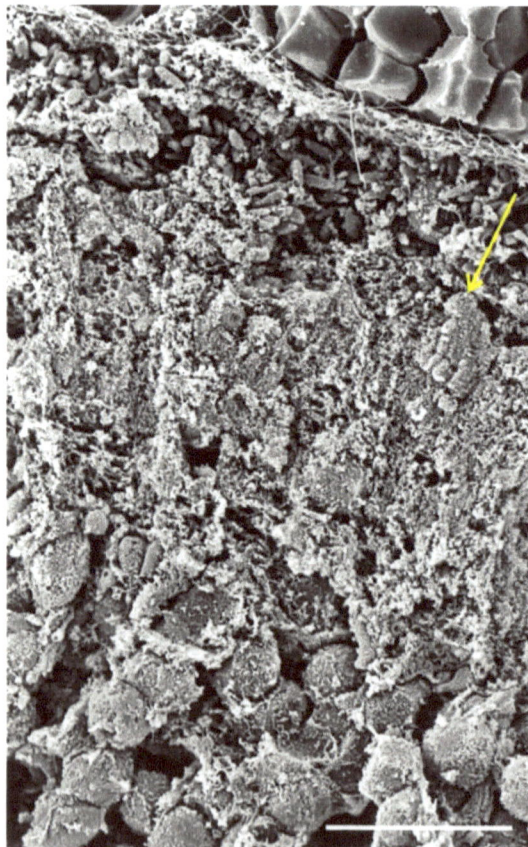

Figure 3.4c. *18 weeks of gestation.*

The human retina at 18 weeks of gestation. Inner segment bulges are still visible sagittally (arrow). Bar = 10 μm.

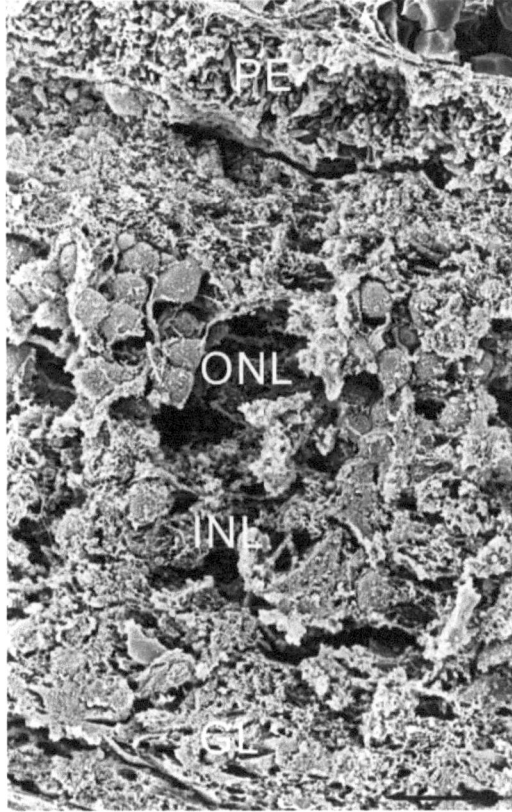

Figure 3.4d. *18 weeks of gestation.*

Most of the other retinal layers are formed by 18 weeks of gestation in human. Bar = 10 μm.

(GL - Ganglion cell layer; INL - Inner cell layer; ONL - outer nuclear layer; PE - Pigment epithelium).

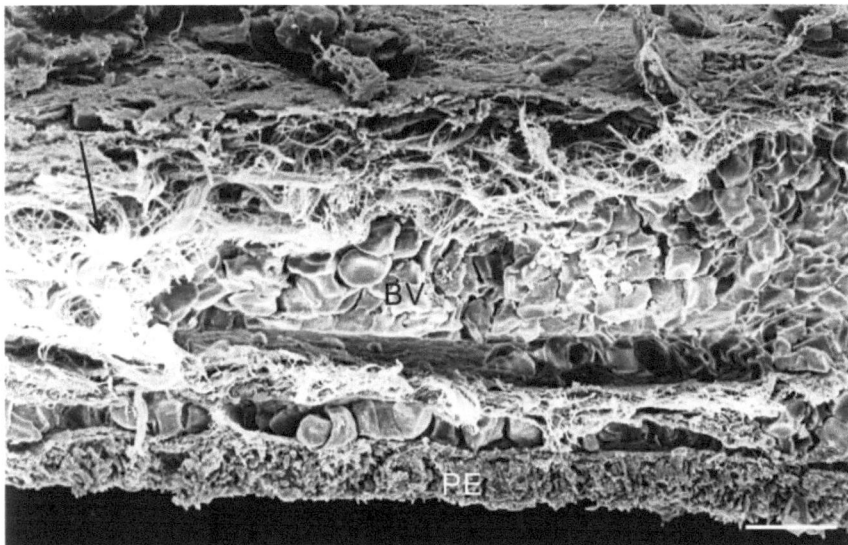

Figure 3.4e. *20 weeks of gestation.*

Human fetal retina at 20 weeks of gestation showing collagen fibers in choroid adjacent to pigment epithelium (PE). "BV" denotes blood vessels. Bar = 10 μm.

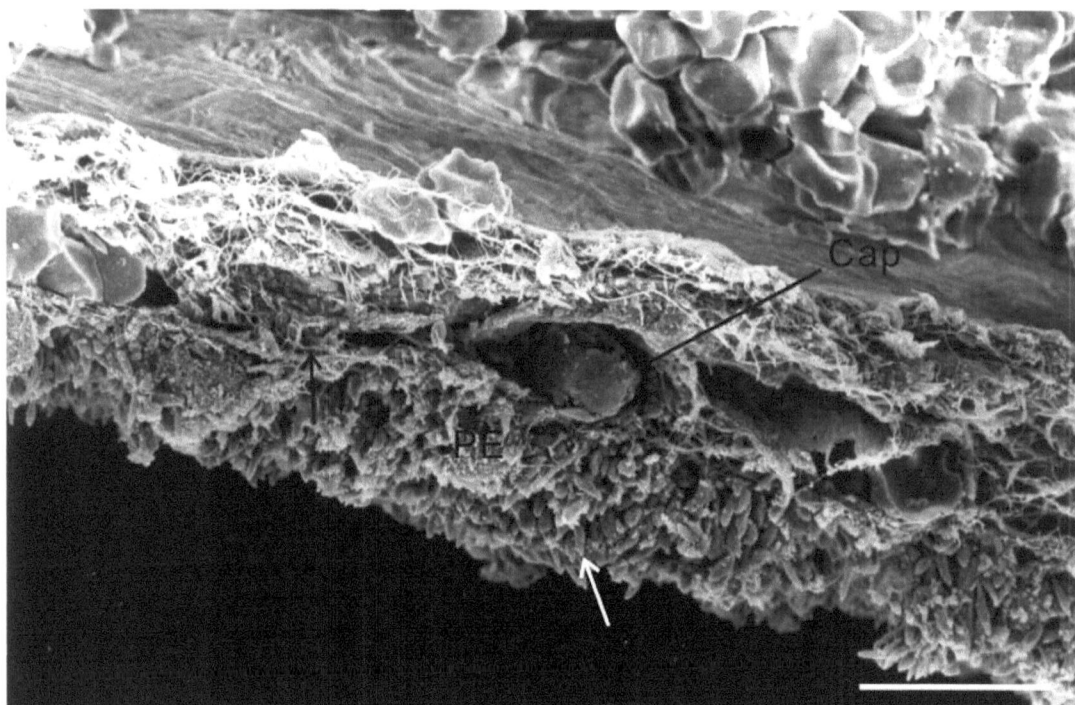

Figure 3.4f. *20 weeks of gestation.*

A high power view of figure 3.4e showing collagen fibers (blue arrow) between the choriocapillaries (Cap) and the pigment epithelium (PE), forming a part of Bruch's membrane. Note the many pigment granules (white arrow) inside the pigment epithelium. Bar = 10 μm.

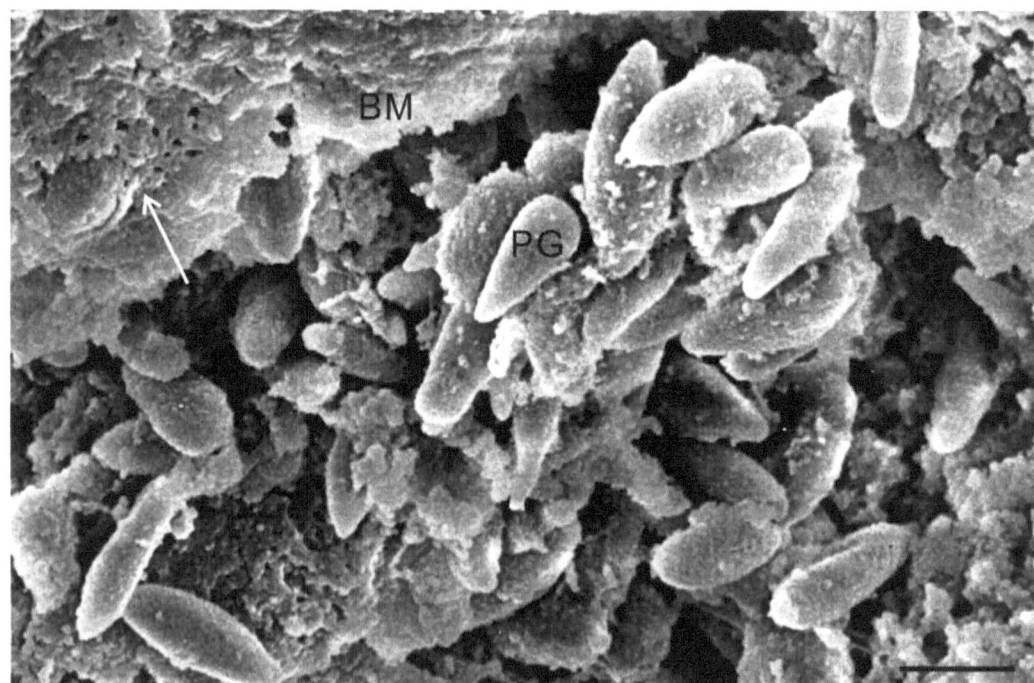

Figure 3.4g. *20 weeks of gestation.*

The arrow points to pores in the wall of choriocapillaries. "BM" denotes the basement membrane of pigment epithelium. "PG" denotes pigment granules inside the pigment epithelium. Bar = 1 μm.

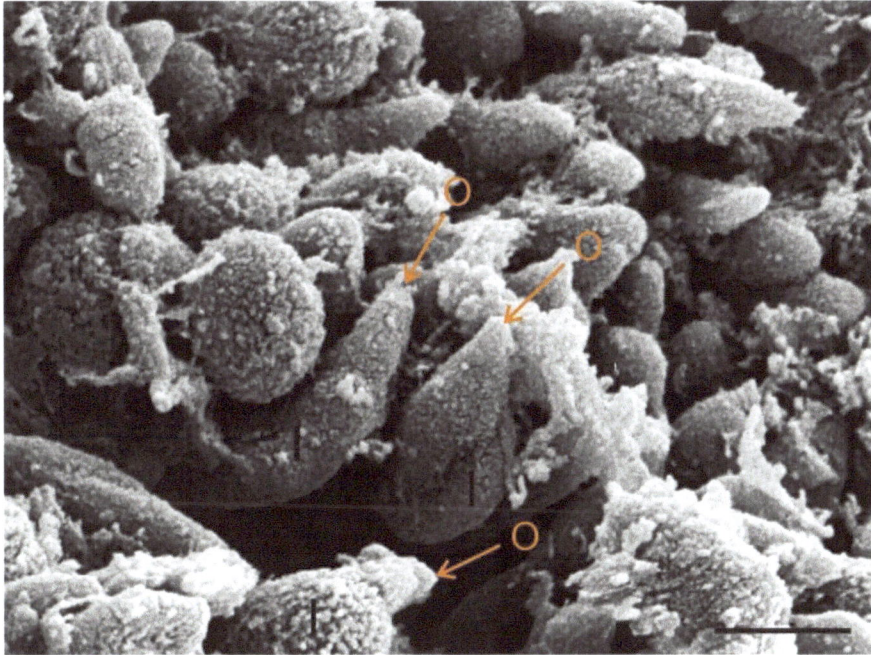

Figure 3.4h. *22 weeks of gestation.*

The human retina at 22 weeks of gestation. Note the presence of small outer segments (O) and inner segments (I) which are either elongated or round. Bar = 1 μm.

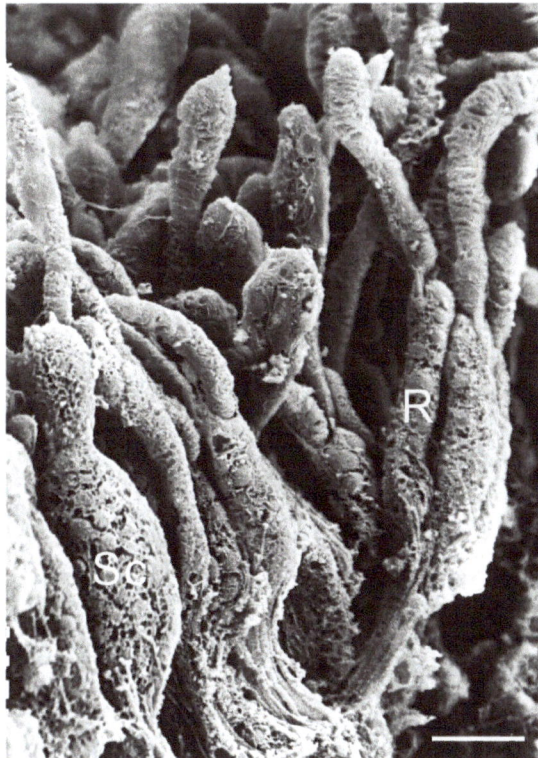

Figure 3.4i. *30 weeks of gestation.*

The human retina at 30 weeks of gestation. Note the structurally well differentiated rod (R) and cone (C) cells protruding from the surface. Bar = 2 μm.

REFERENCES

[1]   Narayanan K, Wadhwa S. Photoreceptor morphogenesis in the human retina: a scanning electron microscopic study. Anat Rec 1998; 252(1): 133-9.

[2]   Hendrickson A, Bumsted-O'Brien K, Natoli R, Ramamurthy V, Possin D, Provis J. Rod photoreceptor differentiation in fetal and infant human retina. Exp Eye Res 2008; 87(5): 415-26.

[3]   Yew DT. The developmental histochemistry of the chicken visual cells. Acta Anat (Basel) 1976; 96(4): 561-7.

[4]   Braekevelt CR, Hollenberg MJ. The development of the retina of the albino rat. Am J Anat 1970; 127(3): 281-301.

[5]   Wai MS, Lorke DE, Kung LS, Yew DT. Morphogenesis of the different types of photoreceptors of the chicken (Gallus domesticus) retina and the effect of amblyopia in neonatal chicken. Microsc Res Tech 2006; 69(2): 99-107.

[6]   Yew DT, Woo HH. The sequential development of the higher visual centers in the C.N.S. of the quail. Anat Anz 1979; 145(5): 493-7.

[7]   Yew DT. Aging in retinae and optic nerves of 2.5- to 9- month- old mice. Acta Anat (Basel) 1979a; 104(3): 332-4.

[8]   Yew DT. Development of the eyes in Agnatha and Chondrichthyes (Elasmobranchia). Anat Anz 1982; 151(3): 231-9.

[9]   Yew DT, Chan Y. The effect of laser on the developing rodent retinas. Acta Anat (Basel) 1977; 99(4): 386-90.

[10]   Wong T, Yew DT, Bau YS. Further studies on the effect of red and far red light on rat retinal development. Experientia 1978; 34(4): 513-4.

[11]   Li WW, Lu G, Pang CP, Lam DS, Yew DT. The eyes of anencephalic babies: a morphological and immunohistochemical evaluation. Int J Neurosci 2007; 117(1): 121-34.

CHAPTER 4

Degeneration

Abstract: Visual degeneration can occur due to different causes, e.g. aging, eye injury, adaptations to the changes in the environment or even alteration in genetics. In this chapter, 6 species of vertebrates are chosen to demonstrate the characteristic degenerative changes in their retinae. The black moore goldfish, which is one of the lower vertebrates that has been reported with severe visual degeneration; and the Royal College of Surgeon rats (RCS rats), which are the frequently used genetic model for the study of degenerative changes in the retina, are included in this chapter. The other examples illustrated are Asian house shrew, Anderson's shrew and human. Their degeneration of retinae is caused respectively by the environmental factors and aging. In the last part of this chapter, degeneration of the retina of ICR mice after receiving chronic administration of ketamine is shown. In humans, some of the most frequently encountered pathological changes of the retina are also included to introduce the readers to these common conditions.

Key Words: goldfish, RCS rat, shrew,degeneration, retina, cystic formation, cell death, merging of inner and outer nuclear layers, invasion of pigment cells, last cones, scanning electron microscopy, light microscopy

INTRODUCTION

Degeneration of the eye may be due to a change in environment, e.g. in the cavefish where the animals have adapted to the dark for long periods of time, consequently inducing regression of an ordinary eye into a degenerative eye. The eyes of a cavefish may range from a perimordium with arrested eye growth that starts in the embryo [1] or they may retain some small visual cells [2]. During evolution, a number of genes are upregulated, including the sonic hedgehog [3], the tiggy-winkle hedgehog [4] and the downregulation of Pax6 [5]. Pax6 affects regeneration in the retina of lower vertebrates [6]. Regeneration occurs daily in the retinae of lower vertebrates, e.g. fish, along with apoptotic degeneration of the older cells [7].

Aging in animals may also affect the visual system. In the 9-month-old rat, compared to those of 2.5 months old, there is a decrease in the ratio of large to small fibers in the optic nerve [8]. Increases in glial cells as well as nerve fiber degeneration are observed in 17-month-old mice [9]. Aging of the retina also has an effect on the photic response. In an experiment using albino mice after photic exposure, decreases in 2 deoxyglucose and dopamine uptake in the retinae of old mice (15 months) are demonstrated [10].

Even for normal animals, vision at night may be different from vision during the day. A vivid example is seen at night when the larval zebrafish downregulates its outer segment activity and synaptic ribbons in the cones disassemble [11].

Degeneration can occur after injury. Upon optic nerve sectioning in the goldfish, the cone cells are the last cells to degenerate [12]. However, on the other hand, when the optic nerve is sectioned while the retina has started to develop in the rat, the development of visual cells continues [13]. Apparently, genetic predisposition has already started to control retinal development and no linkages with the higher centers are necessary at that stage.

Severe eye degeneration is observed in certain lower vertebrates, e.g. the megalophthalmic goldfish [14]. Royal College of Surgeon rats are frequently used as a genetic model to study degenerative changes in the retina, similar to those mutations in the transgenic P347L pigs [15]. In the Royal College of Surgeon rats, a mutation of the receptor tyrosine kinase gene Merk induces changes in the retinal pigment epithelium such that the pigment cells cannot ingest shedded outer segments and subsequently the photoreceptors die, with indications that synaptic changes are present as well15. It has been proposed that cAMP concentration is an "off" signal for phagocytosis in the retinal pigment epithelium [16]. Outer segment shedding and phagocytosis in the retina are correlated phenomena [17] and a malfunction in any one will lead to blindness, e.g. retinitis pigmentosa in the human. There are also other forms of degeneration in human, e.g. those after hemorrhage (*i.e.* ischemia) and secondary degeneration due to tumor invasion, necrosis or subsequent to viral (macula degeneration) or bacterial infection (infectious ophthalmitis oculi).

Degeneration of the retina and the anterior chamber can also happen in susceptible lower species such as fish due to perinatal hypoxia [18, 19]. Moreover, the treeshrew which lives on a high UV exposed plateau commonly has

David T. Yew, Maria S. M. Wai and Winnie W. Y. Li

deteriorated lens. The Asian house shrew, on the other hand, which usually burrows itself in the soil searching for food, is seldom exposure to light, resulting in the degeneration of retinal cells.

BLACK MOORE GOLDFISH *CARASSIUS AURATUS*

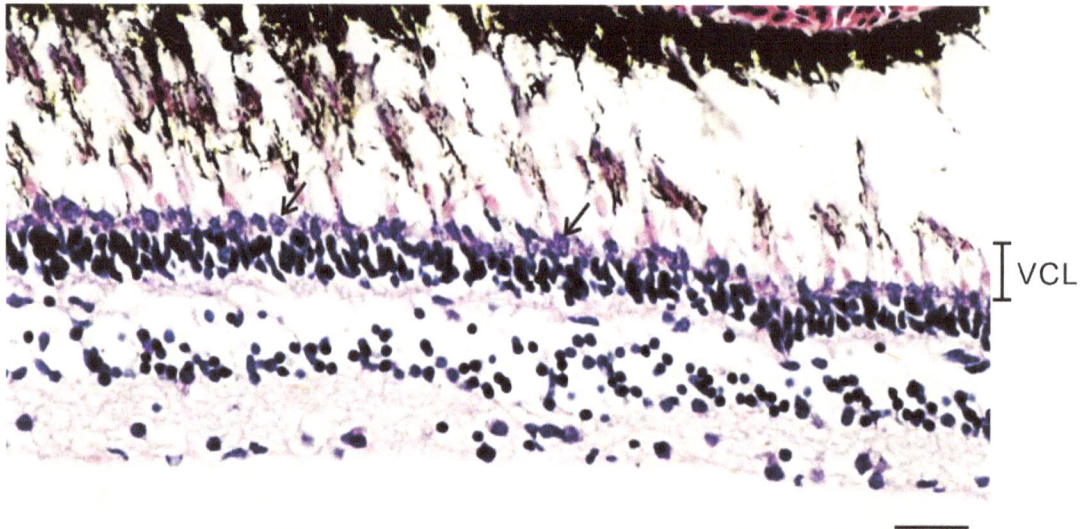

Figure 4.1a.

Peripheral retina. Note that there are very few cells in the visual cell layers (VCL). The first row of the outer nuclear layer (arrow) shows nuclei of lighter contrast which may indicate these are progenitor cells from the margin. Bar = 50 μm.

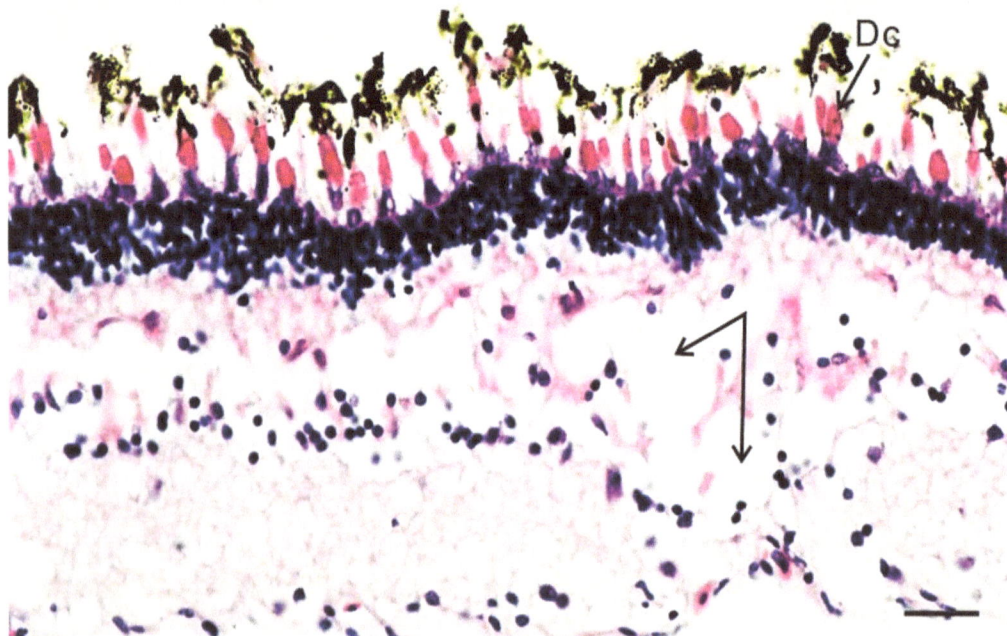

Figure 4.1b.

In the mid-periphery, cone cells are still present. Note a double cone (Dc). Large cystic spaces are also visible (arrows). Bar = 50 μm.

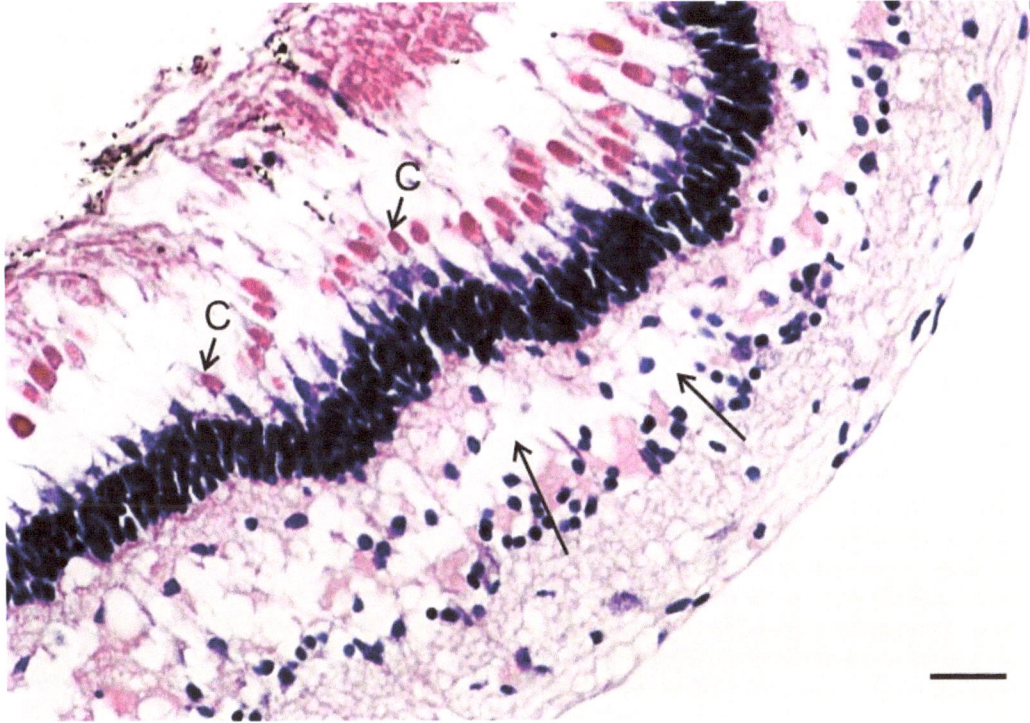

Figure 4.1c.

The central retina still contains cone cells (C). Note extensive cystic spaces (arrow) are present in the inner nuclear layer. Bar = 50 μm.

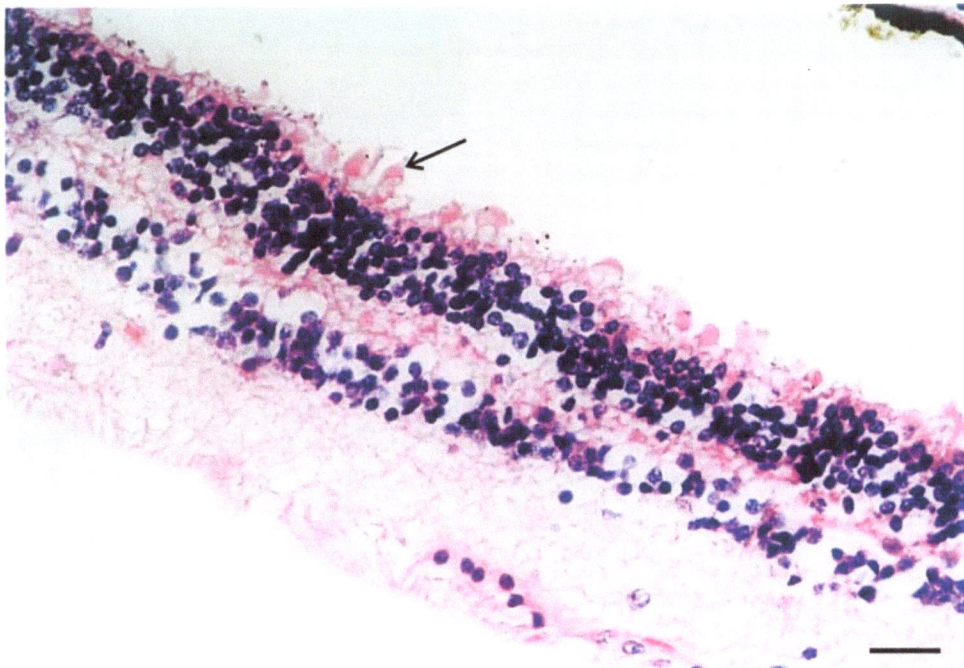

Figure 4.1d.

Some regions of the retina show loss of visual cells. Only cones remain (arrow).

Bar = 50 μm.

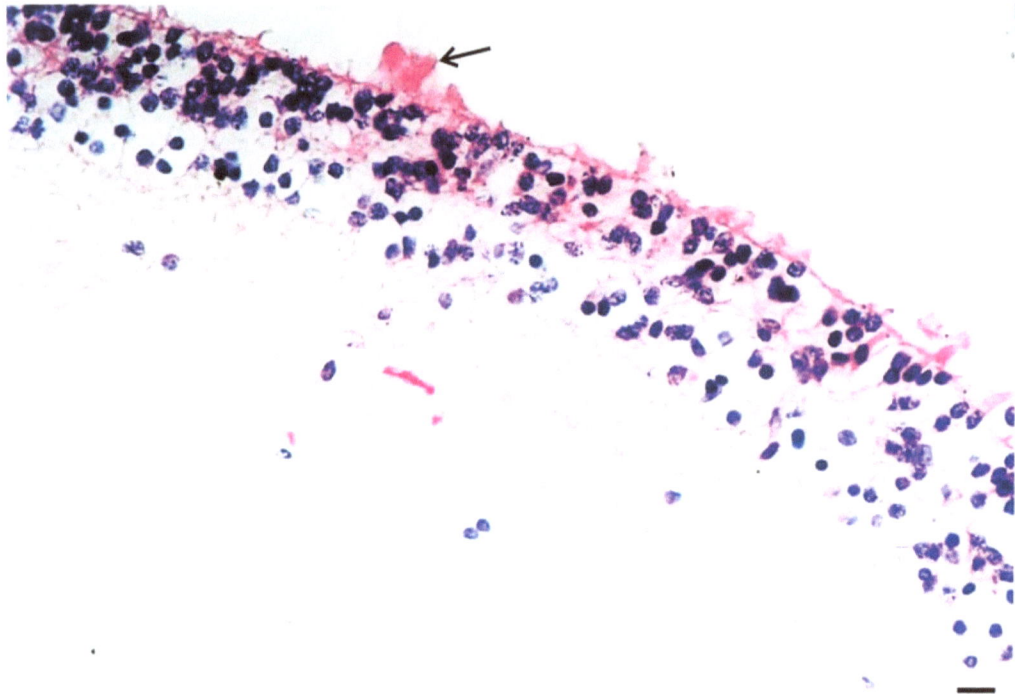

Figure 4.1e.

Merging of the outer nuclear layer & inner nuclear layer is noted in this animal. Very few visual cells remain (arrow). Bar = 50 μm.

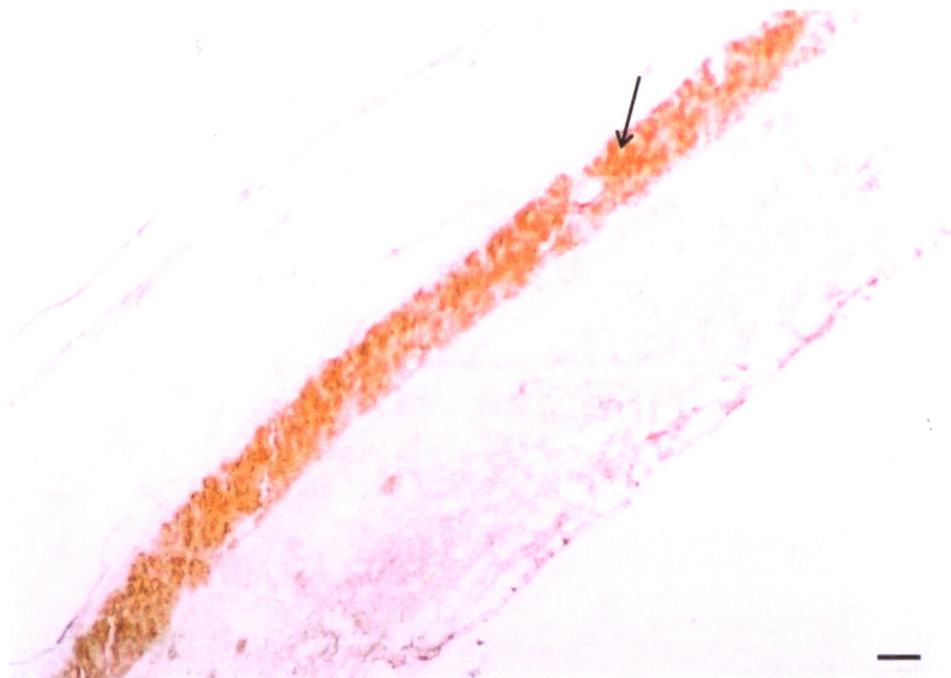

Figure 4.1f.

Activated caspase-3 immunocytochemistry showing apoptotic dying cells in the merged and degenerating nuclear layers. Bar = 50 μm.

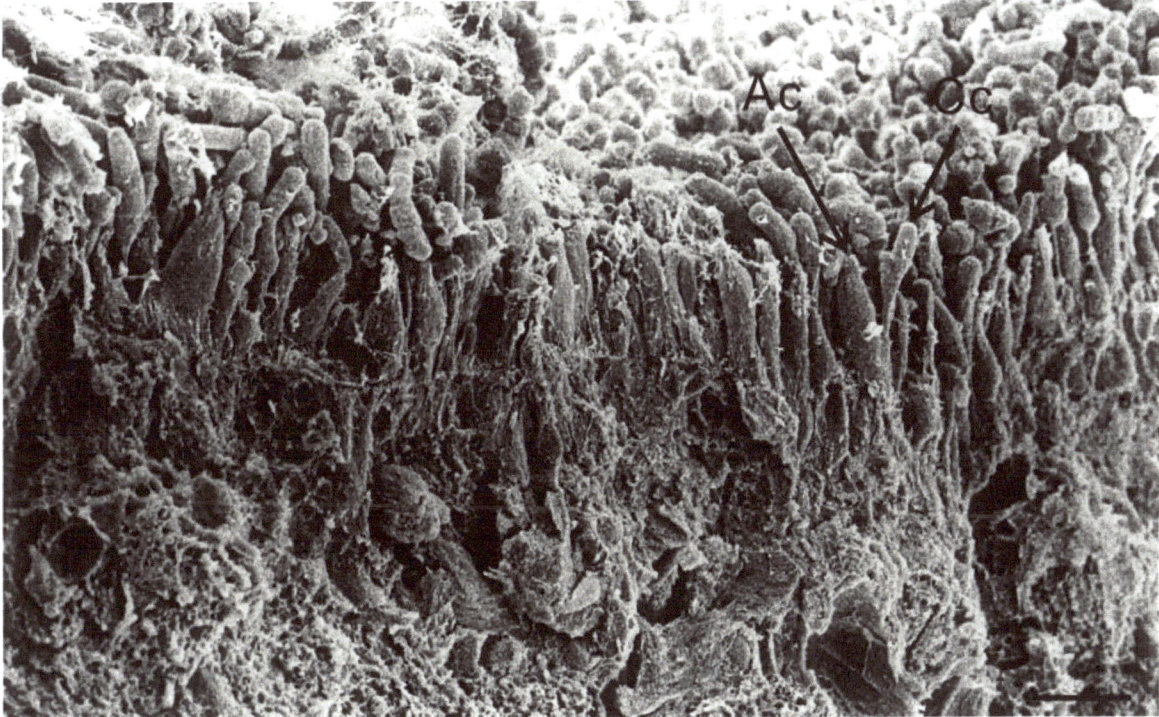

Figure 4.1g.

A rather normal looking goldfish retina. Double cones comprising a chief cone (Cc) and an accessory cone (Ac) are shown. Bar = 10 μm.

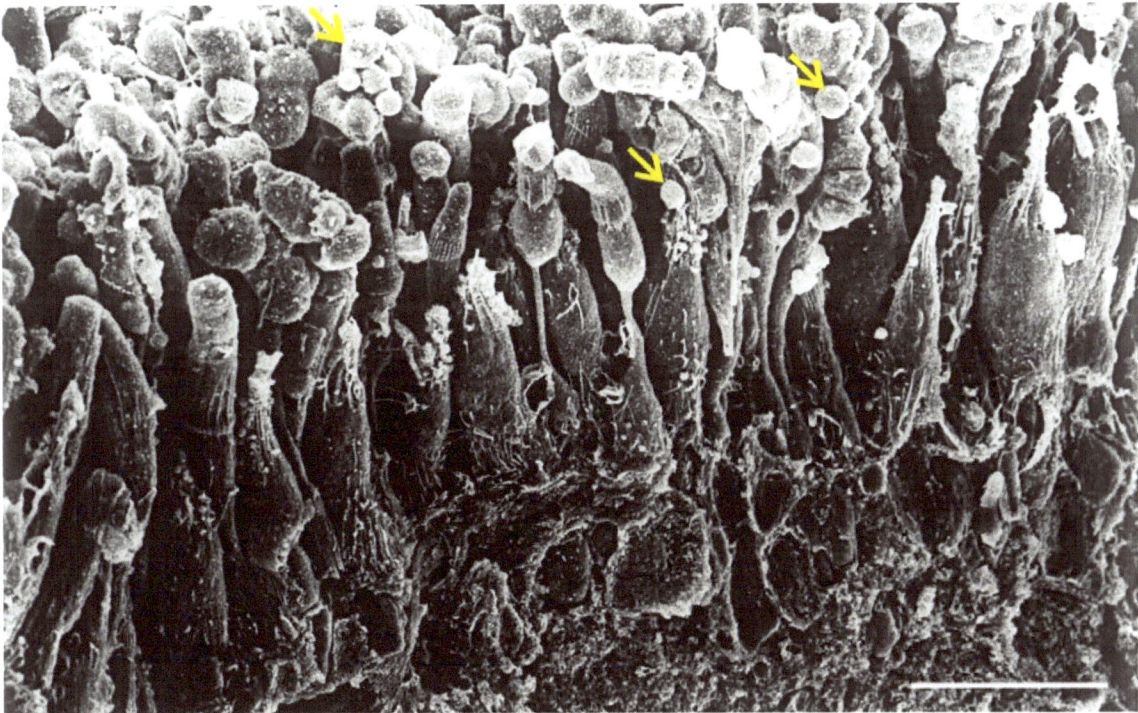

Figure 4.1h.

The first sign of degeneration is the blebbing of the outer segments (yellow arrows). Bar = 10 μm.

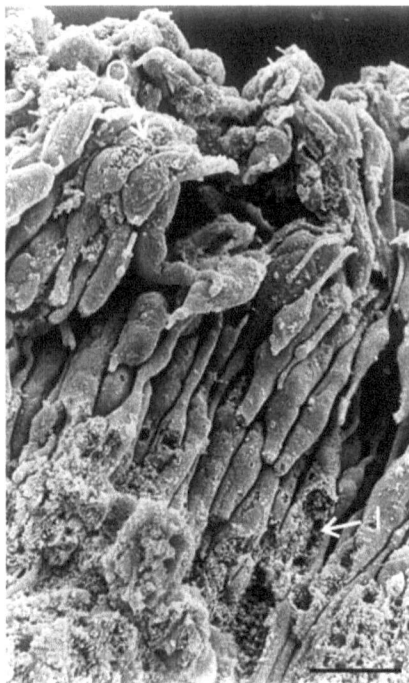

Figure 4.1i.

The second stage of degeneration is the vesiculation of the outer segment (O) and inner segment (I). Bar = 3 μm.

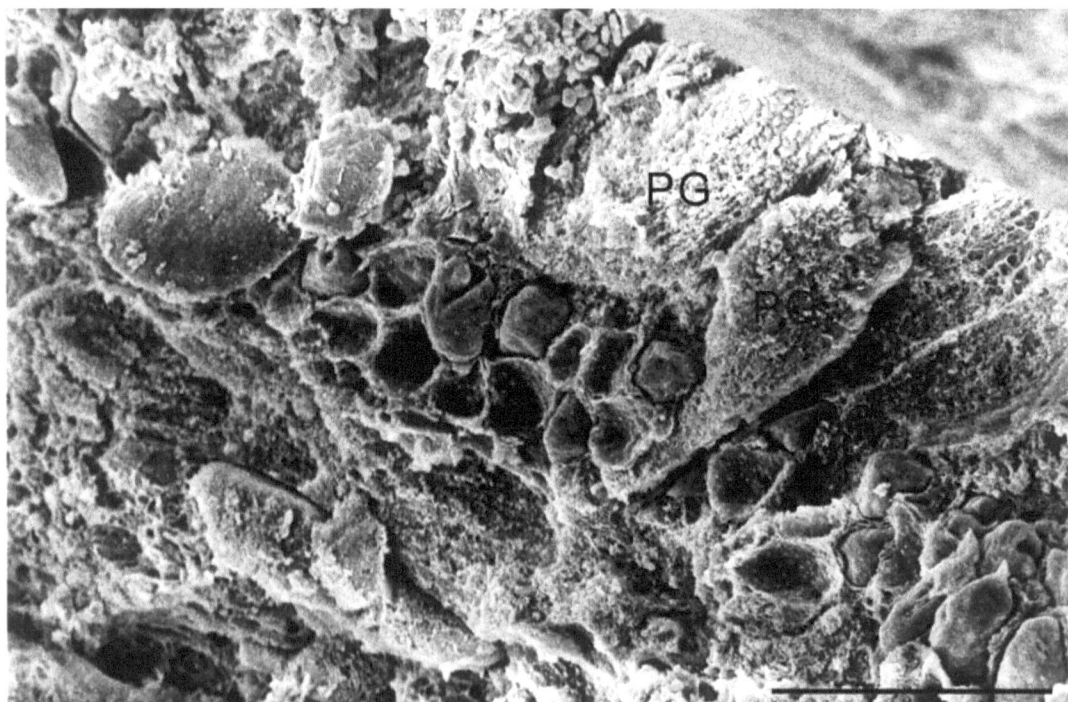

Figure 4.1j.

The third stage involves the invasion of pigment cells (PG) into the nuclear layer.

Bar = 10 μm.

RCS RAT (THE ROYAL COLLEGE OF SURGEONS RAT) *RATTUS NORVEGICUS*

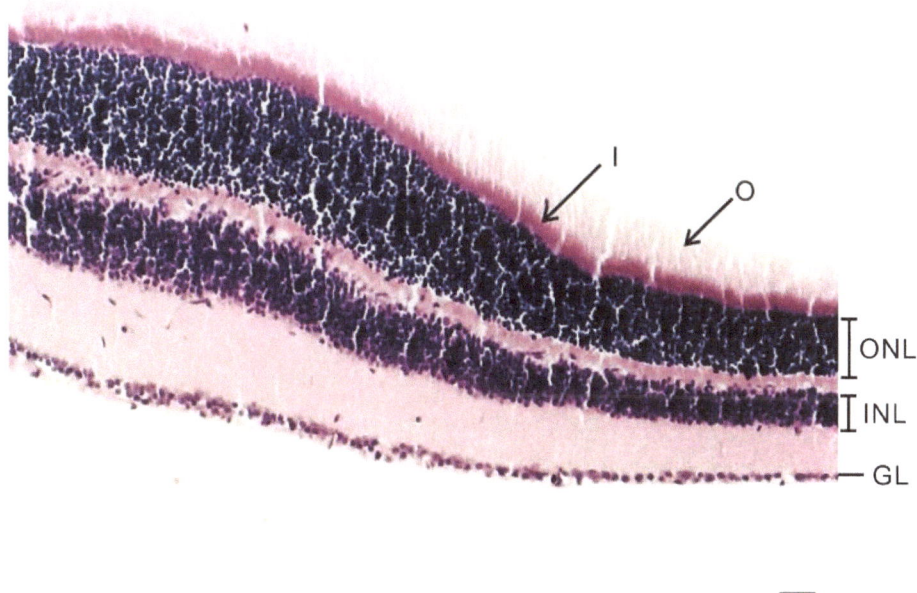

Figure 4.2a.

The retina of the normal strain of RCS rat with normal outer (O) and inner (I) segments. The latter is eosinophilic. Bar = 100 μm.

(GL - Ganglion cell layer; INL - Inner nuclear layer; ONL - Outer nuclear layer).

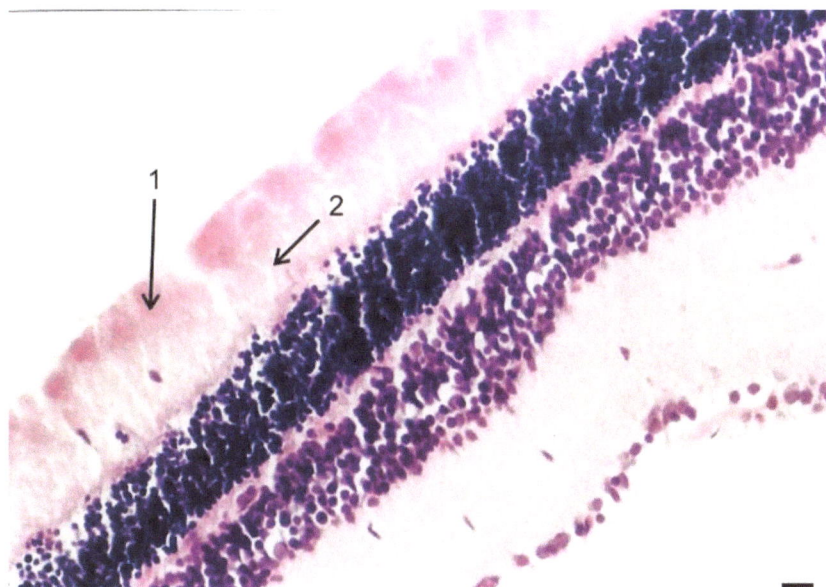

Figure 4.2b

A degenerative RCS rat retina showing a swollen and eosinophilic outer segment (1) and disintergrating inner segment (2). Bar = 50 μm.

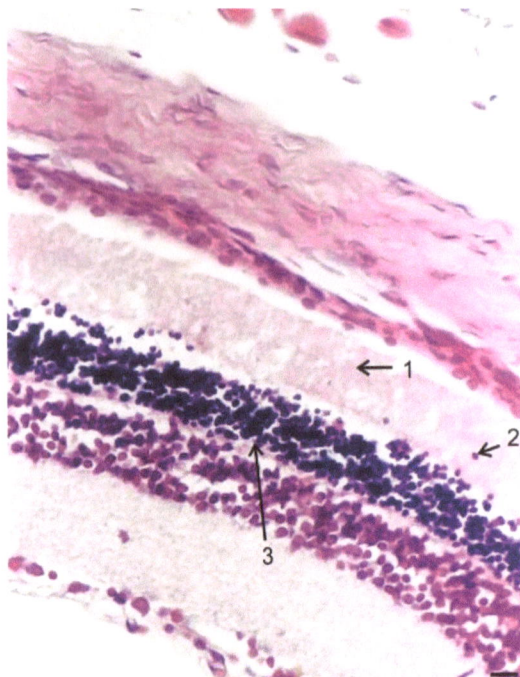

Figure 4.2c.

A totally degenerated visual cell layer with debris (1) and extrusion of nucleus from the outer nuclear layer (2). The region (3) indicating the outer plexiform layer which diminishes in thickness. Bar = 50 μm.

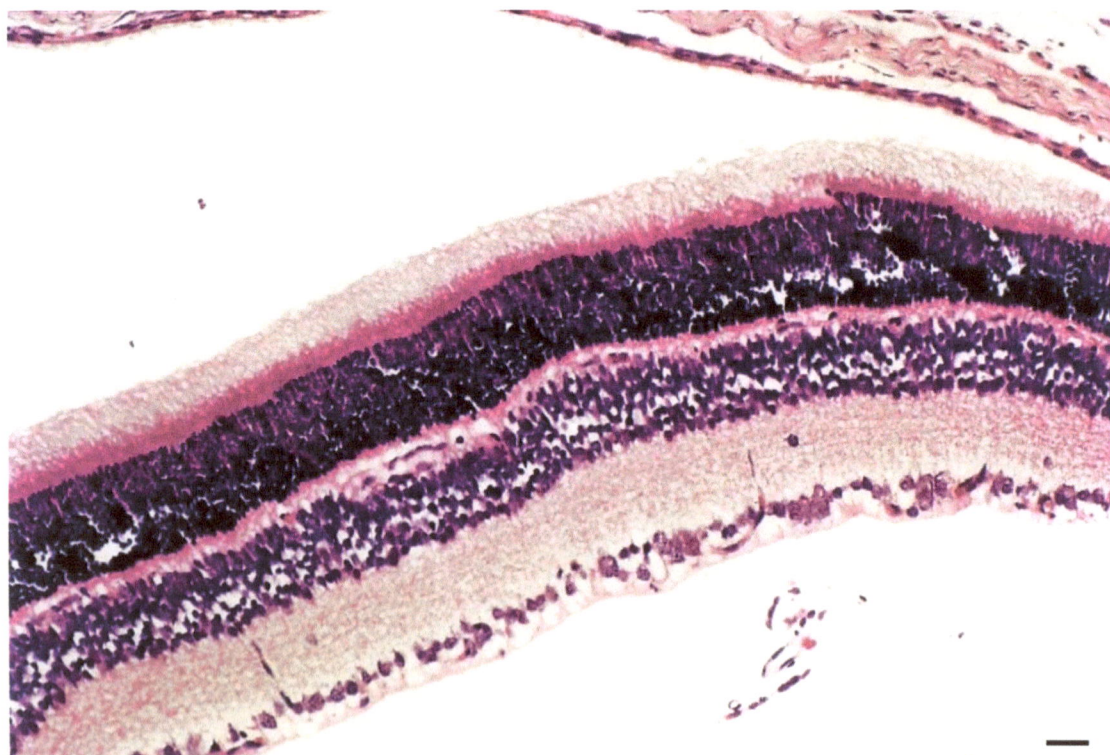

Figure 4.2d.

The control retina in a normal rat. Bar = 100 μm.

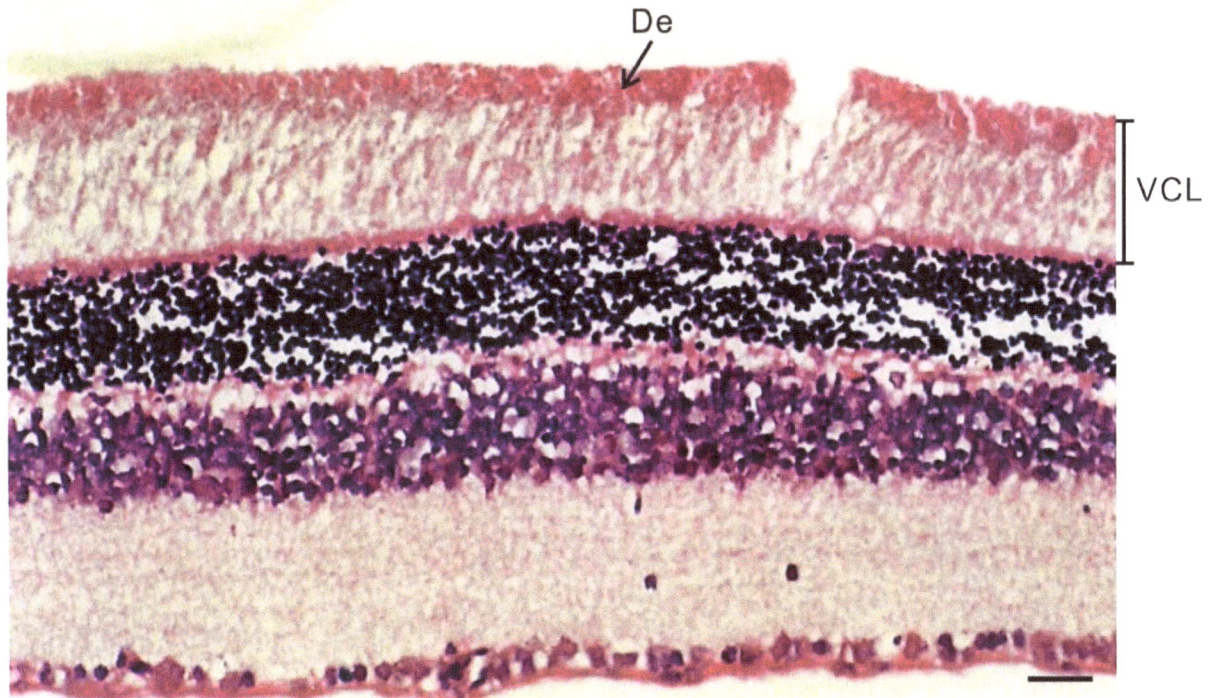

Figure 4.2e.

RCS rat at 35 days showing intense outer segment debris (De) collected in the visual cell layer (VCL). Bar = 100 µm.

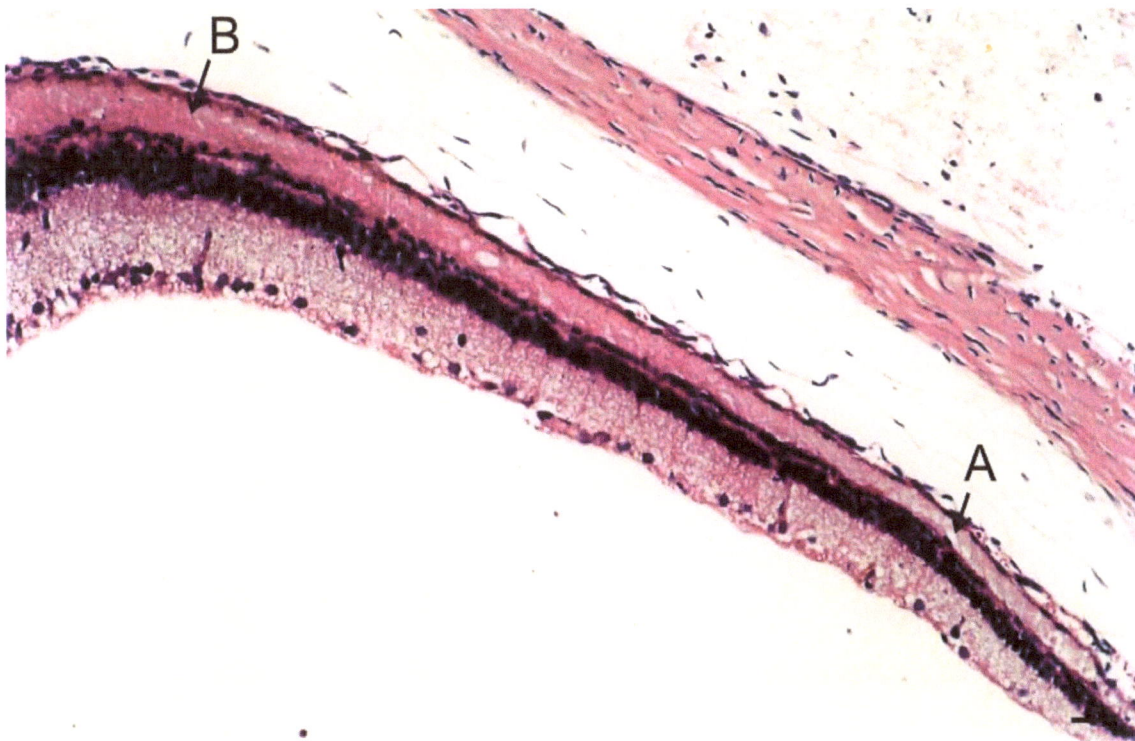

Figure 4.2f.

RCS rat at 40-days showing more severe degeneration at the periphery (A) compared to the centre (B). Bar = 50 µm.

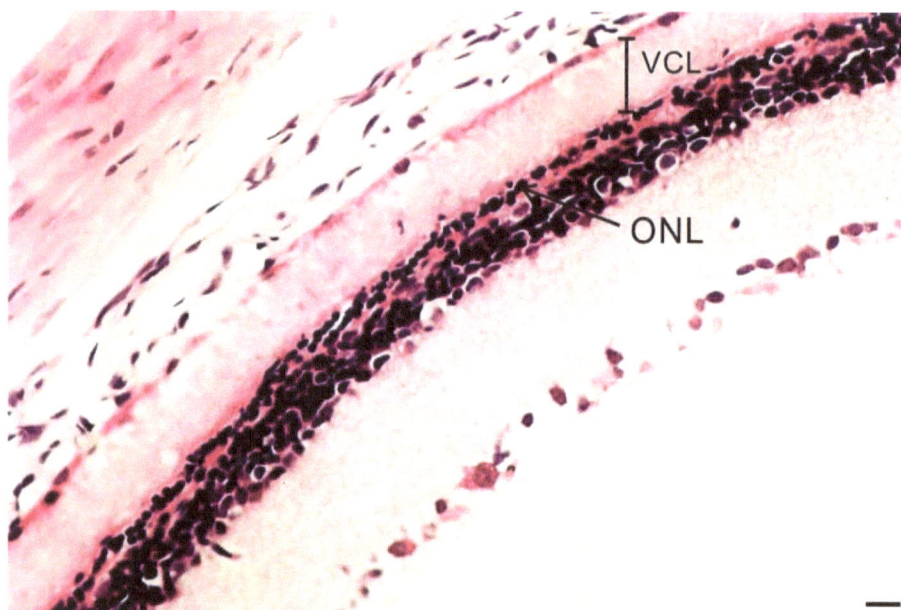

Figure 4.2g.

RCS rat at 40 days old showing total degeneration of visual cells and a thin outer nuclear layer (ONL). Bar = 50 μm.

(VCL - Visual cell layer).

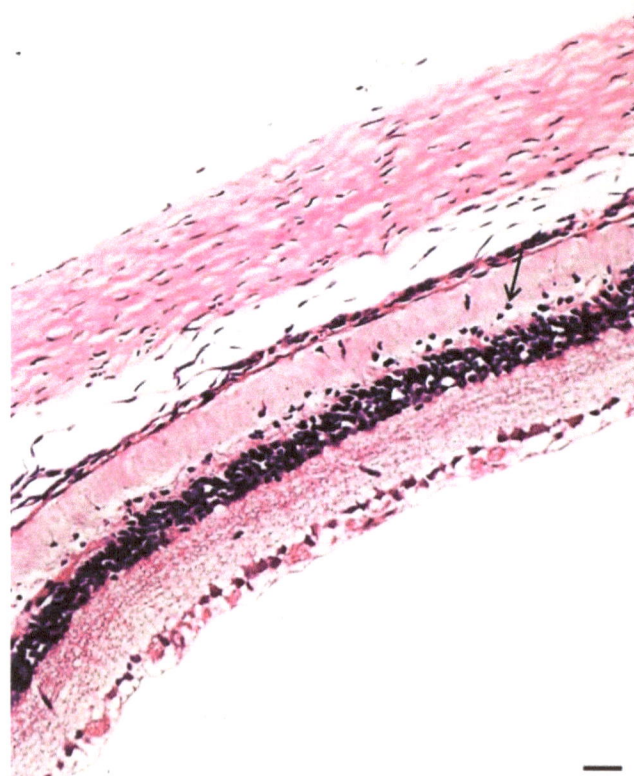

Figure 4.2h.

RCS rat at 60 days showing migration of nuclear cells outwards (arrow). Bar = 50 μm.

ASIAN HOUSE SHREW *SUNCUS MURINUS*

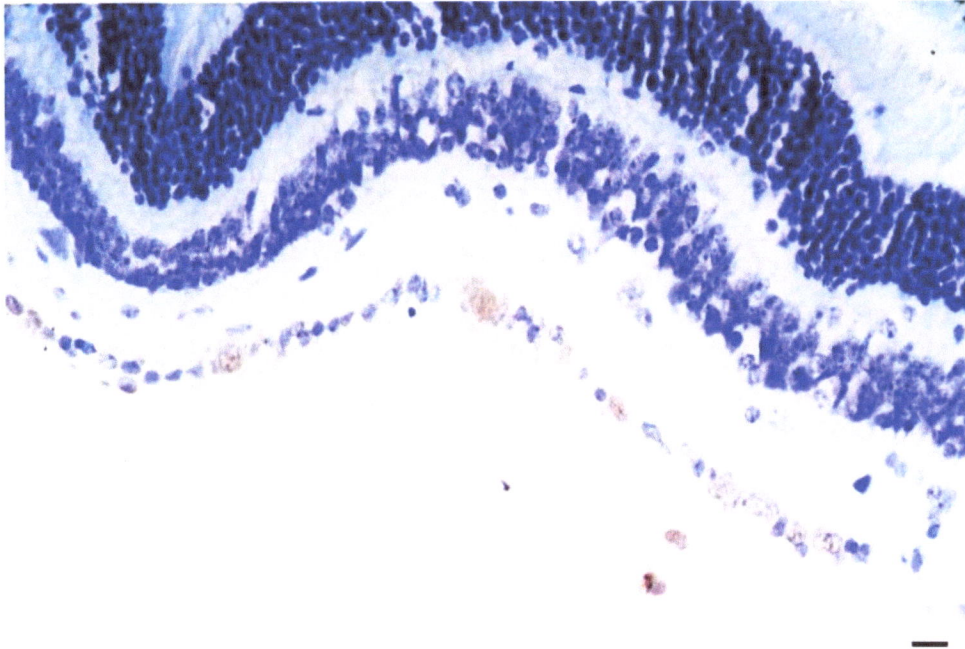

Figure 4.3a.

This section of the retina of a small shrew which is relatively unremarkable with all the retinal layers intact. Bar = 50 μm.

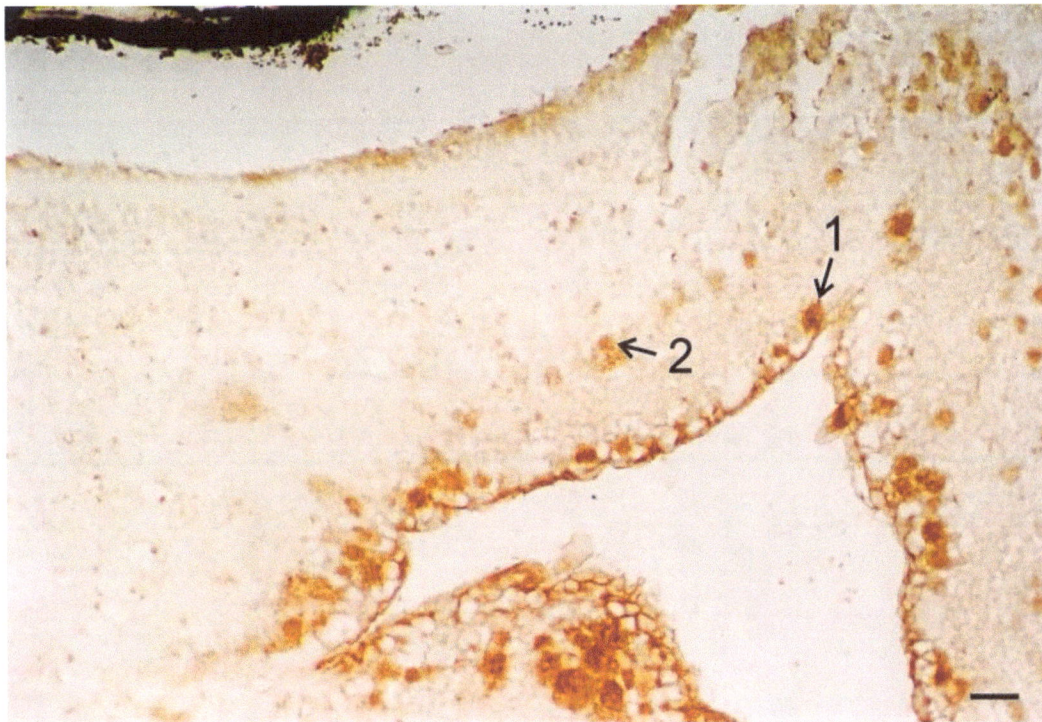

Figure 4.3b.

Activated caspase-3 immunocytochemistry, however, shows some ganglion cells (1) and a few inner nuclear cells (2) which are dying. Bar = 50 μm.

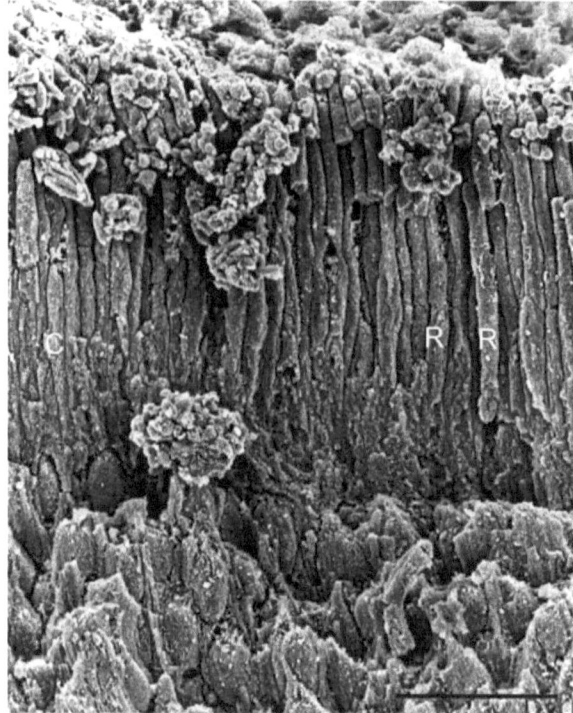

Figure 4.3c.

Most of the visual cells in the retina are rods (R). A few cones (C) are also present. Bar =10 μm.

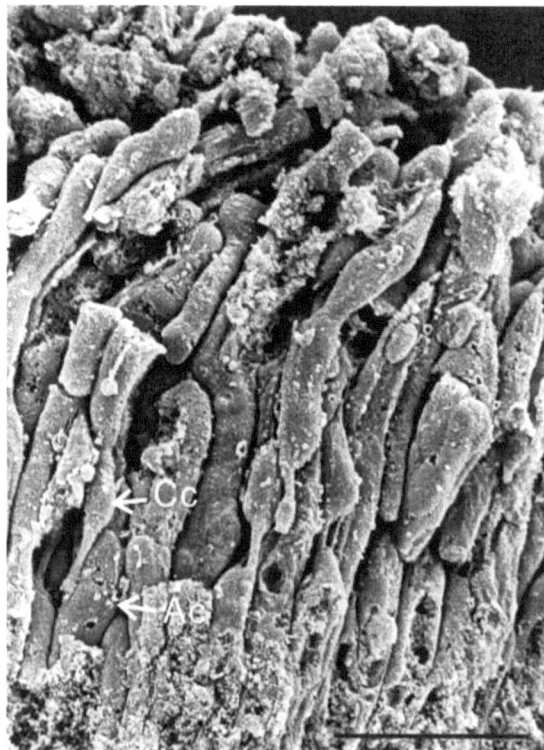

Figure 4.3 d.

This figure shows an accessory cone (Ac) and a chief cone (Cc). Bar = 5 μm.

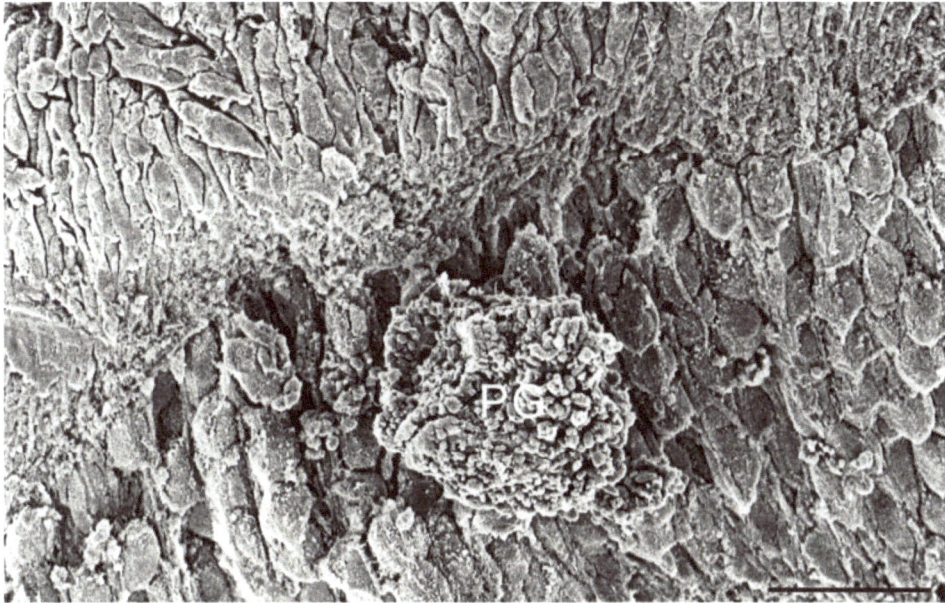

Figure 4.3e.

Pigment cells (PG) are seen to invade into the retina of the small shrew. Bar =10 μm.

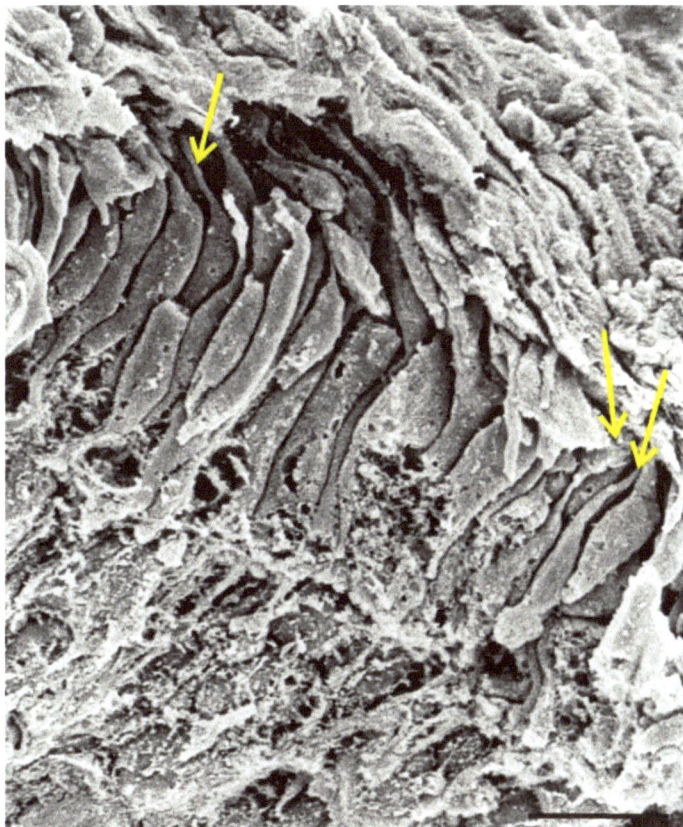

Figure 4.3f

Shrinkage and malformation of the outer segments is also observed at times (arrows). Bar = 5 μm.

ANDERSON'S SHREW (TREESHREW) *SUNCUS STOLICZKANUS*

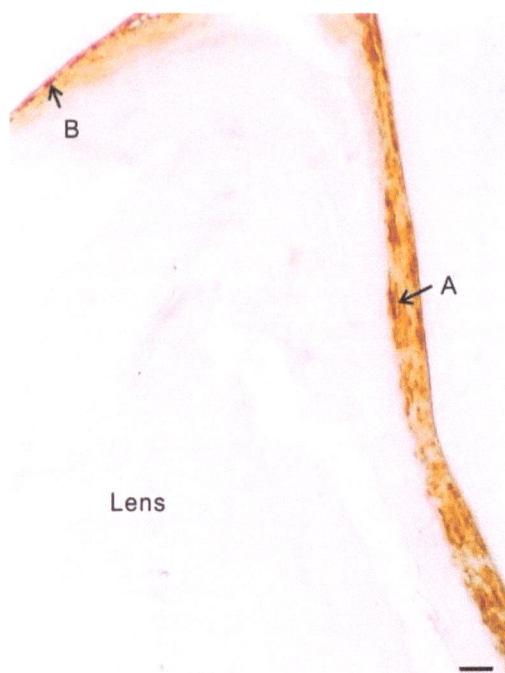

Figure 4.4a.

The natural degeneration of the retina in the treeshrew is related to its habitat. The animals live in the highland where UV irradiation is intense.

This is an activated caspase-3 staining on the lens of the treeshrew's eye. The immunohistochemistry captures apoptotic cells. Young lens fibers (with nuclei) (A) and lens epithelial cells (B) had intense positive reactions, indicating damage to the lens. Bar = 50 μm.

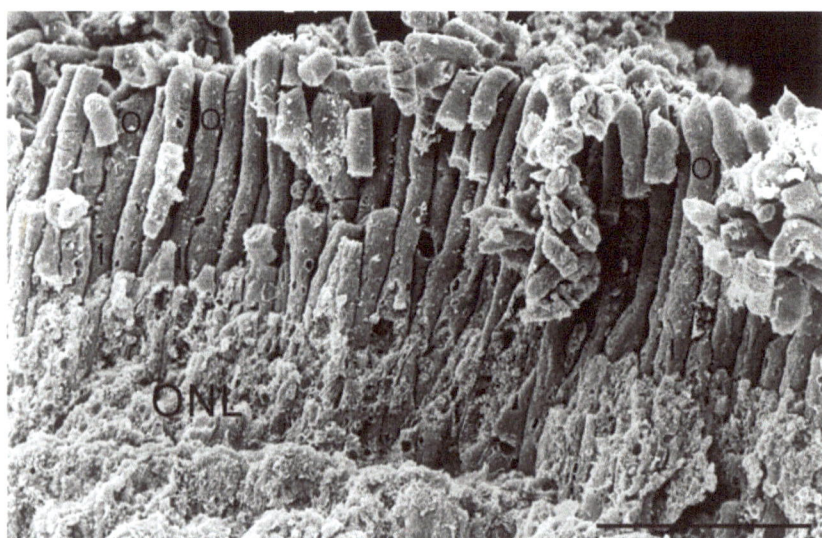

Figure 4.4b.

The treeshrews have relatively normal retina with normal outer (O) and inner (I) segments. "ONL" stands for outer nuclear layer. Bar = 10 μm.

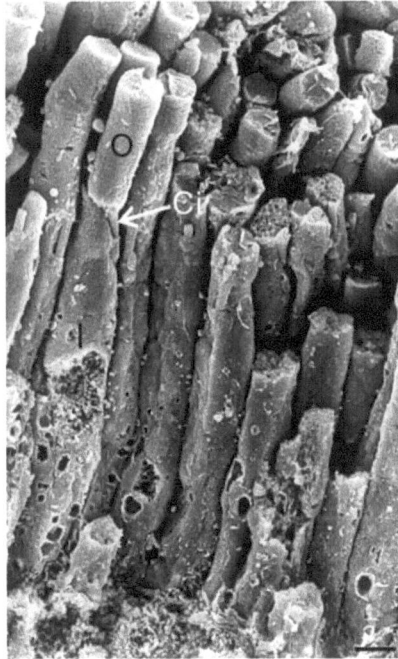

Figure 4.4c.

The treeshrew retina shows the outer segments (O) and inner segments (I) of the cones. There is a cilium (Ci) between the junction of the two segments. Bar = 1 μm.

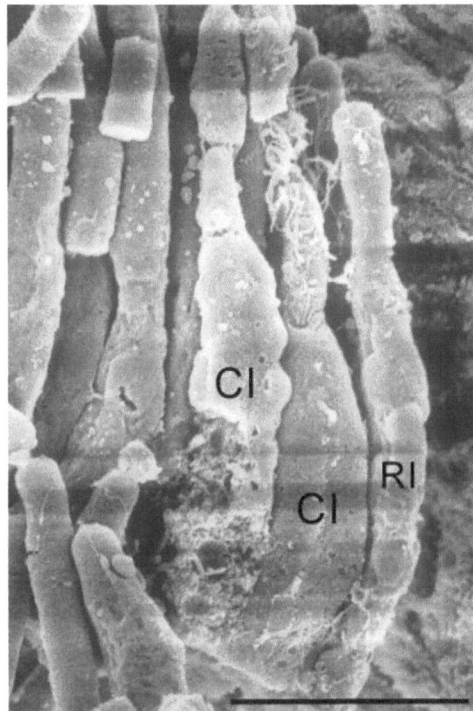

Figure 4.4d.

Another figure of the treeshrew retina showing outer segments and the inner segments of cones (CI) and rods (RI). Bar = 5 μm.

HUMAN *HOMO SAPIENS*

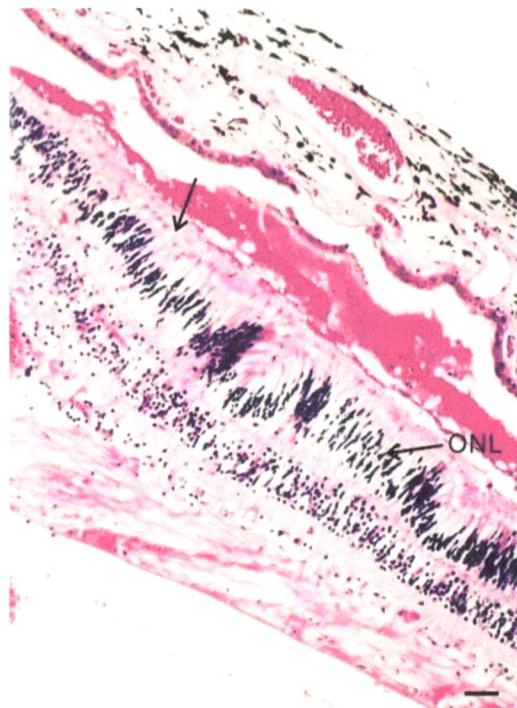

Figure 4.5a.

Degeneration in the human central retina, including degeneration of visual cells (arrow) and the outer nuclear layer (ONL). Bar = 100 μm.

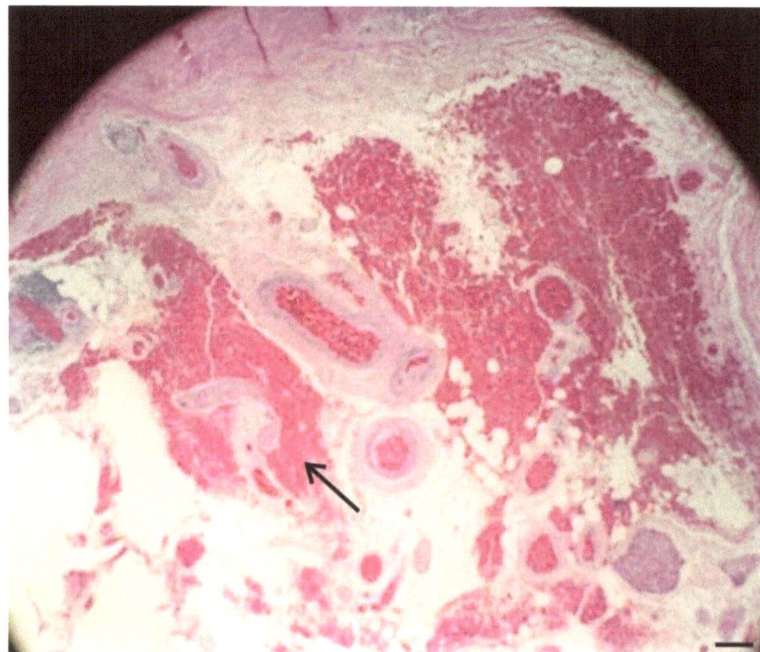

Figure 4.5b

Extensive hemorrhage (arrow) in the optic nerve head of the retina of the human. Bar = 400 μm.

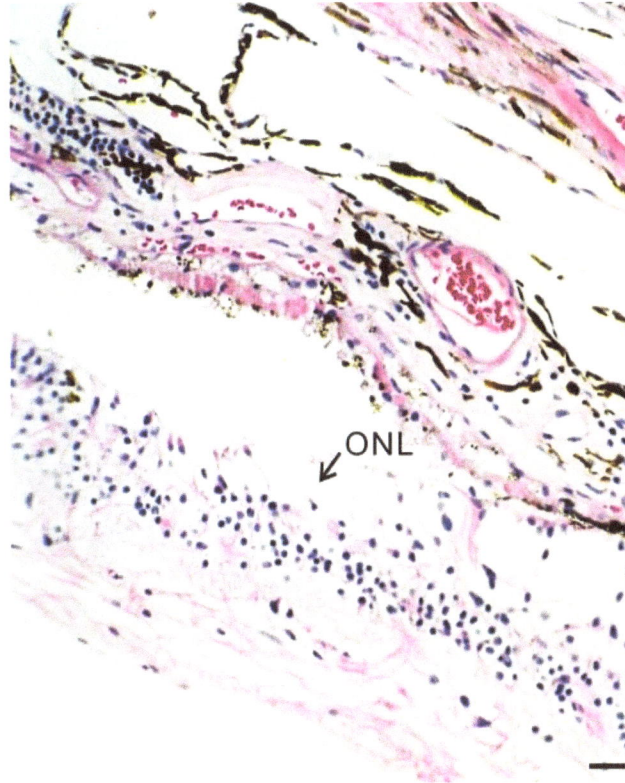

Figure 4.5c.

The event in figure 4.5b leads to degeneration of the retina. In this section, only the outer nuclear layer (ONL) remains. Bar = 100 μm.

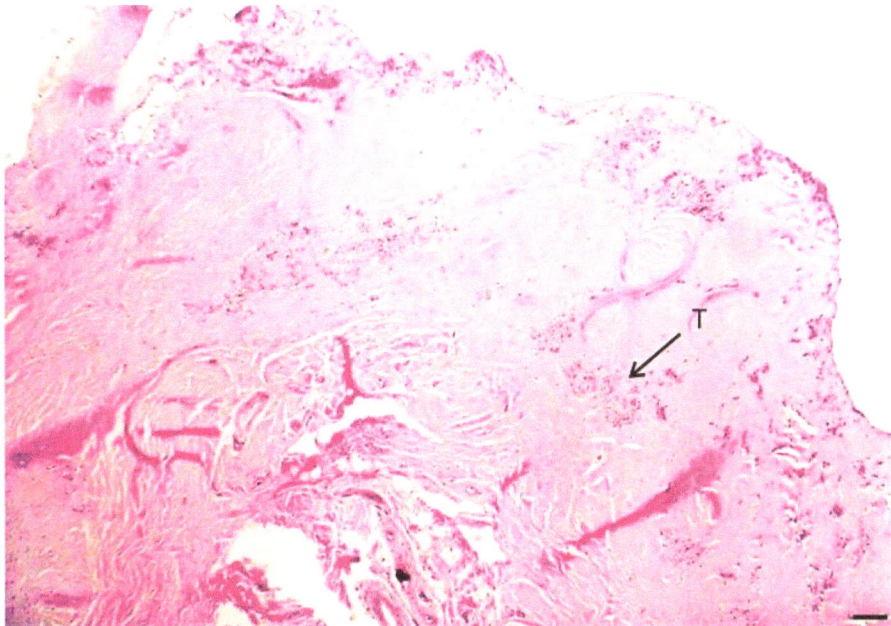

Figure 4.5d.

This figure shows a tumor with tumor cells (T) in the human optic stalk. Bar = 400 μm.

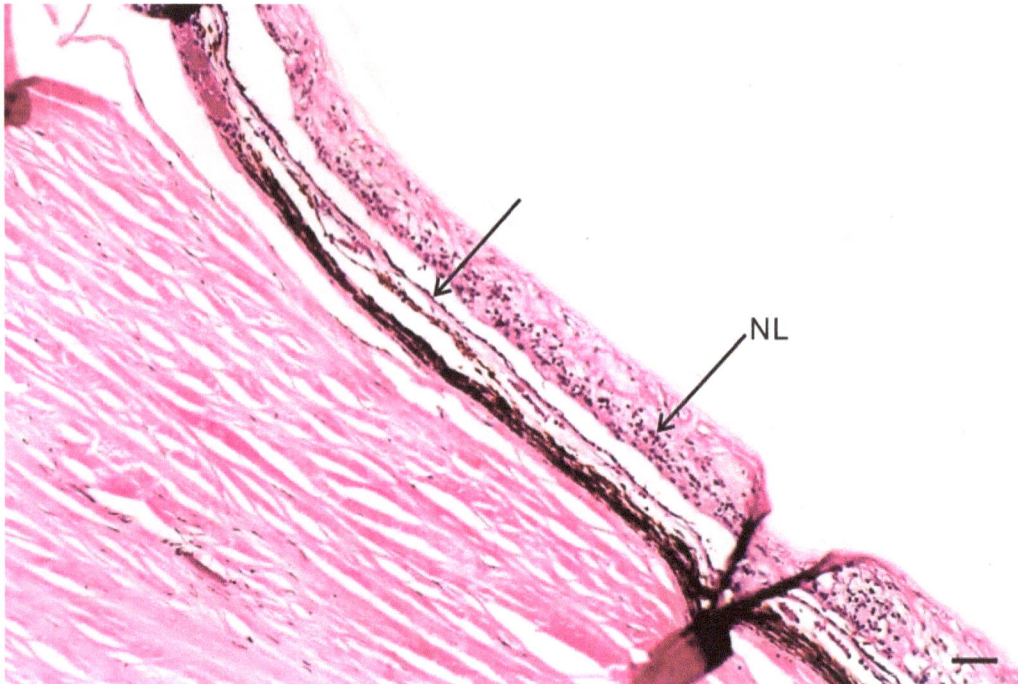

Figure 4.5e.

The central retina of the eye with tumor invasion. Note the disappearance of visual cells (arrow). The nuclear layer (NL) is still present. Bar = 100 μm.

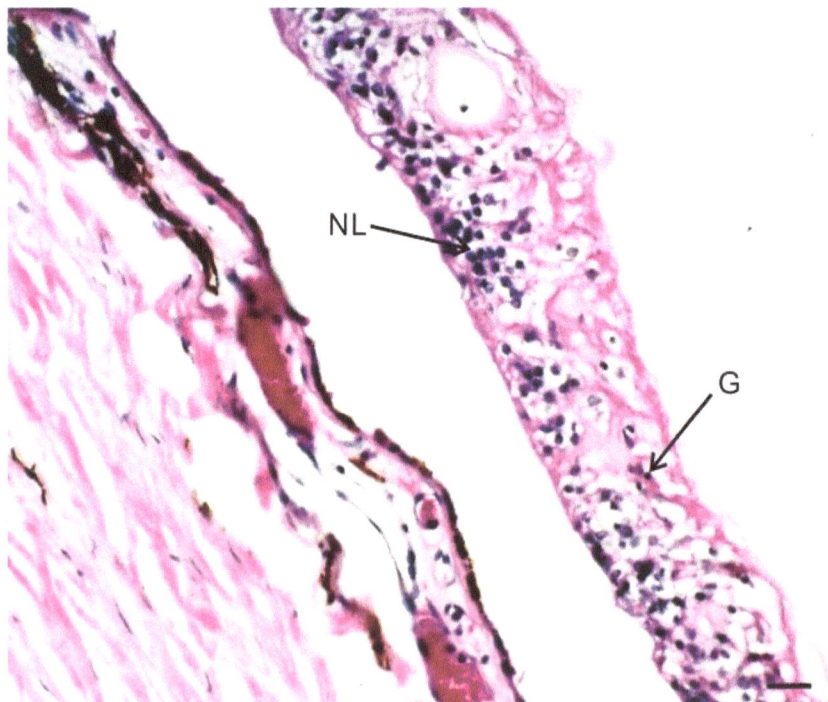

Figure 4.5f.

Higher power of the degenerating retina of the eye with tumor. Note a remaining nuclear layer (NL). Some ganglion cells (G) are also seen. Bar = 50 μm.

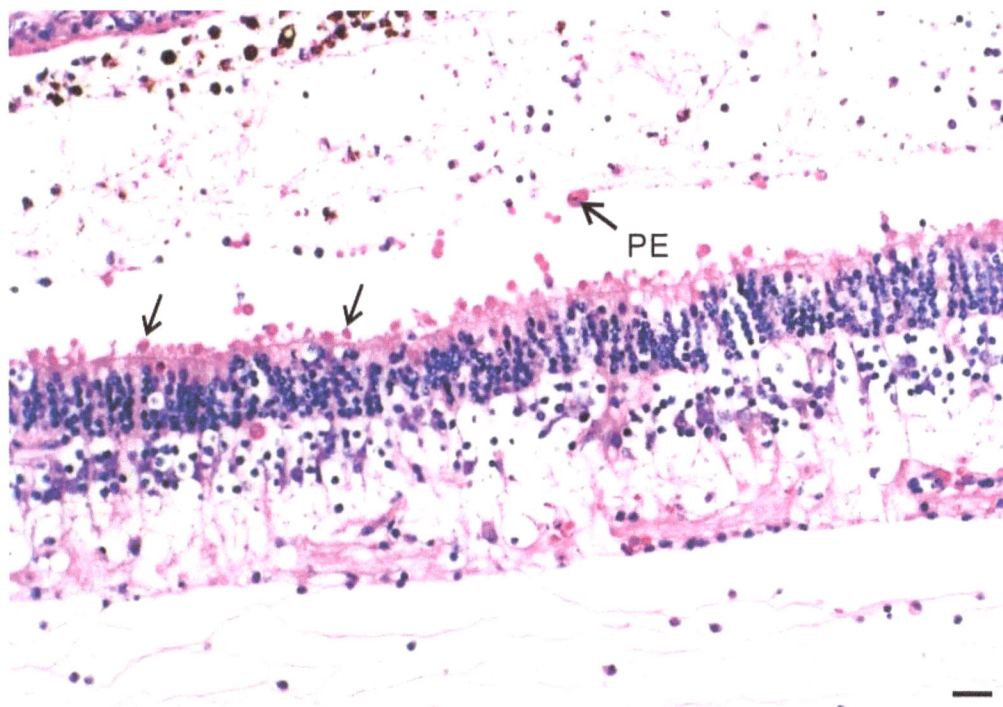

Figure 4.5g.

The degenerating retina of retinitis pigmentosa. Note disintegrating pigment epithelium (PE) and degenerating visual cells (arrows). Bar = 50 μm.

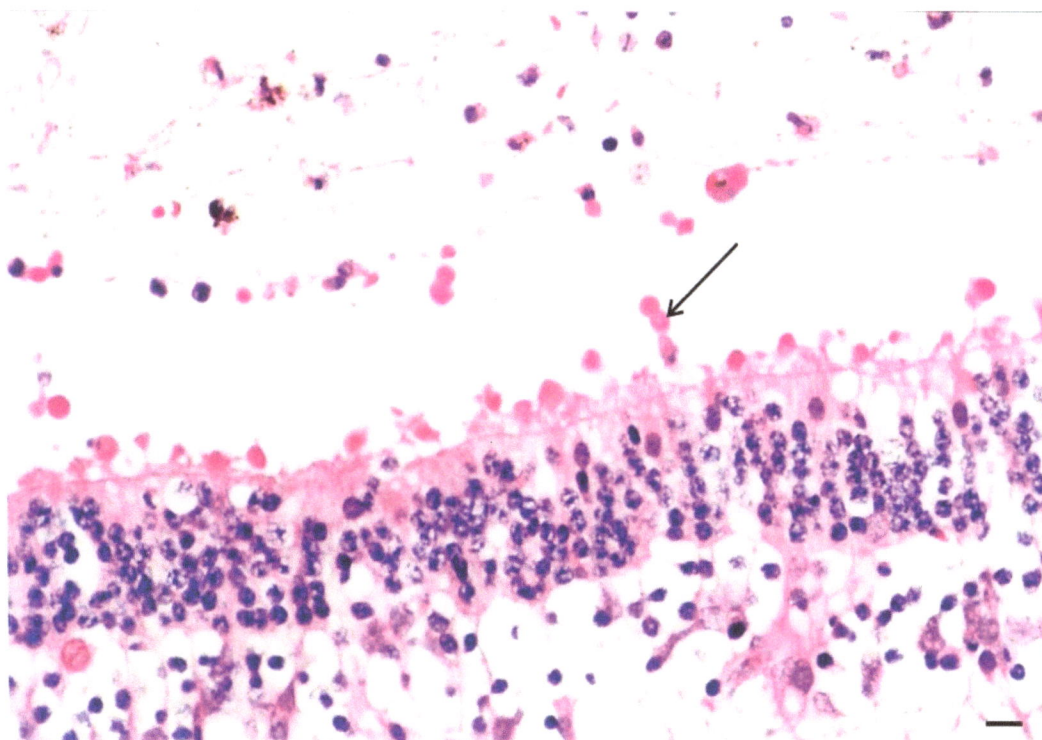

Figure 4.5h.

A higher power figure of figure 4.5g indicating the degeneration of visual cells (arrow). Bar = 50 μm.

DRUG TREATMENT KETAMINE TOXICITY – ICR MICE (INSTITUTE FOR CANCER RESEARCH MICE) *MUS MUSCULUS*

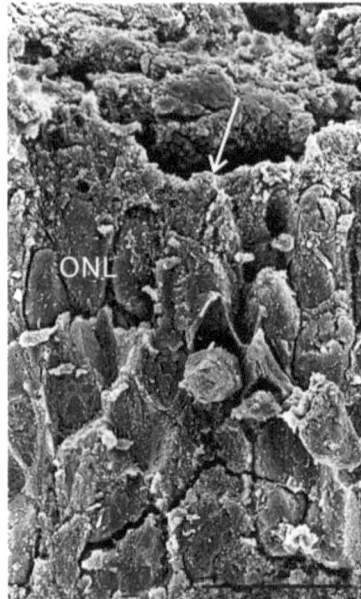

Figure 4.6a.

The retina of a ketamine treated mouse at the age of day 14 neonatally. A single dose of ketamine (1 ml at 0.1 mg/ml concentration) had been given to the eye at day 7 postnatally.

Note the failure of genesis of visual cells above external limiting membrane (arrow). Bar = 10 μm.

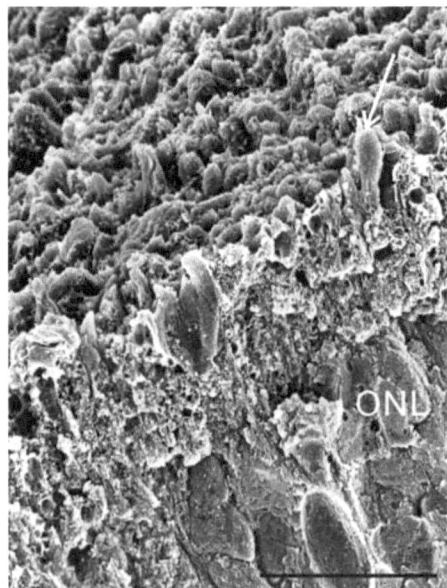

Figure 4.6b.

Other ketamine treated mouse's retina at the age of day 14 neonatal, showing only very small visual cells (arrow). Bar = 10 μm.

(ONL - Outer nuclear layer).

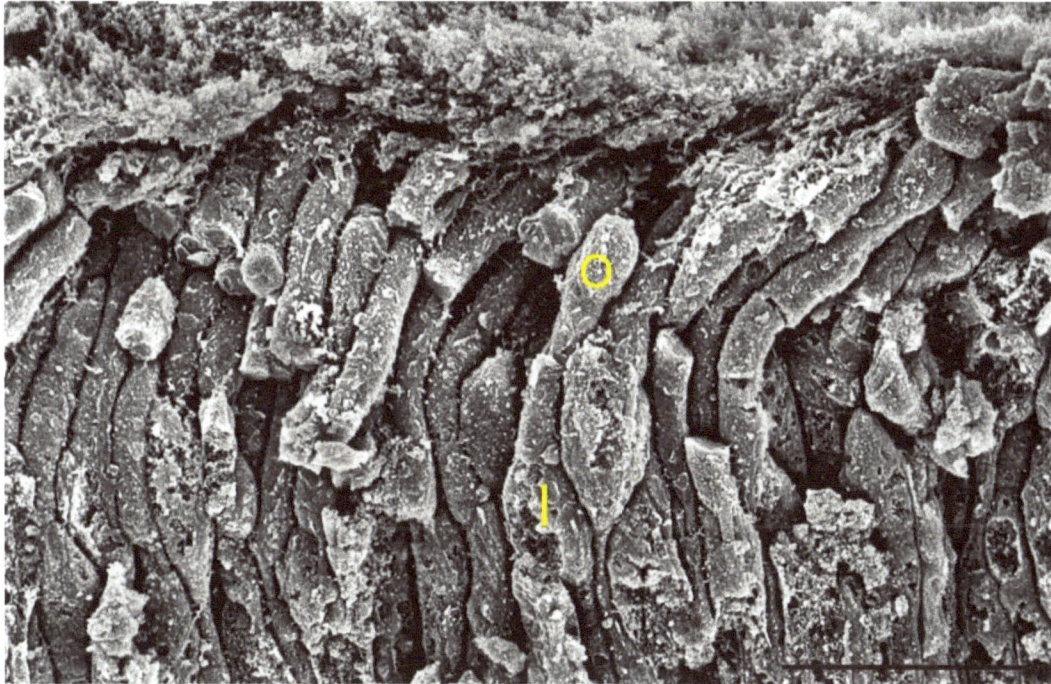

Figure 4.6c.

Normal retina of a 14-day-old neonatal mouse showing outer (O) and inner (I) segments. Bar = 5 μm.

REFERENCES

[1]   Jeffery WR. Chapter 8. Evolution and development in the cavefish Astyanax. Curr Top Dev Biol 2009; 86: 191-221.
[2]   Yew DT, Yoshihara HM. An ultrastructural study on the retina of the blind cave fish (Astyanax hubbusi). Cytologia (Tokyo) 1977; 42(1): 175-80.
[3]   Rétaux S, Pottin K, Alunni A. Shh and forebrain evolution in the blind cavefish Astyanax mexicanus. Biol Cell 2008; 100(3): 139-47.
[4]   Yamamoto Y, Stock DW, Jeffery WR. Hedgehog signalling controls eye degeneration in blind cavefish. Nature 2004; 431(7010): 844-7.
[5]   Tian NM, Price DJ. Why cavefish are blind. Bioessays 2005; 27(3): 235-8.
[6]   Thummel R, Enright JM, Kassen SC, Montgomery JE, Bailey TJ, Hyde DR. Pax6a and Pax6b are required at different points in neuronal progenitor cell proliferation during zebrafish photoreceptor regeneration. Exp Eye Res 2010; 90(5): 572-82.
[7]   Mizuno TA, Ohtsuka T. Caspase-depenedent apoptosis of ON bipolar cells in the goldfish marginal retina. Neuroreport 2009; 20(15): 1330-3.
[8]   Yew DT. Aging in retinae and optic nerves of 2.5- to 9-month-old mice. Acta Anat (Basel) 1979a; 104(3): 332-4.
[9]   Wong SL, Ip PP, Yew DT. Comparative ultrastructural study of the optic nerves and visual cortices of young (2.5 months) and old (17 months) mice. Acta Anat (Basel). 1979; 105(4): 426-30.
[10]   Yew DT, Tsang DS, Chan YW. Photic responses of the retina at different ages: a comparative study using histochemical and biochemical methods. Acta Anat (Basel) 1985; 121(3): 184-8.
[11]   Emran F, Rihel J, Adolph AR, Dowling JE. Zebrafish larvae lose vision at night. Proc Natl Acad Sci U S A. 2010; 107(13): 6034-9.
[12]   Yew DT, Li WW. Early patterns of neuronal degeneration in the retina of the goldfish after optic nerve sectioning. Acta Morphol Neerl Scand 1986; 24(2): 123-32.
[13]   Yew DT, Zhang DR, Hui BS, Li WW. Optic nerve sectioning does not affect the development of the retina. Acta Anat (Basel) 1989; 134(1): 54-6.
[14]   Yew DT, Li WW, Au C, Choi HL, Yang QD, Chan PK. Retinal changes in a mutant form of goldfish with megalophthalmia. Scanning Microsc 1991; 5(2): 585-93.
[15]   Peng YW, Senda T, Hao Y, Matsuno K, Wong F. Ectopic synaptogenesis during retinal degeneration in the royal college of surgeons rat. Neuroscience 2003; 119(3): 813-20.

[16]   Strauss O, Stumpff F, Mergler S, Wienrich M, Wiederholt M. The Royal College of Surgeons rat: an animal model for inherited retinal degeneration with a still unknown genetic defect. Acta Anat (Basel) 1998; 162(2-3): 101-11.

[17]   LaVail MM. Outer segment disc shedding and phagocytosis in the outer retina. Trans Ophthalmol Soc U K 1983; 103 (Pt 4): 397-404.

[18]   Lü LH, Li JC, Wai MS, Lam WP, Forster EL, Fang MR, Yew DT. Perinatal hypoxia induces subsequent retinal degeneration in the offspring of ovoviviparous fish, Xiphophorous maculates. Vet Ophthalmol 2007 Sep-Oct; 10(5): 289-94.

[19]   Chan CY, Lam WP, Wai MS, Wang M, Foster EL, Yew DT. Perinatal hypoxia induces anterior chamber changes in the eyes of offspring fish. J Reprod Dev 2007; 53(6): 1159-67

Index

A

Accessory cone 3, 7-10, 15, 23, 24, 30, 33, 36, 41, 42, 46, 49, 50, 55, 59, 62-64, 66, 67, 74, 75, 77, 82, 85, 93, 95, 98, 99, 101, 102, 104, 108, 118, 119, 124, 126-128, 130, 132, 133, 136-139, 143, 148, 154, 157-159, 167-169, 184, 186-188, 191, 241, 248
Accessory cone nucleus 8, 15, 41, 93
Accessory cone outer segment 184, 186
Acetylcholine 192
Acetylcholinesterase 196, 210, 213
Acid phosphatase 192, 193, 196
Adrenergic 192, 193, 202, 203
Adrenergic ending 192
Adult primate 206
African clawed frog 87-92
Aging 237
Amacrine cell 4, 5,7, 29, 39, 82, 129, 132, 180, 182, 191, 195, 197, 201-207, 209, 212, 216
Amacrine cell process 5, 209
Amacrine-amacrine cell junction 207
Amacrine-amacrine contact 201, 202, 204, 207
Amacrine-amacrine pairing 201
Amacrine-ganglion cell junction 207
Amacrine-ganglion synapse 246, 251
Amphibian 3,5, 202, 212
Anderson's shrew, treeshrew 237, 250, 251
Anencephalic baby 222
Anterior retina 7, 14, 18, 21, 24, 25, 35, 36, 48, 52, 58, 68, 69, 78, 87, 92, 93, 99-101, 109, 110, 114, 120, 122, 125, 126, 130, 131, 134-136, 149, 152, 170, 171, 179, 182
Apoptosis 3
Apoptotic cell 250
Arabian camel 149, 150
Arciform body 212
Ascending fiber 162
Asian house shrew 237, 238, 247-249
Aspartic acid 192
Astrocyte 5,217
ATPase 202
Autolysis 104
Axons 4, 5, 149, 151, 195, 196, 207, 216

B

Bacterial infection 237
Ball-like outer segment 146, 158, 159
Basal nucleus 56
Basement membrane 5, 234
Bipolar 3-6, 29, 39, 82, 102, 103, 132, 143, 157, 180, 182, 191, 195-197, 199, 201, 202, 207, 208, 212
Bipolar axon 5, 207
Bipolar cell contact 201
Bipolar cell layer 196
Bipolar cell process 4, 212
Bird 3, 193, 202
Black moore goldfish 237, 238-242

R

Rabbit 191, 198, 201, 202, 207, 213, 222-225
Ray 193
Receptor tyrosine kinase gene Merk 237
Reciprocal control 207,211
Red light 222
Red rod 3
Regeneration 237
Reptile 3, 4, 92, 102, 112, 120, 210
Retinal differentiation 197
Retinal ganglion cell 213
Retinal layer 4, 18, 21, 53, 57, 58, 62, 69, 78, 83, 104, 109, 110, 116, 121, 134, 150, 179, 191, 192, 233, 247
Retinal oscillation 216
Retinitis pigmentosa 237, 255
Rh1 rod opsin 3
Rh2 cone opsin 4
Ribosome 4, 5, 192, 193, 202, 205, 208, 213, 215
RNA 202, 213
Rod 3, 4,6 7, 11, 13, 16, 17,20, 24-28, 30, 31, 33, 39, 41, 42, 49-51, 60, 64, 70 , 72, 78, 80, 85, 87-95, 100-102, 104,
    111, 116, 118-120, 122, 123, 126-129, 131, 133, 142, 147-150, 152-154, 156, 159-161, 164, 67, 170, 171,
    180-183, 183, 195, 196, 235, 248, 251
Rod bipolar 195, 196
Rod nucleus 41, 93
Rod shaped inner segment 100
Rod spherule 182, 192
Rod terminal 192
Rodent 5, 222
Rough endoplasmic reticulum 4, 5, 192, 194, 195, 198-200, 202-206, 210, 214, 215
Royal College of Surgeon rat (RCS rat) 237, 243-246

S

Salamander 3, 68-77
Stalk of the optic nerve 56
Schwann cell 216
Sclera 181
Scopelarchid retina 3
SD rat (Sprague-Dawley rat) 222, 226-231
Shedding 146, 153, 237
Short wavelength (SWS1) opsin 3
Silver impregnation 202
Silver technique 212, 216
Single cone 3, 4, 6, 9, 22, 23, 27, 30, 31, 33, 36, 39, 41, 44-46, 48, 49, 51, 53, 66-68, 70, 71, 77, 89, 90, 91, 93-99,
    103-105, 108, 113, 118, 119, 122, 126-128, 130, 131, 138-142, 156, 159, 165-167, 172, 175, 192
Single cone nucleus 41, 93
Single layered ganglion cell 5
Snake 3, 4, 109-113
Soma 4, 216
Sonic hedgehog 237
Southern flounder 48-51
Spherule 64, 156, 191, 192
Spotted African lungfish 57-68
Squirrel 201, 207
Stacks of discs 222

www.ingramcontent.com/pod-product-compliance
Lightning Source LLC
Chambersburg PA
CBHW050819220326

41598CB00006B/259